OECD Health Policy Studies

Realising the Potential of Primary Health Care

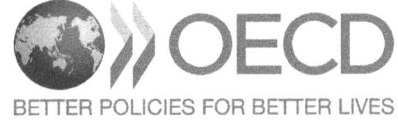

This work is published under the responsibility of the Secretary-General of the OECD. The opinions expressed and arguments employed herein do not necessarily reflect the official views of OECD member countries.

This document, as well as any data and map included herein, are without prejudice to the status of or sovereignty over any territory, to the delimitation of international frontiers and boundaries and to the name of any territory, city or area.

The statistical data for Israel are supplied by and under the responsibility of the relevant Israeli authorities. The use of such data by the OECD is without prejudice to the status of the Golan Heights, East Jerusalem and Israeli settlements in the West Bank under the terms of international law.

Note by Turkey
The information in this document with reference to "Cyprus" relates to the southern part of the Island. There is no single authority representing both Turkish and Greek Cypriot people on the Island. Turkey recognises the Turkish Republic of Northern Cyprus (TRNC). Until a lasting and equitable solution is found within the context of the United Nations, Turkey shall preserve its position concerning the "Cyprus issue".

Note by all the European Union Member States of the OECD and the European Union
The Republic of Cyprus is recognised by all members of the United Nations with the exception of Turkey. The information in this document relates to the area under the effective control of the Government of the Republic of Cyprus.

Please cite this publication as:
OECD (2020), *Realising the Potential of Primary Health Care*, OECD Health Policy Studies, OECD Publishing, Paris, *https://doi.org/10.1787/a92adee4-en*.

ISBN 978-92-64-93333-0 (print)
ISBN 978-92-64-56162-5 (pdf)

OECD Health Policy Studies
ISSN 2074-3181 (print)
ISSN 2074-319X (online)

Photo credits: Cover © Photographee.eu/Shutterstock.com.

Corrigenda to publications may be found on line at: *www.oecd.org/about/publishing/corrigenda.htm*.
© OECD 2020

The use of this work, whether digital or print, is governed by the Terms and Conditions to be found at *http://www.oecd.org/termsandconditions*.

Foreword

Even before the COVID-19 pandemic, health systems in OECD countries faced significant challenges. Citizen expectations about health services are high, societies are ageing, health spending is rising in response to more complex health needs, and fiscal pressures make it difficult to expand allocations of resources to the health sector. The rapid spread of COVID-19 added complexity to these challenges, given both the surge in demand for treatment of the acutely ill and the need to continue to deliver preventive care and manage chronic patients. In this context, primary health care plays a key role for health systems to deliver more and better services. As the first point of contact that is expected to address the majority of health needs, strong primary health care has all the potential to improve health outcomes for people across socio-economic levels and to reduce unnecessary use of more expensive specialised services. But is primary health care across the OECD ready and living up to these expectations?

Realising the Potential of Primary Health Care discusses how primary health care across OECD countries needs to evolve to meet the health challenges that OECD health care systems – and societies more broadly – are facing in the 21st century. It identifies key policy ingredients that countries need to implement to realise the full potential of primary health care. Even in the aftermath of the COVID-19 pandemic, these remain as important as ever, as primary health care is expected to continue to address the majority of health needs. Based on data collected before the COVID-19 pandemic, the report uses a mix of quantitative and qualitative analyses, including information collected through a policy survey covering 26 countries, to suggest key policies and strategies to deliver better primary health care and create stronger primary health care systems. It highlights examples of useful -often local- country experiences.

Realising the Potential of Primary Health Care stresses that there are far too many countries with unrealised opportunities from better primary health care. High-quality primary health care is not always delivered, with avoidable hospital admissions still representing 6% of hospital bed-days across 30 OECD countries for which data are available. Estimates of inappropriate antibiotic prescriptions in primary care range from 45% and 90%. One-quarter of patients suffering from chronic conditions in EU countries did not receive any preventive tests in the past 12 months. Between 29% and 51% of people in 11 OECD countries reported having experienced problems of co-ordination between primary care and specialised care.

New service delivery models, better economic incentives, and broader roles for patients are needed to boost effective, efficient and equitable health systems. Models of organising services that are based on multi-professional teams or networks are being developed in less than half of OECD countries. Better co-ordination among primary care and other providers requires efforts to reward and encourage team work. There is ample scope for further developing the role of primary care nurses and pharmacists, and develop more effective collaboration with general practitioners and other health services. Better use of digital technology, and ability to link datasets across primary care and other part of the health systems is also necessary. Payment instruments linked to outcomes (e.g. for patients with chronic conditions) or desired activities (e.g. vaccination, coordination) are needed to improve care. Better measurement of the inputs, outputs and outcomes of the primary health care sector is vital to improve performance. Patients also need improved ability to access – and interact with – their own records, especially key for those living for many years with chronic conditions.

Countries will certainly conduct thorough reviews of the provision of health care as they seek to draw lessons from the COVID-19 pandemic. Modernising primary health care services is critical to make health systems more resilient to situations of crisis, more proactive in detecting early signs of epidemics and more prepared to act early in response to surges in demand for services.

As this report shows, while the seeds for the future of primary health care are present in local experiences across OECD countries, scaling them up will require both technical leadership and managerial support. It is time to realise the full potential of primary health care.

Acknowledgements

The preparation and writing of this report was co-ordinated by Caroline Berchet and Frederico Guanais. Chapter 1 was written by Caroline Berchet and Frederico Guanais, Chapter 2 by Caroline Berchet, Cristian Herrera and Frederico Guanais, Chapter 3 by Caroline Berchet, Dionne Kringos (Academic Medical Centre, University of Amsterdam), Errica Barbazza (Academic Medical Centre, University of Amsterdam) and Frederico Guanais. Kees van Gool (University of Technology Sydney), Chunzhou Mu (University of Technology Sydney) and Jane Hall (University of Technology Sydney) carried out the statistical work underpinning the analysis of Chapter 3. Chapter 4 was written by Caroline Berchet and Frederico Guanais. Dionne Kringos (Academic Medical Centre, University of Amsterdam) and Erica Barbazza (Academic Medical Centre, University of Amsterdam) provided inputs to the policy analysis presented in Chapter 4. The preparation of Chapter 5 was a joint effort of a team of authors from the Bill & Melinda Gates Foundation (Hong Wang, Brienna Naughton, Ethan Wong, Nicholas Leydon, Caitlin Mazzilli, Susna De and Jean Kagubare) and the Ariadne Labs (Dan Schwarz, Amy VanderZanden and Asaf Bitton).

This report also benefited from the material received from Alexandre Barna and Hélène Colombani (the Fédération Nationale des Centres de Santé), Luc Besançon (pharmaSuisse), Erkkila Eila (Deputy Chief physician – City of Oulu), Mary McCarthy (European Union of General Practitioners) and Lukas Sekelsky (Ministry of Health of the Slovak Republic). The authors are also grateful to the Netherlands Institute for Health Services Research which provided access to the Quality and Costs of Primary Care (QUALICOPC) data, and in particular to Peter Spreeuwenberg for its research assistance. Neither they nor their institutions are responsible for any of the opinions expressed in this report.

At the OECD, Ian Forde, Michael Van den Berg and Niek Klazinga helped shape the overall direction of the report in an early phase. Nick Tomlinson, Francesca Colombo, Mark Pearson and Stefano Scarpetta provided valuable comments and suggestions at various stages of the project. Lukasz Lech, Duniya Dedeyn, Lauren Thwaites, Liv Gudmundson and Lucy Hulett provided vital support in the publication process. Thanks also go to José Bijholt, Frédéric Daniel, and Gabriel Di Paolantonio for their statistical support. The report was edited by Gemma Nellies.

The authors would also like to extend gratitude to all of the delegates of the OECD Health Committee for their responses to the policy questionnaire and for providing valuable comments on a summary document presented to the OECD Health Committee in June 2019 and to a draft version circulated in August 2019.

Table of contents

Foreword 3

Acknowledgements 5

Acronyms and abbreviations 10

Executive summary 11

1 Key findings 14

1.1. Strengthening primary health care offers opportunities to make health systems more efficient, effective and equitable 15
1.2. Primary health care is currently failing to deliver its full potential in many OECD countries 19
1.3. To strengthen primary health care in the 21st century it will be necessary to do things differently 26
1.4. Conclusions: Summary of key policy ingredients to realise the full potential of primary health care 44
References 49
Notes 59

2 Greater efficiency 60

2.1. Primary health care is associated with reduced use of costly hospital and emergency department inputs 62
2.2. Shortcomings in primary health care delivery lead to unnecessary use of more expensive specialised services 63
2.3. Policy options to enable the workforce to deliver more efficient primary health care 72
2.4. Conclusions 95
References 96
Notes 105

3 More effective and patient-centred care 106

3.1. Good quality primary health care improves health system responsiveness, makes health care more patient-centred and can improve health outcomes for the population 108
3.2. Disease prevention and care co-ordination are insufficient in a context of rising health care needs 113
3.3. Policy options to encourage greater effectiveness and responsiveness 118
3.4. Conclusions 142
References 144
Notes 152

4 Less inequalities and more inclusive societies — 153

- 4.1. Strong primary health care can improve the equity of health systems — 155
- 4.2. Accessibility of primary health care services is a challenge in many OECD countries — 158
- 4.3. Leveraging primary health care to reduce health inequalities — 164
- 4.4. Conclusions — 176
- References — 178
- Notes — 181

5 Primary health care in low- and middle-income countries — 182

- 5.1. PHC Governance: Efforts should be stepped up to strengthen PHC governance in LMICs — 184
- 5.2. Measurement of PHC: A more coordinated approach towards measurement of PHC is needed in LMICs — 187
- 5.3. Service Delivery Quality: Efforts must be strengthened to improve service delivery quality — 191
- 5.4. Financing PHC: There are too many gaps in the current understanding of PHC financing in LMICs — 192
- 5.5. PHC Systems Design: Ensuring strong system design capacities for PHC — 196
- 5.6. Conclusions — 199
- References — 201
- Notes — 205

FIGURES

Figure 1.1. The share of generalist medical practitioners continues to drop across the majority of OECD countries, 2000-17 — 20
Figure 1.2. Share of potentially avoidable hospital admissions due to five chronic conditions as a percentage of total hospital bed days, 2016 — 22
Figure 1.3. Inappropriate use of antibiotics in general practice is high — 23
Figure 1.4. One-quarter of patients suffering from chronic conditions in EU Countries did not receive any preventive tests in the past 12 months, 2014 — 23
Figure 1.5. Involvement of primary health care practice in preventive activities has decreased by 13% over the past two decades — 24
Figure 1.6. Problems with care co-ordination between different health care professionals is common across OECD countries, 2016 — 25
Figure 1.7. Prevalence of cervical cancer screening, by income quintile, 2014 (or more recent data) — 26
Figure 1.8. Number of OECD countries using paying for prevention / co-ordination vs pay for performance incentives — 33
Figure 1.9. Eighteen OECD countries have implemented policy measures to collect nationwide performance metrics to monitor the performance of primary health care — 37
Figure 1.10. Less than half of OECD countries implemented concrete policy measures aimed at strengthening the role of primary health care in protecting and improving workers' health — 42
Figure 2.1. Inappropriate use of antibiotics in general practice is high — 64
Figure 2.2. The average volume of opioids prescribed in primary health care is more than 16 DDDs per 1 000 population per day, 2017 — 65
Figure 2.3. Opioid-related deaths in OECD countries have increased by an average of 20% in recent years — 66
Figure 2.4. Share of potentially avoidable hospital admissions due to five chronic conditions as a percentage of total hospital bed days, 2016 — 67
Figure 2.5. On average almost 30% of elderly patients visited an emergency department for a condition that could have been treated in primary health care, 2017 — 69
Figure 2.6. The share of generalist medical practitioners continues to drop across the majority of OECD countries — 71
Figure 2.7. Strategies to develop the primary health care workforce have been implemented in 19 OECD countries in the last five years — 75
Figure 2.8. Seeking health information ranks second in the utilisation of digital technologies — 81
Figure 2.9. Adoption of mHealth programmes by type in 125 countries worldwide, 2015 — 84

Figure 2.10. Percentage of primary health care physician offices using electronic health records in OECD countries, 2016 — 86

Figure 2.11. Number of OECD countries using paying for prevention/co-ordination vs pay for performance incentives, 2018 — 90

Figure 3.1. Evolution and projection of obesity rates in selected OECD countries, 1990-2030 — 114

Figure 3.2. One-quarter of patients suffering from chronic conditions in EU countries did not receive any preventive tests in the past 12 months, 2014 — 115

Figure 3.3. Involvement of primary health care practice in preventive activities has decreased by 13% on average over the past two decades — 116

Figure 3.4. Problems with care co-ordination between different health care professionals are common across OECD countries, 2016 — 117

Figure 3.5. Basic information or test results from general practitioners not communicated to specialists, 2016 — 117

Figure 3.6. Bundled payments and population-based financing are not widely adopted across OECD countries — 129

Figure 3.7. 18 OECD countries have implemented policy measures to collect nationwide performance metrics to monitor the performance of primary health care — 132

Figure 3.8. The percentage of people seeking health-related information online is increasing in all European countries, 2008-17 — 138

Figure 4.1. The probability of a GP visit in the past 12 months differs by only 5 percentage points between the lowest and highest income quintiles, 2014 (or more recent data) — 157

Figure 4.2. In ten out of 33 countries, primary health care services are not affordable for more than 15% of the population, 2013 — 159

Figure 4.3. Prevalence of cervical cancer screening, by income quintile, 2014 (or more recent data) — 160

Figure 4.4. In many European and OECD countries, general practitioners are not available when patients need them, 2013 — 161

Figure 4.5. The density of physicians is consistently greater in urban regions across OECD countries, 2016 (or nearest year) — 162

Figure 4.6. In many European and OECD countries, general practitioners are not easily reached by their patients, 2013 — 163

Figure 4.7. In 20 OECD countries out of 32, patients receive free primary health care services at the point of care — 172

Figure 4.8. Less than half of OECD countries implemented concrete policy measures aimed at strengthening the role of primary health care in protecting and improving workers' health — 174

TABLES

Table 1.1. New models of primary health care delivery have been established in 17 countries — 35
Table 1.2. Summary of findings — 44
Table 2.1. Cost of avoidable hospitalisation for chronic conditions in 30 OECD countries — 68
Table 2.2. Involvement of nurses and assistants in health promotion and prevention — 75
Table 2.3. Indicators used as part of the Estonian pay-for-performance programme — 91
Table 3.1. Impact of primary health care spending on cervical and breast cancer screening uptake in the OECD, 2005-15 — 111
Table 3.2. New models of primary health care delivery have been established in 17 countries — 120
Table 4.1. Gatekeeping systems across OECD countries — 156

Follow OECD Publications on:

 http://twitter.com/OECD_Pubs

 http://www.facebook.com/OECDPublications

 http://www.linkedin.com/groups/OECD-Publications-4645871

 http://www.youtube.com/oecdilibrary

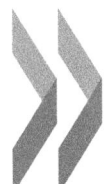 http://www.oecd.org/oecddirect/

Acronyms and abbreviations

ACOs	Accountable Care Organisations
ACSCs	Ambulatory Care Sensitive Conditions
BMI	Body Mass Index
CMS	Centers for Medicare and Medicaid Services
COPD	Chronic Obstructive Pulmonary Disease
CPCF	Community Pharmacy Contractual Framework
CPRD	Clinical Practice Research Datalink
CLI	Combined Lifestyle Intervention
CPTS	Communautés Professionnelles Territoriales de Santé
CCM	Comprehensive Care Management
CPC	Comprehensive Primary Care Initiative
CHF	Congestive Heart Failure
DDD	Defined Daily Dose
eHealth	Electronic Health Systems
EHR	Electronic Health Record
ePrescription	Electronic Prescription
EU	European Union
EBMeDS	Evidence-Based Medicine electronic Decision Support
ENMR	Expérimentations de Nouveaux Modes de Rémunération
GPs	General Practitioners
IDB	Inter-American Development Bank
LMICs	Low- and Middle-Income Countries
mHealth	Mobile Health applications
MMHUs	Mobile Mental Health Units
MyHT	My Health Team
NHS	National Health Service
PHC	Primary Health Care
PHCPI	Primary Health Care Performance Initiative
PREMs	Patient-Reported Experience Measures
PaRIS	Patient-Reported Indicators Surveys
PROMs	Patient-Reported Outcome Measures
P4P	Pay-For-Performance
PIN	Physician Integrated Framework
PHN	Primary Health Network
QALICOPC	Quality and Costs of Primary Care
QOF	Quality and Outcome Framework
RPT	Remote Presence Technology
ROSP	Rémunération sur Objectifs de Santé Publique
SHOPS	Sustaining Health Outcomes through the Private Sector
SDGs	Sustainable Development Goals
UHC	Universal Health Coverage
VSP	Vital Signs Profile

Executive summary

Primary health care can save lives and money while levelling the playing field to achieve more equal access to medical treatment. Such positive outcomes materialise when primary health care is a primary source of care that addresses the majority of their patients' needs, knows their medical history, and helps them to co-ordinate care with other health services as needed. While in most OECD countries primary health care has not yet realised this full potential, several initiatives already show the way forward.

Based on the most promising country experiences, the OECD report *Realising the Potential of Primary Health Care* finds that reconfiguring the delivery of primary health care with multi-professional teams, equipped with digital technology, and seamlessly integrated with specialised care services, could help doctors, nurses, pharmacists and community health workers to provide more effective care. Empowering patients and measuring how primary care services deliver results that truly make a difference to their lives are also key for the provision of high performing care. If anything, the COVID-19 pandemic only makes these messages more relevant. Promising innovations in primary health care can boost the capacity of OECD health systems to contain and manage future health crisis and reduce unnecessary hospitalisation of people that can be effectively treated in the community. In other words, a modern and efficient primary health care system serves as the cornerstone of resilient health systems.

Strong primary health care makes health systems more effective, efficient, and equitable

Interest in primary health care as a path for high performing health systems is not new. The 1978 Alma-Ata declaration recognised the critical importance of high-quality primary health care in the creation of effective and responsive health systems. Since then, the rising costs of medical care, increased citizen expectations from health systems, population ageing, and greater prevalence of chronic diseases have only reinforced the interest in the efficiency of primary health care.

With the share of the population aged 65 and above set to almost double to 28% by 2050, OECD countries must reconfigure their health systems to deliver more effective and high-quality care for people living for a long time with chronic conditions, while avoiding unnecessary use of hospital and specialised services. By providing the main point of contact for patients and especially for those with complex care needs, primary health care can make health systems more efficient, effective, and equitable across OECD countries.

Better, more accessible primary health care results in lower rates of hospitalisations and emergency department use. Primary health care can prevent unnecessary procedures and lower the need for the use of costly and scarce facilities, such as emergency rooms and hospitals.

Robust primary health care can delay the onset of chronic disease and reduce mortality rates. Its role in prevention, from encouraging people to stop smoking to early detection of breast and colon cancer, is critical to patients' lives while quality primary health care is linked to higher patient satisfaction.

Solid primary health care is also associated with lower health inequalities. Across the OECD and EU, 67% of people in the lowest-income group have seen a General Practitioner (GP) in the past 12 months relative to 72% in the top income bracket, a gap of 5 percentage points. Inequalities across income groups are significantly more pronounced when it comes to seeing a specialist (12 percentage points gap), or to have received breast cancer screening (13 percentage points gap). Primary health care can ensure access to vulnerable populations that otherwise can struggle to access medical services.

Most health systems are still failing to reach the full potential of primary health care

So far, primary health care has not always been successful at keeping people out of hospitals. Across 30 OECD countries, hospitalisations for diabetes, asthma, chronic obstructive pulmonary disease, heart failures and hypertension alone – all of them largely avoidable through strong primary health care – correspond to 5.8% of all hospital bed-days. In 2016, these avoidable hospitalisations cost a total of USD 21.1 billion in this group of 30 countries.

Insufficient focus on prevention contributes to these results. Too many patients with chronic conditions still do not receive the recommended preventive care, especially the most vulnerable populations. One quarter of patients across 28 OECD and EU countries suffering with some chronic conditions did not receive any of the recommended preventive tests in the past 12 months.

In most countries, the share of doctors that work in general practice and the proportion of time general practitioners dedicate to preventive care is falling. On average, across OECD countries, generalists accounted for less than three out of ten physicians in 2017. In Australia, the United Kingdom, Denmark, Israel, Estonia and Ireland, the share of generalist medical practitioners decreased by more than 20% between 2000 and 2017.

Patients complain about a lack of communication and co-ordination between different parts of the health care system. In Norway, the United States, and Sweden more than 45% of patients experienced care co-ordination problems linked, for example, to test results, medical histories and receiving conflicting information, while in Germany it was just 29%.

New models of care, more economic incentives, and broader role to patients are needed

Across OECD countries, promising innovations in primary health care are taking place, and the evidence base on how to promote greater effectiveness is growing. However, most of these experiences are at the local level or have small scale, and they have not yet achieved the full potential for a system-wide transformation of care. The report highlights the following necessary changes:

- First, across the OECD, the future of primary health care will be in **new models of care** that are different from the single-practice physician, mostly responding to acute episodes of care, and working in isolation from a network of services. The most promising policy developments in OECD countries are the creation of new configurations of care, which house multiple professionals with advanced skills working in teams, supported by digital technology to enable seamless co-ordination of care, and that are pro-actively engaged in preventive care, tailored to the needs of the population they serve. New models of primary health care based on teams or networks of providers were reported by 17 OECD countries in 2018, including Australia, France, Switzerland, and the United States. Many of those models are focused on improving health care access of low-income or underserved populations, who face barriers to using traditional models of primary health care services, as well as patients with complex needs such as multiple chronic diseases.

- Second, more **economic incentives** are needed to encourage primary health care to work in teams and focus on prevention and continuity of care, especially for patients with chronic conditions, and close attention to care transitions co-ordination. Across OECD countries, policy innovations are taking place to provide better remuneration or economic incentives for the primary health care providers, based on their performance. In 2018, 11 OECD countries, including Israel, Mexico, and the United Kingdom, reported using specific add-on payments to incentivise care co-ordination, prevention activities or active management of chronic disease, and 15 countries, such as the Chile and Netherlands, reported using pay-for-performance mechanisms in primary health care.

- Third, the future of primary health care increasingly depends on giving a **broader role to patients**. In part, this includes involving the patients in the co-production of their health, through better support to self-management of their conditions and exposure to risk factors. Digital tools can play a significant role in this context. In Canada and Finland, for example, patient-provider portals are used to improve communication with primary health care providers to provide patients with access to their own health data and to relevant, curated, health-related information. Listening to the patients through the regular collection of experiences and outcomes of care will be increasingly needed as a tool to improve what matters to them the most. The Patient-Reported Indicators Surveys (PaRIS) launched by the OECD in 2017 will address the need to understand the outcomes and experiences of people with chronic diseases.

These messages are as important as ever in the light of the COVID-19 pandemic which has, in many cases, accelerated the implementation of promising innovations in primary health care to achieve a system-wide transformation of care. Indeed, the coronavirus disease crisis has stimulated many innovative practices at national and local level, such as expanding the roles of nurses and pharmacists, developing digital solutions to monitor health status, ease access to care and using health information infrastructures for disease surveillance. Promoting the continuity of these practices and their wider adoption as health systems move into the pandemic recovery phase is critical for making health systems more resilient to health crisis.

Many of the lessons learned from primary health care experience in OECD countries and the main policy avenues for future developments apply to other contexts, including low- and middle-income countries. The report closes with a discussion of the primary health care landscape in low- and middle-income countries, and the key strategic approaches to ensure the continued development towards high-quality primary health care. Across the many countries where universal health coverage has not yet been achieved, investing in primary health care represents the most feasible roadmap to get there, and in the most affordable way.

Effective primary health care is the cornerstone for efficient, people-centred, and equitable health systems everywhere. Across OECD countries and beyond, investing in primary health care pays off.

1 Key findings

This chapter provides an overview of the publication *Realising the Potential of Primary Health Care*, as well as summarising the main findings. The chapter starts by presenting the evidence base that associates strong primary health care with more efficient, effective and equitable health care systems. The second section shows that primary health care is currently failing to deliver its full potential in many OECD countries, hampered by avoidable hospital admissions, inappropriate antibiotic prescriptions, insufficient preventive care or shortcomings in co-ordination. The third section identifies policy levers to tackle these challenges, and provides an overview of the report's findings on how primary health care could provide more efficient, effective and equitable care. The concluding section presents a summary table of the key policy ingredients that countries will need to address to realise the full potential of primary health care.

1.1. Strengthening primary health care offers opportunities to make health systems more efficient, effective and equitable

In October 2018, health experts and policy makers met in Astana (Kazakhstan) to celebrate the 40th anniversary of the Alma-Ata declaration which recognised the critical importance of quality primary health care in the creation of effective and responsive health systems (see Box 1.1).

The increased recognition of the primacy of strong primary health care is not new: strengthened primary health care systems have the potential to improve health outcomes across socio-economic levels, to make health systems more people-centred, and to improve health system efficiency in the 21st century. This is ever more needed, particularly in OECD countries, where citizen expectations of services are high, societies are ageing, complex cases are costly, and fiscal pressures make it difficult to expand overall allocation of resources to the health sector. The critical role of primary health care has become even clearer during the COVID-19 pandemic. As countries sought to cope with the surge in demand for patients acutely ill with a new, highly infectious disease, while needing to maintain care for chronic patients under difficult circumstances, this pandemic has stimulated many innovative practices at national and local level. Such innovations can be captured with a view to promoting their wider adoption as health systems adapt as they move into the pandemic recovery phase and beyond.

Across the OECD, citizen expectations are high, and a considerable share of the population believe better health services are needed. On average, across the 21 OECD countries surveyed, just over half of the population believe that becoming ill or disabled is one of the top-three social or economic risks facing them or their immediate family in the near future, and in 14 out of 21 countries, this was their top concern. Moreover, 48% of the population identified health care as one of the three top areas requiring additional support from the government to make them and their family feel more economically secure (OECD, 2019[1]).

In addition, populations are ageing and health needs are becoming more complex. The share of the population aged 65 years and over is expected to grow by more than 60% across OECD countries, rising from 17% in 2017 to 28% by 2050. Up to 40% of people in OECD countries live with multi-morbidities, with up to 25% of people suffering from three or more chronic diseases (OECD, 2019[2]). In addition, 20% of the adult population in EU countries is affected by chronic pain (PAE - Pain Alliance Europe, 2018[3]), and around 17% of people in Europe have a mental health problem, such as anxiety or depressive disorders (OECD/EU, 2018[4]). Multiple layers of health problems can accumulate in some people, who form the relatively small group of more complex patients, accounting for a disproportionally large share of health care costs. A recent systematic review found that the top 10%, 5%, and 1% of high-cost patients account for 68%, 55% and 24% of costs respectively within a given year (Wammes, van der Wees and Tanke, 2018[5]).

While needs are on the rise, fiscal space for growth in resources is limited. Many countries have already allowed health to take a larger share of their budgets over time, with health spending now averaging 15% of government spending in OECD countries (Lorenzoni et al., 2019[6]). Increased health spending in the past has been offset by lower public spending in other areas, such as defence and other public services. Continuing such reallocations to health in the future may be increasingly difficult in the face of competing demands for government resources.

In this context, OECD countries are considering strengthening primary health care as a way to address the challenges of the 21st century. However, is primary health care ready to deliver in light of these optimistic expectations? There are unrealised opportunities from better primary health care, however, to reap better efficiency and effectiveness from primary health care, certain things will need to be done differently. This chapter addresses these issues, identifying areas where policy makers need to act so as to better realise the potential of primary health care. This chapter defines primary health care as: the first and the main point of contact of the people with the health system, which provides community-based, continuous, comprehensive, and co-ordinated care (Box 1.2).

Box 1.1. The Astana declaration

In October 2018, health experts and policy makers met in Astana (Kazakhstan) to renew the commitment to comprehensive primary health care for all. The new Astana declaration reaffirms the commitment to the Alma-Ata core principles.

The new Declaration envisions "primary care and health services that are high quality, safe, comprehensive, integrated, accessible, available and affordable for everyone and everywhere, provided with compassion, respect and dignity by health professionals who are well-trained, skilled, motivated and committed". Priority is explicitly given to promotive, preventive, curative, rehabilitative and palliative care; and to the increasing importance of non-communicable diseases which lead to poor health and premature deaths, and to environmental factors such as natural disaster, climate change or other extreme weather events.

Source: Declaration of Astana – Global Conference on Primary Health Care (2018[7]), https://www.who.int/docs/default-source/primary-health/declaration/gcphc-declaration.pdf; Hirschhorn et al., (2019[8]), "What kind of evidence do we need to strengthen primary healthcare in the 21st century?", https://doi.org/10.1136/bmjgh-2019-001668.

Box 1.2. What is primary health care?

Primary health care is expected to be the first and main point of contact for most people with the health care system, focused on the people and their communities. It takes into account the whole person and is patient-focused, as opposed to disease or organ system-focused, and thus recognises not only physical, but also psychological and social dimensions of health and well-being. The most commonly used definitions of primary health care encompass the following characteristics:

- **People and community orientated** – primary health care operates in close proximity with where people live or work, and provides care that is focused on the needs of local people and their families.
- **Continuous care** – primary health care is the first point of contact with the health system, and the people who use it identify it as their main source of care over time.
- **Comprehensive** – primary health care addresses the majority of health problems of the people it serves, providing preventive, curative and rehabilitative services.
- **Co-ordinated** – primary health care helps patients navigate the health system, communicating effectively with the other levels of care. It goes beyond services provided solely by primary health care physicians and encompasses other health professionals such as nurses, pharmacists, auxiliaries and community health workers.

There is extensive discussion about the differences between "primary care" and "primary health care". While primary care has been defined as the more visible and service-oriented core of primary health care, these two definitions are intrinsically linked (Hone, Macinko and Millett, 2018[9]). Given that the concept of "primary health care" typically encompasses "primary care" and places stronger emphasis on health system responsiveness and community orientation, the former it is better aligned with the contents of this report.

1.1.1. Strong primary health care can reduce unnecessary use of more expensive health care resources and improve health system efficiency

There is strong evidence that associates better, more accessible primary health care with lower rates of hospitalisations (Wolters, Braspenning and Wensing, 2017[10]; Rosano et al., 2013[11]; van Loenen et al., 2014[12]) and emergency department use (Huntley et al., 2014[13]; Kirkland, Soleimani and Newton, 2018[14]; Berchet, 2015[15]). Primary health care can avoid unnecessary procedures and lower the need for the use of costly and scarce facilities, such as emergency rooms and hospitals, which contributes to better spending and improving health system efficiency.

The conditions for which primary health care can generally prevent the need for hospitalisation, or for which early intervention can reduce the risk of complications, or prevent a more severe disease from developing are ambulatory care sensitive conditions (ACSCs) (Agency for Healthcare Research and Quality, 2018[16]). Diabetes, chronic obstructive pulmonary disease (COPD), asthma, hypertension and congestive heart failure (CHF) are all ACSCs with an established evidence base that much of the treatment can be delivered by outpatient care at the primary or community care level. Treated early and appropriately, acute deterioration in people with these conditions and consequent hospital admissions could largely be avoided, therefore hospitalisations due to ACSCs are defined as "avoidable hospitalisations" (Purdy, 2010[17]; Nuffieldtrust, 2019[18]) (Starfield, Shi and Macinko, 2005[19]).

In addition to generating avoidable hospitalisations, delays in diagnosis and inappropriate therapeutic interventions in primary health care for these ACSCs are also key sources of patient harm, and can result in emergency department visits (Lin, Wu and Huang, 2015[20]; Sung, Choi and Lee, 2018[21]; Van den Berg, Van Loenen and Westert, 2016[22]; van Loenen et al., 2014[12]). Such emergency department visits are considered "inappropriate" or non-urgent visits, and are characterised by low urgency problems which could be better addressed by other health services than emergency admission including, for example, telephone-based services and primary or community health care services (McHale et al., 2013[23]). According to national definitions and estimates, "avoidable", "inappropriate" or "non-urgent" visits to emergency departments account for nearly 9% of emergency department in Australia (Aihw, 2018[24]), 12% in the United States, between 11.7% and 15% in England, 20% in Italy, 25% in Canada, 31% in Portugal and 56% in Belgium (Berchet, 2015[15]).

As unit costs for treating patients with the same condition in primary health care are lower than those observed in emergency rooms and hospitals, health systems with strong primary health care may attain higher levels of allocative efficiency, which describes a situation where a different combination of inputs could bring better results. Therefore ACSCs are indicators of possible misallocation of resources across different types of goods and services or, in this case levels of care, when comparing primary health care with the alternatives of emergency rooms or hospitals (Cylus, Papanicolas and Smith, 2016[25]).

1.1.2. Strong primary health care can improve population health outcomes and health system responsiveness

The evidence base that associates good primary health care and health outcomes is robust and growing. In a seminal study, Macinko, Starfield and Shi (2003) show the positive contribution of primary health care on health outcomes in 18 OECD countries. The findings show that the stronger a country's primary health care orientation (in terms of continuity of care, co-ordination and community orientation), the lower the mortality rates (Macinko, Starfield and Shi, 2003[26]). The relationship was confirmed for all-cause mortality rates, premature mortality, and cause-specific premature mortality (from asthma and bronchitis, emphysema and pneumonia, cardiovascular disease, and heart disease). The relationship between strong primary health care and decreased mortality rates has also been validated in low- and middle-income countries (Macinko, Starfield and Erinosho, 2009[27]).

More recently, several other studies have shown that countries with strong primary health care performed better on other major aspects of health, including outcomes for patients with chronic diseases. Kringos et. al. (2013[28]), for example, found that both the structure of primary health care (as measured by the governance, economic conditions and workforce development in the primary health care sector) and the co-ordination and comprehensiveness of primary health care were positively associated with the health of people with ischemic heart diseases, cerebrovascular diseases and other chronic conditions including asthma, bronchitis and emphysema. In addition, there is strong evidence that primary health care interventions have a positive impact on measures of mental health indicators, including depression and anxiety (Conejo-Cerón et al., 2017[29]; Trivedi, 2017[30]).

The main positive effect of good primary health care on health outcomes draws from the role it plays in supporting and facilitating the uptake of preventive activities (primary, secondary and tertiary prevention). Primary health care is well placed to carry out preventive interventions not related to any specific disease or organ system. In particular, this hypothesis has been supported in empirical work specific to:

- health counselling regarding smoking cessation (Shi and Starfield, 2005[31]; Saver, 2002[32])
- immunisation (Sans-Corrales et al., 2006[33]; Hartley, 2002[34])
- early detection of breast cancer, colon cancer and melanoma (Campbell et al., 2003[35]).

In addition to better population outcomes, there is evidence that strong primary health care also improves health system responsiveness and makes systems more patient-centred. For example, a study that included 12 OECD countries and 5 other countries in Latin America and the Caribbean found that, on average, patients who had a regular place of care, where there was familiarity with their medical history, where it was easy to communicate with the primary health care team, and where that team helped to co-ordinate care, were 12.1% less likely to say that their health system needs major changes and 29.2% more likely to perceive their usual provider as offering high quality care (controlling for health needs and overall health system characteristics) (Guanais et al., 2019[36]). Moreover, patients who had a physician who explained things in a way that was easy to understand and who spent enough time with them during consultations were 8.6% less likely to say that their health system needs major changes and 69.6% more likely to perceive their usual provider as offering high quality care.

Very recently, Levine, Landon and Linder (2019) have shown that primary health care can offer high value, responsive and patient-centred care. Compared to adults without primary health care, adults with primary health care were more likely to have routine preventive care, to receive high value-care (such as high-value cancer screening, recommended diagnostic and preventive testing, and high-value counselling), and to report better experience with care delivery (Levine, Landon and Linder, 2019[37]).

1.1.3. Strong primary health care can improve the equity of health systems

Primary health care has been described as well placed to support health equity for a number of reasons (Chetty et al., 2016[38]). By definition, it has a broader population coverage than any specialty, therefore it has a better platform for accessing a large number of people. It has direct contact with patients, and most patients will see their primary health care physician as the first point of contact with the health service. In 14 out of the 36 OECD countries that responded to the 2016 OECD Health System Characteristics Survey, patients are obliged to register with a primary health care physician.

Evidence indicates that inequalities in access to primary health care are lower than those of access to specialised care across OECD countries: there are greater opportunities for good primary health care to address the health needs of people, particularly those with chronic care needs, than in other levels of care. Across OECD and EU countries, and accounting for health needs, 67% of people in the lowest-income quintile have seen a general practitioner (GP) in the past 12 months, compared to 72% in the highest-income quintile, which is a rather small difference. Inequalities are significantly more pronounced when it comes to the probability of seeing a specialist: a person with low income is 12 percentage points less likely than a person with high income to see a specialist (OECD, 2019[39]). Systematic reviews of published literature confirm the evidence base that associates strong primary health care and lower health inequalities (Kringos et al., 2010[40]; Salmi et al., 2017[41]).

Evidence also suggests that continuous and comprehensive care provided by the primary health care team can provide effective health education and prevention interventions based on the medical and social needs of the patients (Ruano, Furler and Shi, 2015[42]; Chetty et al., 2016[38]). This helps tackle risk factors and other social determinants of health, which in turn improves equity of health outcomes. In England, for example, strengthening primary health care in underserved areas, notably through the implementation of effective interventions for secondary prevention of cardio-vascular heart disease, diabetes and other chronic conditions, has helped to reduce the absolute socio-economic gaps in mortality amenable to health care from 2007 to 2011 (Cookson et al., 2017[43]).

1.2. Primary health care is currently failing to deliver its full potential in many OECD countries

Despite evidence demonstrating the contribution of primary health care to health systems in terms of improvements in health outcomes, efficiency, and people-centred care, primary health care is not achieving the expected results in many OECD countries. This section presents examples of shortcomings in primary health care performance in terms of:

- **poor efficiency**, as shown by high levels of avoidable hospitalisations and excessive prescriptions of antibiotics
- **ineffective and low responsiveness**, as indicated by low overall utilisation of recommended preventive care, and problems of co-ordination of care between primary health care, specialists, and hospitals
- **inequitable**, as evidenced by inequalities in access to screening tests across different income levels.

These international figures show that primary health care systems are not operating as effectively as they should, whether in terms of keeping people healthy, preventing costly hospitalisations, meeting peoples' expectations or ensuring equal access to quality health services. These shortcomings may partly relate to a shortage and mismatch of skills in primary health care practice, which leads to sub-optimal use of resources in primary health care.

1.2.1. Workforce pressures in primary health care are high

Reductions in the share of generalist medical practitioners and new burdens in workload are putting strain on primary health care teams

While the overall number of doctors and nurses has largely increased, the share of generalist medical practitioners dropped between 2000 and 2017, in the majority of countries (see Figure 1.1). On average across OECD countries, generalists made up about 29% of all physicians in 2017. Between 2000 and 2017, the share of generalist medical practitioners decreased by more than 20% in Australia, the United Kingdom, Denmark, Israel, Estonia, and Ireland (Figure 1.1).

Figure 1.1. The share of generalist medical practitioners continues to drop across the majority of OECD countries, 2000-17

% changes between 2000 and 2017

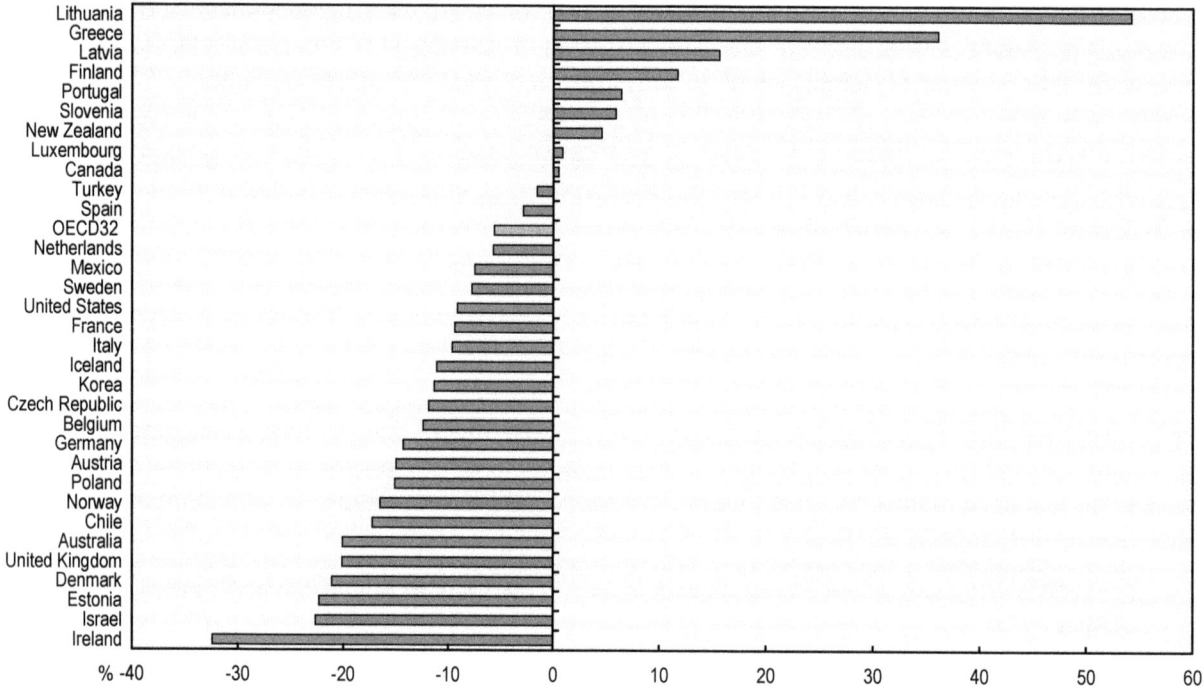

Note: The category of generalist medical practitioners includes general practitioners, district medical doctors, family medical practitioners, primary health care physicians, general medical doctors, general medical officers, medical interns or residents specialising in general practice or without any area of specialisation yet. Generalist medical practitioners do not limit their practice to certain disease categories or methods of treatment, and may assume responsibility for the provision of continuing and comprehensive medical care to individuals, families and communities. There are many breaks in the series for Australia, Estonia, and Ireland over the period. In some countries (Ireland, Israel, Korea and Poland), the share of general practitioners among all doctors has increased over the same period.
Source: OECD Health Statistics 2019, https://doi.org/10.1787/health-data-en.

The reduction in the share of generalist medical practitioners is coupled with an upward trend in both the clinical and administrative workload of general practice. This is observed across several OECD countries, including the United Kingdom (Hobbs et al., 2016[44]; Thompson and Walter, 2016[45]), Australia (The Royal Australian College of General Practitioners, 2018[46]), and Canada. (Grava-Gubins, Safarov and Eriksson, 2012[47]; Medical Association, 2017[48]). In a similar vein, the current workload for primary health care physicians was found to be unreasonable and unsustainable over the longer term in 14 European Countries (Croatia, Hungary, Ireland, Lithuania, Malta, the Netherlands, Norway, Poland, Portugal, Romania, Slovenia, Spain, Sweden, Turkey)[1]. This growing workload might adversely affect the quality of patient care, and is inadequate to meet patients' needs (Fisher et al., 2017[49]).

The current distribution of skills and tasks among primary health care teams is inefficient

Across OECD countries, there is a mismatch of skills and tasks within primary health care teams to population and patient needs (Frenk et al., 2010[50]; OECD, 2016[51]). Previous estimations show that more than three-quarters of doctors and nurses reported being overskilled for some of the tasks they have to do in their day-to-day work. Nurses having a master's level or equivalent are, for example, twice as likely to report being overskilled for some of the work they do than those qualified up to bachelor's degree level. The mismatch of skills and tasks represents a dramatic waste in human capital given the significant length of training of doctors and nurses. In the United Kingdom, up to 77% of preventive care and 47% of chronic care could be delegated to non-physician team members (Shipman and Sinsky, 2013[52]), while in the United States the amount of administrative work doctors have to do is increasing. For example, for every hour physicians were seeing patients, they were spending nearly two additional hours on administrative work (including electronic health records [EHRs] and deskwork) (Sinsky et al., 2016[53]). Many primary health care systems aim to improve care co-ordination and it may be that the increase in paperwork and other administrative tasks relates to these increased responsibilities. This is not a bad thing per se, but such non-medical tasks should be delegated to appropriate staff, thereby reducing administrative workload for medical staff and improving time for patient care and communication.

At the same time as being overskilled for some tasks, physicians and nurses also report being underskilled for others. Across OECD countries, 51% of doctors and 43% of nurses reported being underskilled for some of the tasks they have to do. A systematic review found that, on average, clinicians have more than one question about patient care for every two patients (regarding drug treatment, symptoms or diagnostic results), and nearly half of these questions are not pursued (Del Fiol, Workman and Gorman, 2014[54]). Further, primary health care teams might not have important soft skills to deliver people-centred care, such as shared communication, collaboration and partnership (Ranjan, Kumari and Chakrawarty, 2015[55]). Primary health care teams seem ill-prepared to meet growing and complex health care needs given technological progress, new ways of delivering services and the rapid pace of medical knowledge development. The need for change in the training and development of primary health care teams is thereby evident.

1.2.2. There are several shortcomings in primary health care performance across OECD countries

Avoidable hospitalisations for chronic conditions remain high

Avoidable hospitalisations are a prime example of inefficient use of resources at the health system level, and this indicator has been used for years across OECD countries (Auraaen, Slawomirski and Klazinga, 2018[56]). Analysis of hospital admission data for five chronic conditions (diabetes mellitus, hypertensive diseases, heart failure, COPD and asthma) across OECD countries for which data were available, shows that in 2016, just over 5.6 million hospitalisations with a principal diagnosis of one of these five conditions took place (see Chapter 2 for methodology). This suggests that primary health care is not always successful at keeping people out of hospitals. In total, in 2016, over 47.5 million bed days were consumed by admissions for these five chronic conditions alone across OECD countries, amounting to 5.8% of the total hospital bed day capacity (Figure 1.2).

Using the 2011 WHO CHOICE model, which estimates the "cost per hospital bed day", it is possible to give a rough estimation of the opportunity cost associated with avoidable hospitalisation for ACSCs across OECD countries. Only the "hotel" component of hospital costs (including costs such as personnel, capital and food costs) is considered here, excluding the cost of drugs, treatment and diagnostic tests. This means that the opportunity cost related to avoidable hospitalisations for these five chronic conditions is largely underestimated. Moreover, several countries have developed lists of causes of hospitalisation that are potentially avoidable, including more conditions than the five listed in this estimation (for example angina, influenza and other vaccine preventable diseases, illnesses resulting from nutritional deficiencies, etc.) (Fleetcroft et al., 2018[57]). Therefore, the total number of avoidable hospitalisations is also significantly underestimated.

With these limitations in mind, on average, the cost generated by avoidable hospitalisations for these five chronic conditions is estimated to be USD 21.1 billion in 2016. With better organisation and focus, good primary health care can avoid many of these hospitalisations, increasing efficiency of health systems and improving people's well-being.

Figure 1.2. Share of potentially avoidable hospital admissions due to five chronic conditions as a percentage of total hospital bed days, 2016

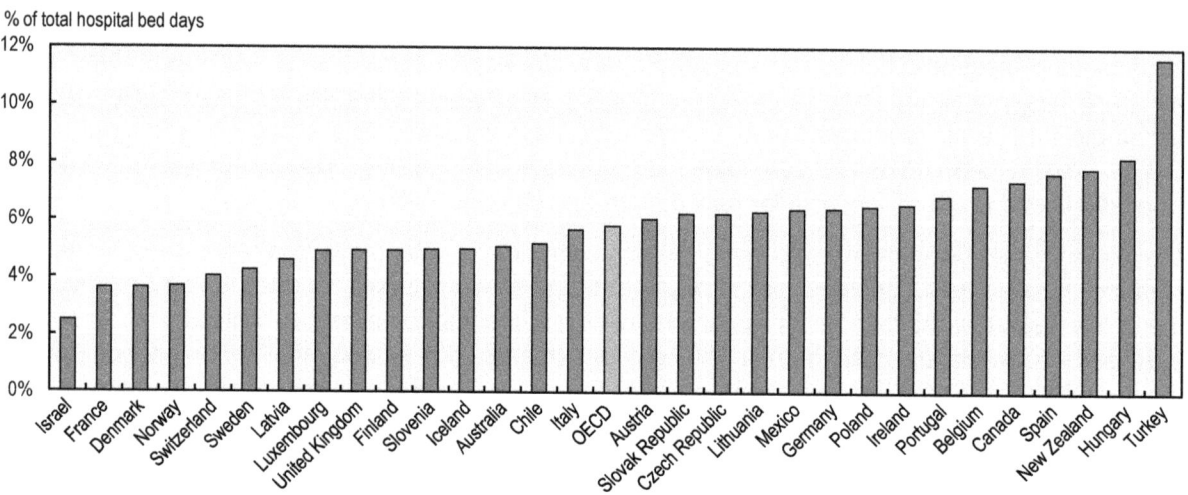

Note: The data includes only admissions with a minimum of one night's hospital stay. Not counted are 'same-day' admissions (e.g. a patient with acute on chronic conditions admitted for observation but discharged a few hours later). These "same-day" admissions consume hospital resources. In addition, the share of avoidable hospital admissions is also largely underestimated as there are more causes of hospitalisations that are potentially preventable. In Australia for example, potentially avoidable hospitalisations for 22 conditions accounted for 9% of all hospital bed days in 2016-17 (AIHW, 2019[58]). Cross-country comparisons of potentially avoidable hospital admissions should also be interpreted with caution, as many other factors, beyond better access to primary health care, can influence the statistics, including data comparability and the prevalence of these chronic conditions. These are crude data and are not age-standardised.
Source: OECD estimates based on OECD Health Statistics 2018, https://doi.org/10.1787/health-data-en.

Inappropriate prescribing, such as for antibiotics, is excessive in general practice

Appropriate prescribing is a good marker of primary health care quality, but also of allocative efficiency, because it indicates inappropriate use of resources. One example is the appropriate use of antibiotics in primary health care. Antibiotics should be used only when there is evidence that they are needed to address infections. However, recent evidence shows that general practice services are an area of concern, as consistently high levels of inappropriate use are reported. The inappropriate use of antibiotics in general practice ranges between 45% and 90% (Figure 1.3). The volume of all antibiotics prescribed in primary health care in 2017 was 19 defined daily doses per 1 000 inhabitants per day across OECD countries, but ranged from 10 in Estonia and Sweden to 36 in Greece (OECD, 2019[59]).

Too many patients with chronic conditions still do not receive the recommended preventive care

Insufficient preventive care throughout the course of life increases the probability that old age will be marked by health problems and disabilities. This has the potential to create future financial liabilities for health systems, particularly in OECD countries, since societies are ageing and the burden of chronic disease is growing.

Figure 1.3. Inappropriate use of antibiotics in general practice is high

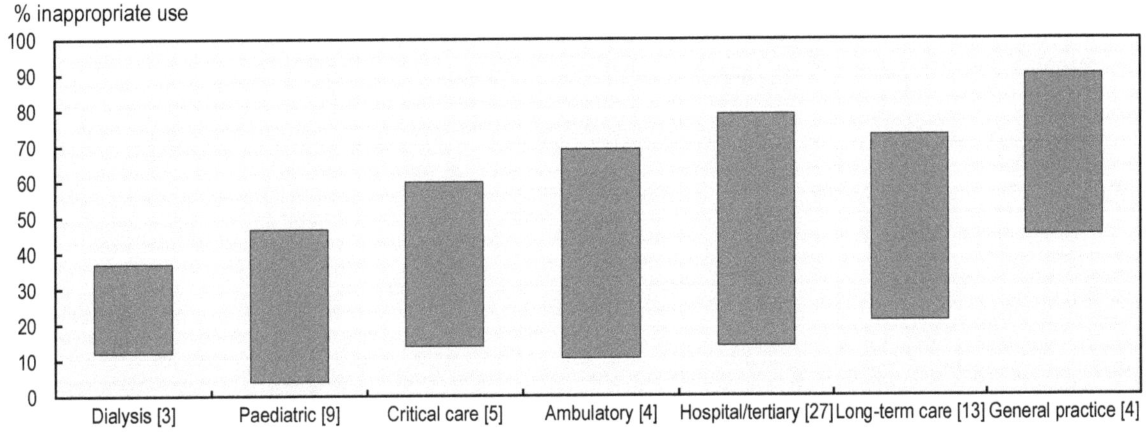

[Bar chart showing % inappropriate use across: Dialysis [3], Paediatric [9], Critical care [5], Ambulatory [4], Hospital/tertiary [27], Long-term care [13], General practice [4]]

Note: Numbers in brackets indicate the number of studies used to determine the range of inappropriate use.
Source: OECD (2017[60]), *Tackling Wasteful Spending on Health*, https://doi.org/10.1787/9789264266414-en.

As the first point of contact with the health care system, and as a trusted source of information, primary health care teams are in a unique position to advise patients on healthy lifestyles and behaviour, to administer screening tests, and to manage and control the progress of chronic conditions. However, recent data shows that too many patients with chronic conditions do not receive the recommended preventive care. In 2014, across EU countries, 26% of patients suffering from certain chronic conditions did not receive any of the recommended preventive tests in the previous 12 months (Figure 1.4). This proportion reaches nearly 50% in Iceland, followed by Finland, Norway, Sweden, Romania, and Slovenia, where more than a third of people with chronic conditions did not receive the recommended tests in the previous 12 months. At the lower end of the scale, in Spain, Belgium, the Czech Republic, Luxembourg and Portugal, less than 20% of people with chronic conditions did not receive the recommended tests in the previous 12 months.

Figure 1.4. One-quarter of patients suffering from chronic conditions in EU Countries did not receive any preventive tests in the past 12 months, 2014

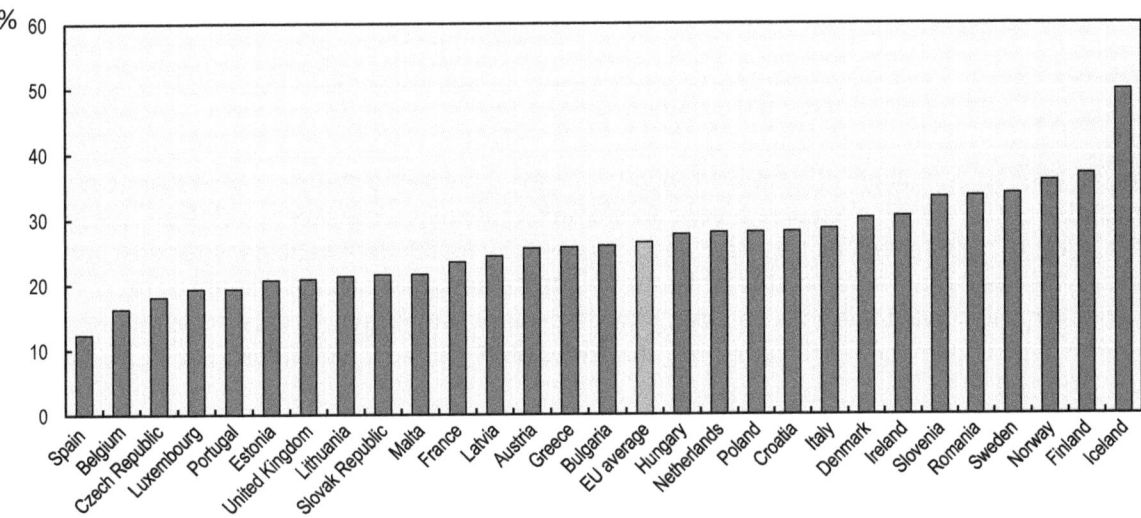

Note: The data refer to the proportion of people suffering from hypertension, myocardial infarction (or chronic consequences of myocardial infarction), stroke (or chronic consequences of stroke) or diabetes, who did not receive any blood pressure measurement, blood sugar measurement or blood cholesterol measurement in the previous 12 months. Data corresponds to the year 2014, in which the United Kingdom was member of the European Union and therefore part of the EU average.
Source: OECD estimates based on EHIS-2.

Figure 1.5. Involvement of primary health care practice in preventive activities has decreased by 13% over the past two decades

% relative change in disease treatment (▲) and in prevention (■) between 1993 and 2012

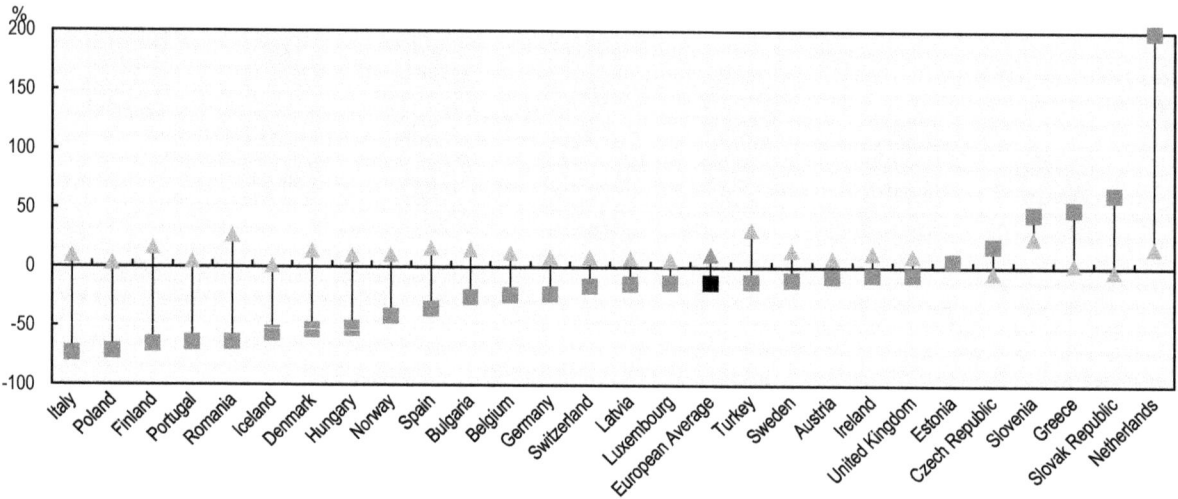

Note: Involvement in prevention includes the measurement of blood pressure, the measurement of cholesterol, and providing health education.
Source: Adapted from Schafer et. al., (2016[61]), "Two decades of change in European general practice service profiles: Conditions associated with the developments in 28 countries between 1993 and 2012", https://doi.org/10.3109/02813432.2015.1132887.

Previous work suggests a decrease in preventive care by primary health care teams (Figure 1.5) (Schäfer et al., 2016[61]). Involvement of primary health care practice in curative care has increased all over Europe over the past decade, while involvement in preventive activities has decreased by 13%, on average, over the same period (Schäfer et al., 2016[61]). Italy, Poland, Finland, Portugal, Romania, Iceland, Denmark and Hungary saw the most significant decreases of more than 50% (Figure 1.5). By contrast, the increase in primary health care practice involvement in treatment of disease is particularly marked in Turkey (+32%), Romania (+26.7%) and Slovenia (+25.2%). Increased participation in treatment may be one of the reasons why preventive care is not being delivered properly.

Patients report significant co-ordination problems between primary health care, specialists and hospitals

Integration and co-ordination of care correspond to an important dimension of patient-centred care (Santana et al., 2019[62]). This requires a good flow of information and consistency of decisions across the different levels of care in the health system, including primary health care settings, specialist settings and hospitals. When care is not co-ordinated, patients have to repeat information or diagnostic tests, conflicting instructions are given, and transitions between providers – for example at hospital discharge when patients are referred back to primary health care – may be associated with adverse effects (Couturier, Carrat and Hejblum, 2016[63]).

Evidence from patient-reported data indicates that there are high levels of care co-ordination problems between primary health care, specialists and hospitals. Figure 1.6 shows that between 29% and 51% of the people surveyed in 11 OECD countries in 2016, reported having experienced problems of care co-ordination. These co-ordination problems refer to: medical tests not being available at the time of appointment or that duplicate tests were made; specialist did not have basic information from GP or GP not informed about specialist care; or received conflicting information from different providers.

Figure 1.6. Problems with care co-ordination between different health care professionals is common across OECD countries, 2016

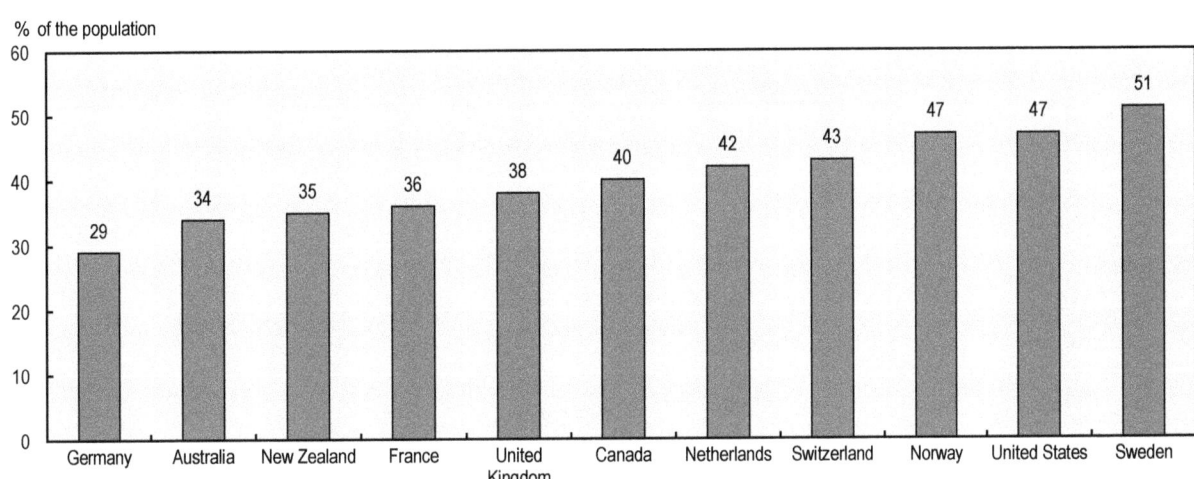

Note: Care co-ordination problem is defined as: test results/records not being available at appointment or duplicate tests ordered; specialist lacked medical history or regular doctor not informed about specialist care; and/or received conflicting information from different doctors or health care professionals in the past two years. The Swedish response rate in the Commonwealth Fund International Health Policy Survey is low, so cross-country comparability is low. The proportions are controlled for age, gender and health status.
Source: Commonwealth Fund International Health Policy Survey 2016.

People with lower incomes have a lower probability of undergoing screening

Despite fairly low inequalities in access to a GP, people with a lower income consistently have lower utilisation rates of preventive services in virtually all EU and OECD countries (OECD, 2019[39]). This indicates that primary health care may not be succeeding in delivering recommended preventive care across different socio-economic levels.

For cervical, breast and colorectal cancers, the probability that those in the target population and in the lowest-income quintile will have undergone screening in the recommended period are significantly lower than that of people in the highest-income quintile. For instance, only 61% of women with a low income had cervical cancer screening, compared to 78% of women with high income. Figure 1.7 presents the rate of cervical cancer screening, showing large income-related inequalities in screening uptake in many EU and OECD countries.

Figure 1.7. Prevalence of cervical cancer screening, by income quintile, 2014 (or more recent data)

Share of women aged 20-69 years who had a pap smear test in the past 3 years in 32 European and OECD countries

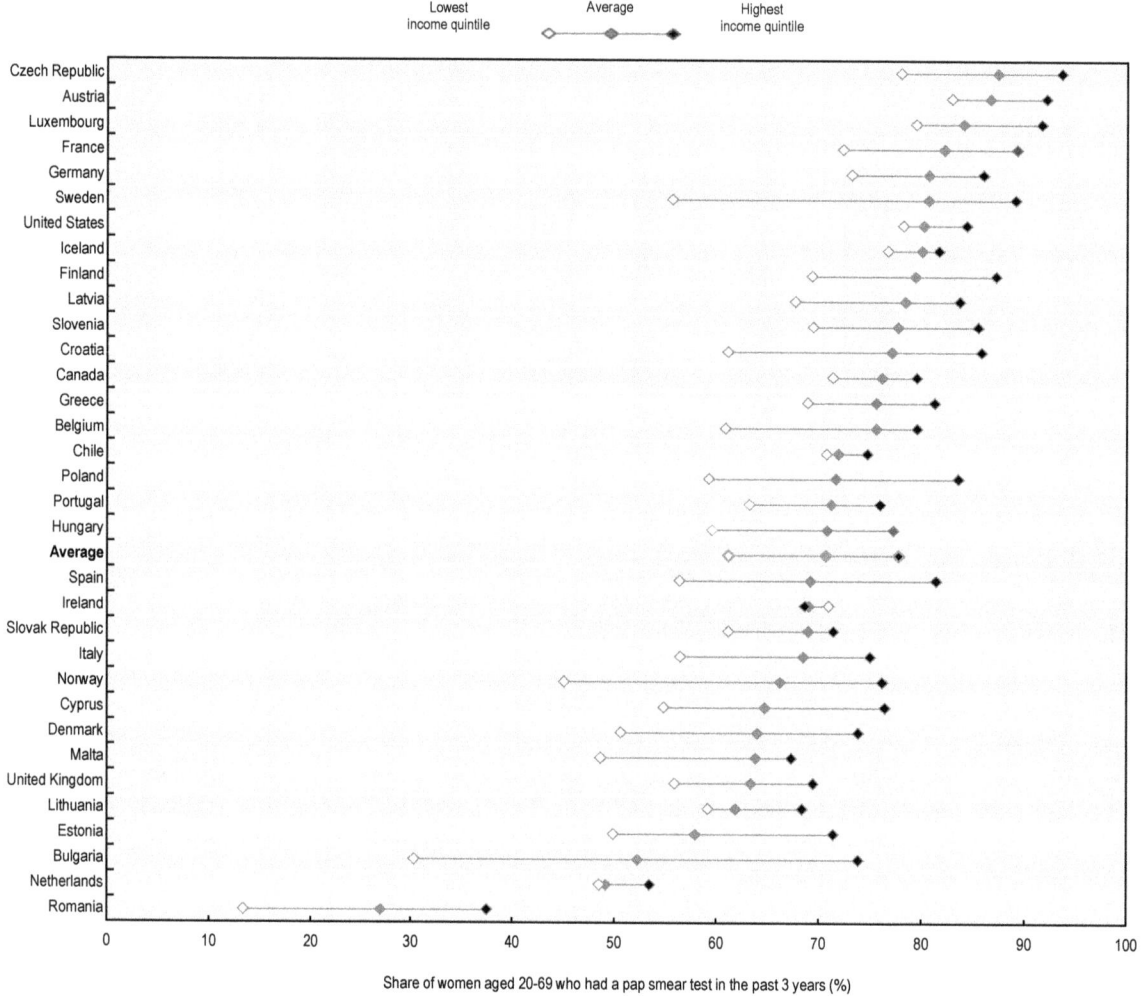

Share of women aged 20-69 who had a pap smear test in the past 3 years (%)

Note: Small sample size in Bulgaria (about 300 individuals per income group for this analysis). Screening rates in the Netherlands are higher based on national surveys.
Source: OECD (2019[39]), *Health for Everyone?: Social Inequalities in Health and Health Systems*, https://dx.doi.org/10.1787/3c8385d0-en.

1.3. To strengthen primary health care in the 21st century it will be necessary to do things differently

There are many contributing factors that can help explain why primary health care is not delivering to its full potential.

In part, it may be linked to the fact that primary health care physicians are not doing the right things, for example, not doing enough preventive medicine, or not co-ordinating care to help avoid hospitalisation or unnecessary complications. Several countries have sought to encourage improved allocative efficiency of primary health care tasks through, for example, different payment schemes and non-financial incentives, or an improved matching of doctors' skills to tasks.

Another reason could be the lack of resources in primary health care relative to other sectors. More evidence is needed to fully assess whether reallocation of resources to primary health care would be a way to improve the delivery of health care output. However, the declining share of GPs, due in part to the lower attractiveness of general practice relative to specialist care, mean that fewer primary health care physicians are asked to deliver care to a growing number of people with complex care needs. A number of countries have sought to counter the increasing trends towards specialisation through training and task delegation.

A third reason, could be that the organisational model of primary health care still mostly relies on face-to-face consultations with a physician who works in a solo practice. Better use of teamwork, inclusion of other health professionals and electronic communication could potentially increase the pool of patients that every primary health care physician oversees, while effectively improving the quality of services provided (Green, Savin and Lu, 2013[64]). Moreover, better integration of health and social care services could offer opportunities to better address social determinants of health and reduce the need for health care services.

Overcoming these problems will require new models for the delivery of primary health care, extensive use of digital tools and financing mechanisms that reward performance. This section discusses policy levers that can be used by OECD countries, in the 21st century, to improve the efficiency, effectiveness, responsiveness and equity of their health systems, through more effective and stronger primary health care.

1.3.1. Improving the efficiency of primary health care

New mechanisms for workforce recruitment and training are needed to improve allocative and technical efficiency

Changes in training are more important than ever, given the challenges and opportunities introduced by digital technologies and new ways of delivering services

With technological progress and new ways of delivering services, primary health care systems are changing rapidly. Professional education in primary health care may not be aligned with these changes, and may not match increasing citizen expectations and rising health care needs. As illustrated by Schafer et al (2016[61]), primary health care practices do not engage sufficiently in preventive care and mostly deliver care that focuses on disease treatment, often targeting one illness at a time (Schäfer et al., 2016[61]) (see also Chapter 3). Such an approach is not appropriate in today's climate and changes are needed to realise the required efficiency gains.

To improve technical efficiency, the primary health care team needs to have expertise on a wide range of areas, which go beyond treating infectious diseases, and include: nutrition, addiction, mental health and healthy ageing. Consistent with a people-centred approach, "soft" and transversal skills are also needed when engaging in prevention and disease management activities, such as behaviour counselling, shared communication, collaboration and partnership (Ranjan, Kumari and Chakrawarty, 2015[55]).

Providing initial and continuing training programmes in all these areas is critical in providing the tools and knowledge that allow primary health care teams to engage in these activities properly. Initial and continuing education should prepare primary health care teams to:

- Manage and control chronic diseases and associated risk factors. Screening assessment tools, individual counselling, and behavioural change programmes should be the main priority of training programmes in primary health care, at least to the same extent as diagnosis and treatment of diseases.
- Recognise the importance of environmental and social determinants of unhealthy behaviour and the factors that impact behavioural change.

- Use technological resources effectively. Primary health care teams need to learn how to use digital tools, such as technology-enabled consultation, clinical data coding and IT-based quality improvement.
- Achieve skills for person-centred communication. It is vital to expand attention to patients' personal and social situations in order to improve diagnosis and tailor care plans, and to practice shared decision making to address patients' goals and values.
- Achieve skills for effective teamwork and interprofessional collaboration, notably to break down professional silos and enable effective working both with, and through other health and social care professionals.

Several health care systems are working toward these goals. For example, to strengthen providers' competencies in IT-based quality improvement tools, England has developed the NHS Digital Academy. In a similar vein, Canada, Germany and the United States have introduced modules in the medical curricula to ensure health care professionals achieve skills for data-driven quality development, digital literacy and interprofessional collaboration. In France, the Ministry of Health, jointly with the Ministry of Education, recently announced that the primary health care workforce will have to perform a public health rotation (see Box 1.3).

Box 1.3. The public health rotation in France

The Ministry of Health, jointly with the Ministry of Education, recently announced that students in the health field will have to perform a public health rotation (called "*service sanitaire*"). The new curricula for medical doctor, nurse, pharmacist and physiotherapist students consists of going to public places, such as universities and high schools, to undertake prevention activities on four priority areas: diet, physical activity, addictions, and sexual health (see also Box 2.2). It is estimated that from 2019 around 50 000 students per year will undertake the public health rotation.

Source: OECD (2018[65]), Policy Survey on the Future of Primary Care.

The efficiency of primary health care in the future will also depend on the use of community-based teams

New support role for nurses, community pharmacists and community health agents have the potential to reduce the workload of primary health care physicians, without undermining the quality of care and patient satisfaction (Green, Savin and Lu, 2013[64]). Ensuring that the primary health care workforce has sufficient professionals with the right mix of skills will be key to making sure new models of primary health care delivery meet local health needs. Nurses, community pharmacists and community health agents frequently have all-important soft skills and relevant knowledge about their communities. OECD health care systems need to harness the full capacity of these community-based teams by setting up appropriate training and ensuring that legislation is adequate, whilst not being unnecessarily restrictive.

However, the majority of nurses or assistants independently provided immunisation, health promotion or routine checks for chronically ill patients in less than half of OECD countries in 2016 (OECD, 2016[66]), and only 19 OECD countries (OECD, 2018[65]) reported strategies to develop the primary health care workforce (see Chapter 2).

New roles of care co-ordinators, care planners and patient navigators, are progressively being introduced to focus on providing continuous care across different specialties. These co-ordination functions often extend beyond the traditional health care boundaries, and include close working relationships with social services and long-term care teams. Currently, many of these new functions are being carried out by expanding the scope of practice of existing health professionals, for example, nurse practitioners taking the lead in patient planning and care co-ordination, whilst also promoting healthy living and preventing and managing disease. In Canada, registered nurses and nurse navigators have an important role in improving co-ordination and continuity of care in the MyHealthTeam model of primary health care. Nurses with a navigator role ensure that patients move swiftly through the system, and that they receive the appropriate care in the appropriate place. Australia, Estonia, Ireland, Latvia, Mexico, Sweden and the United Kingdom are increasing the role of nurses in primary health care.

In some OECD countries, notably Belgium, England, Finland, Italy and Switzerland, community pharmacists are taking a greater role in health promotion and prevention, thereby improving access to primary health care services in remote or underserved areas where there is a shortage of primary health care physicians (see Section 3.3.3). During the COVID-19 pandemic, several countries have made efforts to mobilise pharmacists and care assistants. In Austria, Canada, Ireland, Portugal and the United States, pharmacists have been allowed to extend prescriptions beyond what they were previously allowed to do and to prescribe certain medications to allow doctors to focus on the more important cases and minimise the number of medical consultations (PGEU, 2020[67]; OECD, 2020[68]). In France, community pharmacists were given an exceptional authorisation to renew prescriptions of drugs for chronic diseases. In the United Kingdom, there was a proposal to scale up and use community health workers to provide support for the elderly in the context of the COVID-19 crisis (Haines et al., 2020[69]).

Other health care systems are working towards the development of community health workers. In the United Kingdom, the GP contract five year framework provides funding to contribute towards an extra 20 000 non-GP roles in general practice including clinical pharmacists, social prescribing link workers, physician associates, first contact physiotherapists and first contact community paramedics. These roles have been chosen to meet strong practice demand, and because the tasks they perform can help reduce GP workload, improve practice efficiency and better meet health system objectives (NHS, 2019[70]).

As a greater use of community based workforce has all the potential to increase efficiency in primary health care practice, health care systems need to ensure that their community based workforce is able to take on different roles where it benefits a patient, such as person-centred communication, co-ordinator role, or involvement in prevention (Shipman and Sinsky, 2013[52]; Matthys, Remmen and Van Bogaert, 2017[71]; Green, Savin and Lu, 2013[64]). In the future, it would be vital to allow nurse practitioners and other primary health care staff to practice to the fullest extent of their training and ability, and remove restrictions that limit their scope of practice (Buerhaus Peter, 2018[72]; Maier and Aiken, 2016[73]). This would allow health systems to boost their health workforce capacity in case of future pandemic crises.

Better use of digital technology is key to improving efficiency in the delivery of primary health care services

An efficient primary health care system needs to leverage all the functionalities offered by digital technologies (also called eHealth) to support health outcomes and health-related activities. Key objectives shaping digital technologies include: improved efficiency, productivity and quality of care (OECD/IDB, 2016[74]; Shaw T, Hines and Kielly-Carroll, 2017[75]).

In Europe, a recent report found that in all of the 27 countries surveyed, eHealth adoption in primary health care has increased between 2013 to 2018, with the highest levels of implementation in Denmark, Estonia, Finland, Spain, Sweden and the United Kingdom, while in Greece, Luxembourg and the Slovak Republic uptake remains relatively low (Valverde-Albacete et al., 2019[76]). While full-scale use of digital technologies is still not the norm across all OECD countries, there are several important experiences that should be noted:

- **EHR systems**, particularly those that are well structured and portable (Australia, Canada, Israel and the United States), can generate clinical reminders to help physicians track preventive and ongoing care services for patients with chronic diseases. EHRs can have major effects on patient safety and the overall quality of the care delivered, by increasing compliance with guidelines, lowering the number of medication errors and reducing the risk of adverse drug effects (Chaudhry et al., 2006[77]; Campanella et al., 2016[78]). In Finland, the POTKU model provides primary health care physicians with the locally developed Evidence-Based Medicine electronic Decision Support (EBMeDS) system, which is matched with patient records to provide personalised care guidance (Hujala Anneli et al., 2016[79]). The system also generates automated reminders and warnings. As a medical support tool, EHR has been associated with improved workflow, policy, communication and cultural practices, as recommended for safe patient care in primary health care settings (Tanner et al., 2015[80]).

- **Electronic prescription** (ePrescription) allows prescribers to write prescriptions that can be retrieved by a pharmacy electronically, to assess a patient's medication regimen at the point of care or to identify non-adherence. ePresciption, as implemented in Estonia and Sweden, can improve the accuracy and efficiency of pharmaceutical drug dispensing (Khan and Socha-Dietrich, 2018[81]). ePrescription programmes have been associated with a reduction in prescribing of potentially inappropriate medications (Iankowitz et al., 2012[82]) and efficiency gains have been found for prescribers and dispensers (Deetjen, 2016[83]).

- **Telemedicine**, which includes telemonitoring, store and forward[2], and interactive telemedicine, may contribute in several ways to providing care in the right place at the right time, for instance, by improving the process and appropriateness of referrals. Teleconsultations are one of the most used telemedicine interventions in primary health care, notably to improve access to care for people living in underserved areas. Such systems are already in use in Belgium, Canada, Costa Rica, Estonia, France, Germany, Korea, Norway, Switzerland and the United Kingdom. There should be careful oversight and regulation of digital services in order to maximise benefits and avoid harm, but used effectively, telemedicine makes health service delivery more efficient (Pecina and North, 2016[84]).

- **Home monitoring, ePatient portals and self-management applications** are key levers to improving care quality and the delivery of people-centred primary health care. There is an increasing body of evidence about the effectiveness and economic assessment of mobile health applications, otherwise known as mHealth. For example, three digital applications in the areas of diabetes, depression, and anxiety have been found to improve the management of chronic diseases (Kitsiou et al., 2017[85]). Patients have also been found to perceive greater awareness of their condition, to be better able to make health-related decisions and be considered as co-producers (Morton et al., 2017[86]). The use of digital health applications has also been shown to reduce acute care utilisation in the United States (IQVIA, 2017[87]). Such policy options already exist in Canada (miHealth), Denmark (telerehabilitation service), Finland (Oulu Self Care Service) or the United States (HealthConnect).

- **Clinical algorithms bringing external and patient-derived data** into the clinical decision-making process can create personalised predictions of disease status and generate more appropriate treatment, thereby increasing the efficiency of health service delivery (Bell, Gachuhi and Assefi, 2018[88]; Shaw T, Hines and Kielly-Carroll, 2017[75]). The data used could include social, environmental and behavioural patient information, as well as financial, clinical, and administrative records, as in the United States with Kaiser Permanente and HealthConnect, or the risk stratification model used in Spain. Models based on clinical algorithms could be used to identify relationships between multiple behavioural factors to enable the assessment of opportunities and risks associated with a particular set of conditions. This could, for example, be used to flag patients at risk of avoidable hospital (re)admission, or to conduct specific targeted preventive actions towards disadvantaged or high-risk populations.

The critical role of digital technology has become even clearer during the COVID-19 pandemic. Telehealth has been used to monitor the health and wellbeing of people who have been diagnosed with COVID-19, including both less severe patients who are able to stay at home and the more critical cases who need to be hospitalised. Korea and Israel use wearables and communication technologies to remotely monitor patients with COVID-19 at home, catching signs of possible deterioration, and adding to health researchers' understanding of how the disease develops (OECD, 2020[68]). Other than that, telehealth has many potential benefits in the context of COVID-19, as people with mild symptoms can consult from their homes – avoiding potentially infecting others and reserving physical capacity in health care units for critical cases and people with serious health conditions. England, France, Germany, Japan and the United States have relaxed regulatory barriers to encourage the use of teleconsultation (OECD, 2020[68]). In France for instance, patients are authorised to consult remotely with any doctor that uses telemedicine, whether or not they have consulted that doctor face-to-face in the past. In Germany, the Federal Joint Committee eased regulations outside of traditional face-to-face outpatient practice. In an effort to protect providers and patients from catching the virus while ensuring access to health care, a temporary provision was introduced to allow physicians to issue or renew prescriptions, referrals, or sick notes digitally or by phone, and to offer video consultations. Intensifying the implementation of digital technologies in primary health care practice will make primary health care teams more efficient to make smarter use of scarce health care resources and make health systems more resilient to health crises. In the aftermath of the pandemic, policy makers should ensure that these tools are made available to all primary health care teams, patients and communities.

In a modern and efficient primary health care system, primary health care teams would follow clinical reminders and guidelines produced by EHR to deliver high quality primary health care, and would proactively integrate targeted preventive action towards high-risk patients. Prescriptions would be automatically renewed. A patient could easily describe a condition via a health app, which in turn would recommend the most accessible primary health care team or organise an appointment. Patients could also benefit from mobile tools and apps to communicate with primary health care teams, and to achieve personalised prevention plans. Patients' medical histories could be instantly transferred from one care facility to another, removing the need for paper forms that previously passed through several hands and often went missing.

Shifting services from hospitals to new settings for the delivery of primary health care

At a time of great fiscal constraint, primary health care systems will have to assume a greater role in taking care of patients who no longer need acute care. Several health care systems are working towards these goals, by developing intermediate care facilities or home-based programmes to improve care continuity, and reduce the use of expensive hospital inputs.

Intermediate care facilities

Intermediate care facilities provide short-term care for patients who no longer require acute hospital care, but nevertheless require a level of support that they could not obtain if they were discharged directly home. Intermediate care facilities can also deliver non-urgent care and a mix of post-acute, rehabilitation and nursing care, 24 hours a day, 7 days a week. The overarching objective is to strengthen the role of the primary health care system, improving experiences with care for patients, while reducing hospital costs.

There is already a large body of evidence confirming that using intermediate care following a hospital admission may reduce the need for further hospital admissions, and reduces the number of emergency department visits. In Norway, for example, studies have shown that intermediate facilities significantly reduce the number of hospital readmissions for the same disease, increase the quality of life for patients, and did not result in an increased risk of mortality (Dahl, Steinsbekk and Johnsen, 2015[89]; Garåsen, Windspoll and Johnsen, 2007[90]). In the Netherlands, van der Brug (2017) found that the use intermediate care facilities was associated with reduced hospital readmission rates (van der Brug, 2017[91]). Recently, intermediate care facilities have been established in four countries: Costa Rica (interdisciplinary outpatient units for people with mental health issues and health hostels for patients with chronic conditions), France (local hospitals), Ireland (community intervention teams) and Mexico (CESSAS).

Early discharge home-based programmes

Early discharge home-based programmes allow patients to return home when they might previously have stayed longer in hospital or been referred to a nursing home. Such programmes provide post-discharge care at home, but also associated with counselling and health education, and with support from social care and digital technologies (Zhu et al., 2015[92]). The overarching objective is to curb hospital costs and to reduce delays in hospital discharge due to a lack of primary health care options, while improving patient experience and health outcomes.

Previous empirical work show that discharge home-based programmes are associated with reduced length of hospital stays, a lower risk of readmission and good clinical outcomes (Zhu et al., 2015[92]; Hernández et al., 2018[93]). Some health care systems are increasingly providing post-discharge care at home as an alternative to hospital-based care, such as Canada and the United Kingdom with the use of virtual wards. Such systems have been developed to reduce hospital readmissions, by providing short-term transitional care to high-risk patients with complex needs who have recently been discharged from hospital. In Germany, since 2017, mental health care following discharge from psychiatric hospital can be delivered within the patient's home.

Providing economic incentives can aid favourable developments in primary health care services

Adapting existing models of payment for primary health care is key to improving technical and allocative efficiency. When properly designed and implemented, add-on payments to remunerate specific activities and paying-for-performance (P4P) programmes can encourage desirable behaviours at specific points of the care continuum. Add-on payments can, for example, target the management of chronic diseases, care co-ordination or early discharge from hospitals, while P4P are expected to reward high quality and performance outcomes. Such economic incentives are designed to maximise health care outputs and health outcomes through better care processes, and to reduce the use of expensive inputs by moving care out of the hospital sector. They are useful ways to encourage primary health care teams to operate differently.

Across OECD countries, add-on payments are mainly used to incentivise care co-ordination, prevention activities or management of chronic disease. In 2018, 11 OECD countries used this type of payment (Figure 1.8). In Canada, additional fees are offered to physicians to compensate for time spent communicating with other health care providers involved in the patient's care and for sharing information with other providers to better manage complex needs. In Israel, the payment system rewards providers for taking care of chronic patients in multi-disciplinary teams. In Australia, the Practice Incentives Programme Quality improvement supports general practice activities that encourage continuing improvement, quality care, enhance capacity and improve upon access and health outcomes for patients, including improving health outcomes relating to chronic disease.

Economic incentives can also be employed to encourage reductions in delayed hospital discharge and to improve care transitions out of hospital. These often take the form of negative incentives[3], where hospitals or municipalities are fined for excessive delays in discharge from hospitals, as seen in the Czech Republic, Denmark, Norway, Sweden and the United Kingdom.

P4P programmes in primary health care are implemented in 15 countries (Figure 1.8), including for example Chile, the Czech Republic, Estonia, Sweden and the United Kingdom. New forms of P4P programmes are currently being developed to expand the role of community pharmacies in the delivery of primary health care services as seen in the United Kingdom and the United States (see Box 1.4)

To be effective, these economic incentives need to encourage the delivery of appropriate services in primary health care settings that can be directly influenced by the level of the primary health care team's efforts. However, and as shown by systemic reviews, evidence on the impact of P4P on health outcomes remains limited or inconclusive (OECD, 2016[94]). In the United Kingdom, for example, there is no evidence that P4P has a sustainable impact on health outcomes (Ryan et al., 2016[95]), and some researchers argue that P4P schemes go in the opposite direction of goal-oriented care (see Chapter 2) (De Maeseneer and Boeckxstaens, 2012[96]). P4P programmes and related quality and performance targets should therefore focus on outcomes that matter the most to patients, such as improving quality of life and daily life activities through better management of chronic conditions, and on patient-centred care processes, such as care co-ordination. P4P programmes, and value-based payments more generally, need to be properly designed and blended with other payment schemes. Appropriate information systems is also required to monitor and follow up process- and outcome-indicators.

Figure 1.8. Number of OECD countries using paying for prevention / co-ordination vs pay for performance incentives

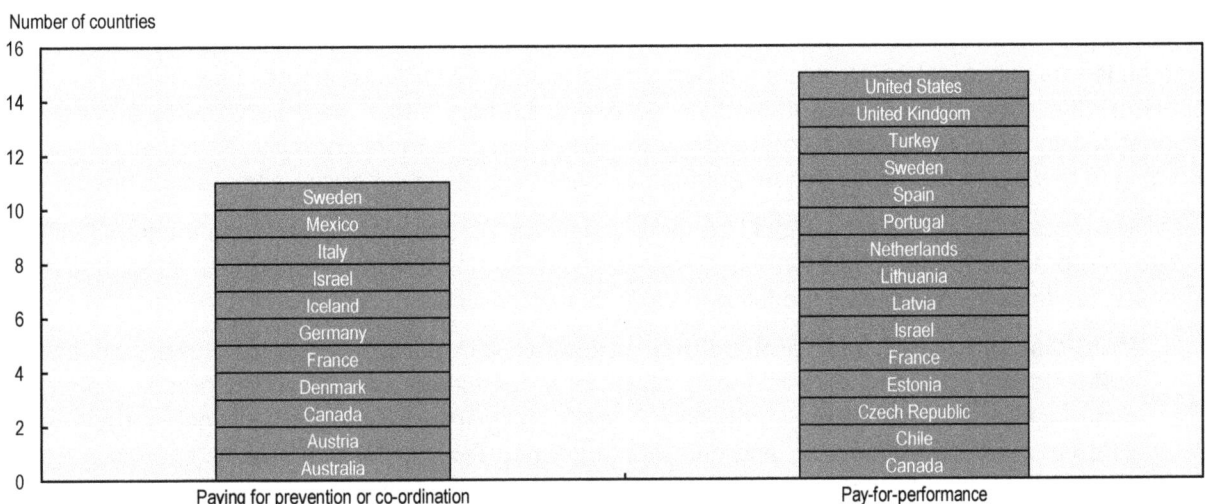

Source: OECD (2018[65]), Policy Survey on the Future of Primary Care, and OECD (2016[66]), Health System Characteristics Survey, http://www.oecd.org/els/health-systems/characteristics.htm.

Box 1.4. Pay-for-performance programmes outside of GP practice

The Community Pharmacy Quality Payments Scheme in the **United Kingdom** was established in 2016. The scheme rewards community pharmacies for delivering quality criteria in three dimensions: clinical effectiveness, patient safety and patient experience. Among the defined criteria to be met are: public health, clinical efficacy for certain chronic conditions, and workforce development. As part of the new Community Pharmacy Contractual Framework for 2019/2024, a new Pharmacy Quality Scheme will be introduced to replace the Quality Payment Scheme.

In the **United States**, a pay-for-performance (P4P) programme for pharmacists is run by the Inland Empire Health Plan (IEHP), a non-profit Medicare and Medicaid health plan in Southern California. Among the quality measures that pharmacies must meet include proportion of days covered (PDC) for diabetes, PDC for hypertension, PDC for statins or use of high-risk medications in older people and the generic dispensing rate.

Source: Based on OECD (2018[65]), Policy Survey on the Future of Primary Care, (Bonner, 2016[97]), and (NHS, 2019[98]).

1.3.2. Improving the effectiveness and responsiveness of care

Reorganisation of primary health care based on teams and integrated networks can deliver more co-ordinated and comprehensive care

Developing new models of people-centred primary health care based on teams and networks is both a matter of striving for better health outcomes and an economic necessity:

- From a **population health perspective**, people-centred primary health care models based on teams and networks are expected to better meet population health needs by offering both medical and social services (Borgermans et al., 2018[99]). They have a higher capacity than traditional solo-practices to meet patient needs by offering a broad range of health care and social services. This is particularly important for people who have several risk factors or are suffering from more than one chronic condition.
- From an **economic perspective**, people-centred primary health care models based on teams and networks are found to offer economies of scale (Mousquès, 2011[100]). Integrating the primary health care workforce within a single organisation lowers transaction costs and reduces the health production cost because of shared use of inputs, such as equipment, human resources, and ICT.

The 2018 Policy Survey on the Future of Primary Care indicates that new models of primary health care based on teams or network of providers are being developed in 17 OECD countries (see Table 1.1). Such models of care steer patients from immediate access to primary health care services to a continuous relationship with the primary health care team when needs become more complex. Patients are stratified according to risk, so that services can be adapted to meet their particular social and medical needs.

These new models of organisation should be more widely adopted to move away from the traditional and reactive solo-practice model. While there is no one-size-fits-all model of organisation, an integrated model of primary health care often meets the following four characteristics:

- **Multi-disciplinary or inter-professional practices** with a various mix of primary health care professionals (including GPs or family physicians, registered and advanced nurses, community pharmacists, psychologists, nutritionists, health counsellors, and non-clinical support staff), different models of teamwork, and different target populations (for example as seen in Australia, Canada, the United Kingdom and the United States) (Socha-Dietrich, 2019[101]).
- **Comprehensive health services in the community,** (for example in Costa Rica), including disease prevention and health promotion, curative services, rehabilitation and management of chronic diseases. Care co-ordination between health professionals is key to enabling the early detection of disease, reducing the exacerbation of diseases, avoiding duplication of services, and increasing provider and patient satisfaction.
- **Population health management**, generally based on risk stratification using sophisticated IT systems (for example in Canada and Spain), is implemented to better understand the health and risk profiles of the community and to undertake proactive management of patients' needs. Patients are stratified to identify opportunities for intervention before the occurrence of any adverse outcomes for individual health status.
- **Engagement of patients in shared decision making,** (for example in Israel). The overarching objective is to incorporate patients' values, needs, and preferences.

Among the countries developing new models of primary health care delivery, the United States (with the patient-centred Medical Home, and the more recent Comprehensive Primary Care Plus), Australia (with the Health Care Home and Primary Health Network), and Canada (with My Health Team) appear to be at the leading edge of this practice. These models of primary health care are highly integrated, team-based practices and promote patient-centred care through patient engagement and better access to primary health care. This allows for a co-ordinated, whole system approach, spanning primary health care, community services, hospital care and social care. The common denominator to achieving high levels of integration, across the care team and care continuum, is the extensive use of EHR, integrated with functionalities such as electronic scheduling of appointments, secure communication between patient and clinical team, reference information on self-management of chronic conditions, and electronic prescriptions and dispensing of drugs.

While it is too early to evaluate the impact of integrated primary health care teams in Australia and Canada, several studies in the United States show positive results. Primary health care medical homes have been found to improve care quality for a number of chronic conditions (Friedberg et al., 2015[102]; NCQA, 2017[103]; Schuchman, Fain and Cornwell, 2018[104]; Bates and Bitton, 2010[105]), improved patient experience and increased staff satisfaction (NCQA, 2017[103]). They have also been linked with reduced costs, lower emergency department visits and fewer hospitalisations for patients with chronic conditions (Schuchman, Fain and Cornwell, 2018[104]; Bates and Bitton, 2010[105]; NCQA, 2017[103]).

In line with these findings, a recent literature review of 20 studies shows that inter-professional practice was associated with improved health outcomes and quality of life (notably for patients suffering from chronic diseases and cancer), decreased length of stay and admission rates, and has demonstrated cost-effectiveness (NAP, 2019[106]).

There is also emerging evidence suggesting that advanced care teams in primary health care is more satisfying to clinicians and primary health care staff, when compared to more traditional single practice models (Sinsky and Bodenheimer, 2019[107]; AHRQ, 2016[108]). Reviewing evidence from four interventions, Sinsky and Bodenheimer (2019) for example show that implementation of primary health care teams has led to a reduction in the number of after-hours work for family physicians, has increased physician satisfaction and resulted in a drop in physician burnout (from 56% to 28% in one year of implementation). Therefore, a new model of organisation based on teams or networks of providers is an improvement for primary health care staff, since it may save time, improve care quality and physician satisfaction notably by decreasing stress and improving work-life balance.

Implementing team-based delivery of primary health care is not a simple undertaking given the traditional divisions of professional silos: it requires effective support from policy makers. This includes adjusting the training of health care professionals, changes in governance framework, in reimbursement practices and in the use of digital technologies (Socha-Dietrich, 2019[101]).

Table 1.1. New models of primary health care delivery have been established in 17 countries

Panel A. Name of primary health care organisations across OECD countries	
Countries	Name of the primary health care organisation recently established
Australia	Health Care Homes; Primary Health Networks
Austria	Primary care units
Canada	My Health Teams working with community health centres
Costa Rica	Basic Teams of Comprehensive Health Care (EBAIS)
Estonia	Primary care centres
France	Centres de Santé, Communautés Professionnelles Territoriales de Santé
Greece	Primary care facilities
Ireland	Primary care centres
Italy	Complex Primary Care Units (UCCPs)
Mexico	Health Centres with Extended Services
Norway	Intermediate care facilities
Slovak Republic	Integrated Primary care Centres
Slovenia	Primary care centres
Switzerland	Ambulatory Network
Sweden	Primary care centres
Turkey	Healthy Life Centres
United States	Patient-Centred Medical Home and Comprehensive Primary Care Plus

Panel B. Examples of services delivered and health professionals included	
Examples of services delivered	Examples of health professionals included
Prevention	General practitioners or family physicians
Health education	Registered or advanced nurses
Patient education	Community pharmacists
Self-management support	Psychologists
Curative services	Nutritionists
Disease management	Social workers
Specialist referral	Health counsellors
Care co-ordination	Other allied health professionals

Note: There is a lot of variation on the degree to which these health care services are delivered, and also a large heterogeneity in the combinations of health professionals included.
Source: OECD (2018[65]), Policy Survey on the Future of Primary Care.

Bundle payments and population-based payments have been effective in improving care co-ordination and care quality

Bundle payments and shared saving models have the potential to support new models of care that are better equipped to achieve people-centred care stretching across several health providers and different levels of care, including primary health care centres, specialist clinics and hospitals.

Bundled payments, which consist of one payment per patient, per chronic illness, covering the cost of all health care services provided by the full range of providers during a specific defined time period, are currently being implemented in six OECD countries (Australia, Belgium, Canada, France, Italy and the Netherlands). Bundled payment programmes have been found effective at: containing rising costs, increasing the quality of care, enabling higher patient satisfaction and better adherence to medication and treatment protocols (OECD, 2016[94]; Hussey et al., 2012[109]). This was particularly evident in the Netherlands, where bundle payments for diabetes showed improvements in care quality for most process indicators (HbA1c, BMI checked, blood pressure checked, improvement in kidney function and cholesterol tests). The bundle payment also led to more effective collaboration among health care providers and better adherence to care protocols (Struijs and Baan, 2011[110]; de Bakker et al., 2012[111]). Although the design and characteristics of bundled payments differ between these health care systems, the models developed in Australia and Canada are valuable initiatives that could guide other OECD countries. In these countries, the bundled payment accounts for patient complexity, which is an important prerequisite to encourage the participation of primary health care providers (Stokes et al., 2018[112]).

Population-based payments are made to groups of health providers, such as independent primary health care physicians, specialists, practice networks, hospitals, as well as management companies, and cover most health care services for a defined group of the population. The innovation with these schemes is the possibility for providers to share the savings generated if they are able to reduce treatment costs while still meeting pre-defined quality requirements. A prospective budget for a population is defined, and providers are financially rewarded if they can keep total costs below the benchmark value. This provides an incentive for providers to collaborate to reduce health care costs. As seen with bundled payments, population-based payments require sophisticated IT systems, and also add administrative burden to providers. Such innovative payment models are still uncommon across OECD countries. Several population-based payments with a shared saving approach have been operating in the United States since the 2010 Affordable Care Act, and in Germany with the introduction of the Gesundes Kinzigtal GmbH population-based integrated care model. Pimperl et al (2017), show that in 11 years, the integrated model of care in Germany resulted in sustained improvements in health outcomes (such as lower hospitalisation rates and higher life expectancy), increased patient satisfaction and cost reduction of 7% per insured person since 2014 (Pimperl et al., 2017[113]).

A good information system is vital to ensure that primary health care is effective

Compared to the hospital sector, health care systems know little about the quality and outcomes achieved within primary health care. The data generated in most health care systems remains concentrated on inputs and activities. Although nearly all OECD countries report structure indicators, such as the number of primary health care physicians and the number of consultations, only a handful of OECD countries systematically report primary health care quality measures at the national level. Robust reporting information systems are needed to detect, measure and learn from inappropriate and poor primary health care quality. A rich information system is a prerequisite to achieving a good understanding of how, where or why inappropriate and poor primary health care quality exists. These measurements will be developed into actions for quality improvement.

The 2018 OECD Policy Survey on the Future of Primary Care indicates that 18 OECD countries reported having implemented policy measures to collect nationwide performance metrics to monitor the performance of primary health care (Figure 1.9).

Figure 1.9. Eighteen OECD countries have implemented policy measures to collect nationwide performance metrics to monitor the performance of primary health care

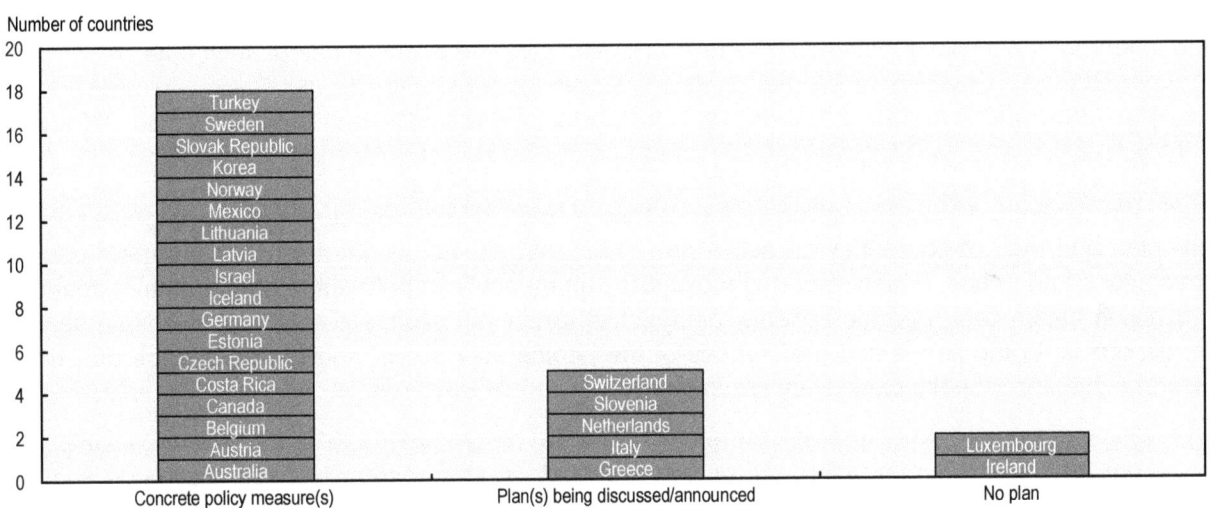

Source: OECD (2018[65]), Policy Survey on the Future of Primary Care.

To ensure primary health care is effective, it is necessary to collect data on clinical performance and efficiency at individual provider level. This can then be used to provide feedback to providers, who may be able to compare themselves to their peers and access tools for performance improvement (OECD, 2017[114]).

Indicators could, for example, focus on:
- defined daily doses of antibiotic use in ambulatory care per 1 000 inhabitants
- prescription or referrals in accordance with guidelines
- percentage of individuals with COPD or asthma who have had a lung function measurement during the last 12 months
- percentage of diabetic population with blood pressure above 140/90 mmHg observed in the last 12 months.

Evidence shows that such clinical performance and efficiency indicators are available in only a limited number of OECD countries. Canada, Denmark, Estonia, Finland, France, Israel, Italy, Latvia, Lithuania, the Netherlands, Portugal, Slovenia, Spain, Sweden, the United Kingdom and the United States, are among these countries (Reynders et al., 2018[115]; OECD, 2017[114]; Chipman, 2019[116]). Ideally, the information collected should be used systematically to identify inappropriate or poor primary health care and undertake actions for quality improvement (as is already done in some regions of Italy and Spain). In the region of Lazio, for example, primary health care quality indicators are systematically used by the Health Plan Directorate to evaluate clinical performance for chronic conditions, and to set clinical and organisational objectives for health care providers. Similarly, in Spain, performance indicators help to target strategic areas of improvement in health centres, which has resulted in slight improvements in some of the health problems which were prioritised (Reynders et al., 2018[115]).

Other than that, a strong health information infrastructure (notably though standardised national electronic health records) is required for disease surveillance, clinical trials and health system management which can help through the COVID-19 crisis and future public health crises. Effective use of such data would assist health professionals, researchers, and policy makers to understand the severity of pandemic disease, analyse trends and transmission patterns, and ensure preventive measures (Carinci, 2020[117]). Currently, only Finland, Estonia, Israel, Denmark, Austria, Canada, the Slovak Republic and the United Kingdom, as well as Singapore, have high technical and operational readiness to generate information from EHRs (Oderkirk, 2017[118]). To face future public health emergencies, there is a critical need to strengthen health information infrastructures and promote effective use of such data.

Collecting patient-reported measures at the primary health care level is an opportunity for monitoring and improving the effectiveness of issues that matter most to patients

Health care systems still know relatively little about how primary health care contributes to improve people's well-being and their ability to play an active role in society, as well as whether services meet people's expectations and needs. Patient-reported indicators can measure both health status and the experience of receiving health care from the patients' perspective. Such indicators are essential to ensure services are responsive to the needs and preferences of the people they serve, and to improve the quality and outcomes of primary health care. They are defined as:

- Patient-reported experience measures (PREMs), which capture the patient's view on health service delivery (e.g. communication with nurses and doctors, staff responsiveness, discharge and care co-ordination); whereas
- Patient-reported outcome measures (PROMs), provide the patient's perspective on their health status (e.g. symptom burden, side effects, mental health and social functioning).

It is vital to consult patients on the primary health care aspects that matter most to them. As primary health care is often the first point of contact with the health care system, taking into account patients' perspectives on their experiences with services, their values and perceptions, are all crucial elements for performance assessment. Yet, there is little effort nationally and internationally to survey patients' self-reported outcomes and experiences, which makes it very difficult to gauge what improvements are necessary from patients' perspectives. Very few countries survey PROMs within primary health care, while PREMs are collected in 18 OECD countries at national level. England and the United States are among the few OECD countries collecting PREMs at practice level. In 2017, the OECD launched the Patient-Reported Indicators Surveys (PaRIS) to address the need to understand the outcomes and experiences of people with chronic diseases; preparation for the survey instruments is ongoing (Box 1.5).

> **Box 1.5. The PaRIS survey**
>
> In 2017, the OECD launched the Patient-Reported Indicators Surveys (PaRIS) to address the need to understand the outcomes and experiences of people with chronic diseases. PaRIS offers an opportunity for gathering the evidence necessary to transform health care systems into patient-centred systems based on the needs of the people they serve.
>
> The initiative includes:
>
> - the collection of validated, standardised, internationally comparable patient-reported indicators in three areas: hip and knee replacements, breast cancer care and mental health care
> - the collection of a new set of internationally comparable measures which focus on patients with one or more chronic conditions, who are living in the community, and who are largely treated in primary health care or other ambulatory care settings.

Counselling in primary health care and the use of mobile health apps have great potential to improve patient self-management

A range of services can be provided in primary health care that support individuals to gain access to necessary information, develop technical skills, such as techniques for self-administration of medication or to practice new exercises, and ultimately, ensure a high level of self-efficacy and behaviour change. There is a growing body of evidence showing that patients who are more involved in their care have better health outcomes and care experiences (Hibbard and Greene, 2013[119]). Clinical and non-clinical services to support self-management are varied. Such services include personalised care planning, one-on-one coaching and counselling in primary health care.

Health coaching or counselling offers self-management support enabling a patient to be an active participant in the self-management of a chronic condition. Evidence shows that such strategies, most often offered as part of combined lifestyle interventions, achieve sustained behavioural change, including improved nutrition, physical activity, weight management and medication adherence (DeJesus et al., 2018[120]). In the Netherlands, for example, the Coaching on Lifestyles (Cool) intervention and the SLIMMER diabetes prevention lifestyle intervention in Dutch primary health care have been effective in improving body weight, dietary intake, physical activity and quality of life over the long term (van Rinsum et al., 2018[121]; Duijzer et al., 2017[122]). Canada, the Czech Republic, Estonia, Germany, Italy and Japan are among the relatively few other OECD countries offering counselling in primary health care.

In addition, mobile health and technology-based platforms offer a wide range of smart modalities for self-management support and by which patients can interact with health professionals on health-related activities, ranging from prevention to diagnosis, treatment and monitoring (OECD, 2017[123]). Patient-provider portals (as developed in Estonia, Finland and Turkey), smartphone applications (as developed in Australia and the United Kingdom) and telehealth interventions to support self-management (as in Denmark) show promise for improving self-efficacy, health behaviours and clinical outcomes (Whitehead and Seaton, 2016[124]; Ormel et al., 2018[125]; Payne et al., 2018[126]; Chandrashekar, 2018[127]; Guo and Albright, 2018[128]; Hanlon et al., 2017[129]).

1.3.3. Improving access and equity through primary health care

Expanding coverage of primary health care services should be a priority

Financial barriers to primary health care, including co-payments or cost-sharing arrangements, are still too significant in some OECD countries. As of 2016, user charges or other types of cost sharing for using primary health care exist in 12 out of 32 countries. In Finland, Iceland, Japan, Latvia, Norway, Portugal, Slovenia and Sweden patients pay user fees or co-payments, while in Belgium, France, Luxembourg and Switzerland patients have to pay the full cost and get reimbursed for covered services afterwards. For example, across OECD countries, co-payment per visit ranges from EUR 1 in France, EUR 1.42 in Latvia, to around EUR 14 in Norway (NOK 136) and Finland (FIM 82). In Australia, Medicare data show that patient out-of-pocket contributions continue to increase each year. Between 2016-17 and 2017-18, out-of-pocket costs to visit a GP increased from AUD 35.86 to AUD 37.39, and there has been a 20% increase in these costs since 2013-14 (The Royal Australian College of General Practitioners, 2018[46]).

Previous work shows that covering health care costs for populations not previously covered increases their use of health care services, which also improves health outcomes, particularly among the poorest populations and for children (Bourgueil, Jusot and Leleu Henri, 2012[130]). Several OECD countries are taking steps to remove financial barriers that impede access to primary health care. These strategies range from making primary health care free at the point of care (as seen in Greece in 2016), to reducing the amount of out-of-pocket payments or setting a ceiling (as seen in Belgium and Iceland in 2017). Specific measures associated with the response to the COVID-19 crisis were introduced to cover diagnostic testing for the disease and regulate their prices, for example, in the United States, Germany and France (OECD, 2020[68]). Efforts in this direction should be stepped up universally to ensure that no one is left behind.

New configurations for bringing health care delivery closer to communities can improve continuity of care and reduce health inequalities

Digital consultations can improve timely and geographical access to primary health care

Telemedicine, through digital consultations for example, makes primary health care services available to patients closer to their home or work. This allows communication between patients and medical staff, as well as the transmission of medical records and other data between different locations. Teleconsultation is a very promising way to improve access – both in respect of time and geographic location – and to relieve pressure on primary health care physicians. Liddy et al (2019) show that patients were highly satisfied with teleconsultation in terms of met expectations and confidence, and patients rated the service "high" for quality of care, timeliness, improved access, and safety (Liddy et al., 2014[131]). Several other reviews show evidence associating telemedicine with improvements in access to care, reduced travelling costs and better equity for rural and indigenous populations (Caffery et al., 2017[132]; Atherton et al., 2018[133]; Caffery et al., 2017[132]; Atherton et al., 2018[133]; Cravo Oliveira Hashiguchi, 2020[134]).

In the majority of countries, digital consultations (set up either in the public or private sector) have been deployed to improve access to health care services for patients living in remote areas (Canada, Costa Rica, the Czech Republic, Finland, France, Korea, Norway and Sweden). The Saskatchewan region of Canada started a pilot programme in 2017 called Remote Presence Technology (RPT). Accordingly, a physician, nurse or pharmacist will be "present" in several Northern communities to give patients the ability to access these services without leaving their own community. The RPT initiative shows promise in reducing travel and time costs for patients. As demonstrated by the Ontario Telemedicine Network, patients in the Canadian Network avoided travelling 270 million kilometres in 2017 and the network saved CAD 71.9 million in travel grants (OTN, 2018[135]).

Mobile clinics provide high quality primary health care to high-risk populations

Low-income and minority groups often suffer with poorer health, have multiple risk factors for diseases and face a higher number of barriers in accessing health care services (OECD, 2019[39]). Transforming primary health care services to better reach out to vulnerable population groups is vital at a time when inequalities are persisting across OECD countries.

Developing mobile health clinics is a policy option with the potential to alleviate health disparities for the most vulnerable populations (Peritogiannis et al., 2017[136]; Yu et al., 2017[137]). Mobile health clinics provide a wide range of primary health care services (including preventive care, mental health or dental services) from a bus or a van equipped with all of the necessary technology to provide clinical services in underserved or disadvantaged areas. Such facilities provide community-tailored care to vulnerable populations, both in urban and rural areas, to overcome barriers of time, money, or distance, and are particularly effective in providing urgent or preventive health care, and for initiating chronic disease management.

International experience shows that mobile primary health care clinics are able to gain the trust of vulnerable populations. Moreover, they also contribute to better health outcomes through improved access to screening (as seen in Latvia), better management of chronic diseases such as mental health (as seen in France), and by addressing social determinants of health (as seen in Mexico and the United States). In Germany and Portugal, mobile health clinics are being implemented in some rural areas to guarantee adequate primary health care and help alleviate workforce shortages.

Engaging primary health care action in the workplace will promote more inclusive societies

Connecting primary health care and occupational health is critical for better prevention of chronic conditions (such as musculoskeletal or mental health disorders) that lead to absenteeism or early departure from the labour force (James, Devaux and Sassi, 2017[138]). In 2017, exposure at work to injuries, noise, carcinogenic agents, airborne particles and ergonomic risks accounted for a substantial share of the burden of chronic diseases at global level (for example 37% of all cases of back pain and 11% of asthma) (WHO, 2017[139]).

Through closer integration between primary health care and work, health policies can play an important role in reducing the detrimental labour market impact of ill-health, contributing to reducing social health inequalities for better lives and more inclusive economies (OECD, 2017[140]). Primary health care could take a more proactive role in this direction. However, in 2018, only 10 countries out of 24 implemented concrete measures aimed at strengthening the role of primary health care in protecting and improving workers health (Figure 1.10), this is despite evidence suggesting the effectiveness of such interventions (Nicholson and Gration, 2017[141]).

Among OECD countries, the few positive examples include Germany and Sweden, where plans focus on prevention of mental distress at work and on easing the return to work for people who have suffered a disabling experience. Sweden, for example, has recently developed a new function within primary health care called "the rehabilitation co-ordinator" to enhance return to work outcomes in patients with common mental disorders.

Figure 1.10. Less than half of OECD countries implemented concrete policy measures aimed at strengthening the role of primary health care in protecting and improving workers' health

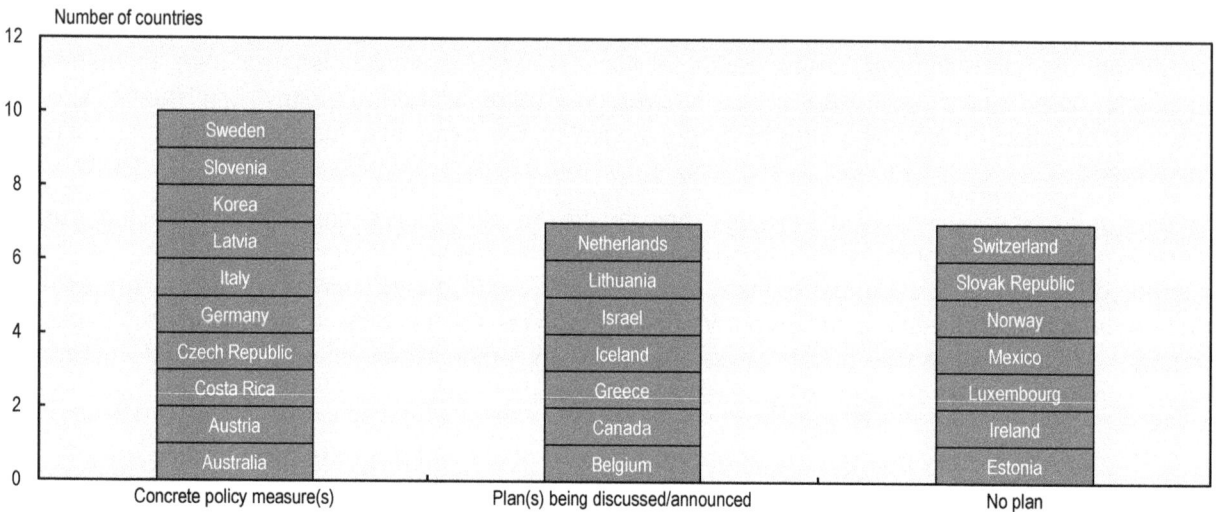

Note: Countries were asked whether policy measures aimed at strengthening the role of primary health care in protecting and improving workers' health were introduced in recent years.
Source: OECD (2018[65]), Policy Survey on the Future of Primary Care.

Revisiting the roles of health care professionals to better serve needs in remote areas

Revisiting how health care professionals are utilised and changing their scope of practice can improve access to primary health care services in remote or underserved areas where there is a shortage of primary health care physicians. This is widely recommended to help manage the increasing demands for health care, while reducing geographical inequalities in access to care. A positive trend that is apparent in some OECD countries is the growing role of nurse practitioners, community pharmacists and community health workers to carry out patient education, prevention, chronic disease management and immunisations traditionally carried out only by doctors.

In France, for example, extending the roles of nurses and pharmacists is part of the National Plan Ma santé 2022 to improve access in underserved areas. The new decree, released in June 2018, established the profession of Advanced Nurse Practitioner (Infirmière en Pratique Avancée). The Advanced Nurse Practitioner will work within a primary health care team and is expected to manage patients with chronic conditions and take the lead in prevention and co-ordination. In addition, the role of community pharmacists is being gradually increased in France. They are allowed to undertake vaccination and perform three rapid diagnostic orientation tests: the capillary blood glucose test (diabetes screening), the oropharyngeal tests for influenza and the group A streptococcal tonsillitis test. In Switzerland, the Swiss Pharmacist's Association (pharmaSuisse) has developed the Netcare programme to face a relative shortage of GPs. Participant community pharmacists provide primary triage using a structure decision tree for 24 common conditions, and if exclusion criteria are not met, the community pharmacist can manage the care (see Box 1.6). Recent evaluation shows positive results (Erni et al., 2016[142]), with pharmacists able to resolve around three-quarters of the cases presented to them. The Netcare programme is now rolled-out nationally. In 2017, 309 pharmacies were enrolled in the NetCare project, and they are being progressively introduced in some health insurance schemes. In Australia, Belgium, Canada, Italy and the United States, community pharmacists also carry out patient education, disease prevention, chronic disease management and immunisations traditionally carried out only by doctors.

> **Box 1.6. Collaboration between physicians and pharmacists in primary health care in Switzerland: The NetCare programme**
>
> Assessment of a patient's medical condition consists of a two-step process. The first step consists of checking for the exclusion criteria, which relates to patients with severe co-morbidities, unclear clinical situations, or alarming symptoms. The second step consists of assessing the patient's medical condition with the specific decision tree, which can result in:
>
> - Management by the pharmacist (counselling and dispensing of over the counter drugs), the pharmacist will also make a follow-up call to check the patient's condition three days after the assessment.
> - Management by the pharmacist with physician backup via the telemedicine centre with a secure video consultation. If appropriate, a prescription is sent to the pharmacist.
>
> Referral to either an emergency room or GP for a face-to-face consultation.
>
> Source: OECD (2018[65]), Policy Survey on the Future of Primary Care and Erni et al (2016[142])', "netCare, a new collaborative primary health care service based in Swiss community pharmacies", https://doi.org/10.1016/j.sapharm.2015.08.010.

Tools are needed to improve health information for underserved populations

Providing clear information about rules for access to care and about available services helps patients from different social and economic backgrounds access and use primary health care services in a more timely and appropriate way (OECD, 2018[143]). The provision of sufficient information about health care entitlements and available primary health care services is a key element in making primary health care services more approachable by improving health literacy skills. It is important that these initiatives reach their target audience, such as certain population groups (the migrant population for example) or people suffering from specific conditions, (such as mental health or other chronic conditions).

There are good examples across OECD countries of how to improve transparency on available primary health care services through online tools (for example, Symptom Checker or HealthDirect in Australia, *Santetresfacile* in France) and information sessions or education courses (as in Sweden which targets the migrant population, and Spain with the Network of Health Schools for Citizenship).

Developing specific training or tools for health professionals to best tailor information to high-risk or priority population groups is another key policy option. In Ireland, the ENGAGE initiative has worked to equip primary health care providers with the skills and resources to best engage and work with men (Jakab et al., 2018[144]). This initiative was launched in response to higher rates of poor lifestyle behaviours among men and low-utilisation of primary health care services. ENGAGE has been found to boost community outreach and uptake of primary health care prevention and health promotion services among this target group (Jakab et al., 2018[144]). In the Netherlands, to increase access and use of health information, PHAROS – the Dutch Centre of Expertise on Health Disparities – in co-ordination with other stakeholders, has developed specific tools for primary health care providers to optimise the delivery of primary health care services to migrant groups (EuroHealthNet, 2016[145]). Resources include a website for GPs with frequently asked questions on the provision of services to immigrant patients, a teaching toolkit for education in the prevention of girls' circumcision, and a programme for refugee children aged 10-12 years (EuroHealthNet, 2016[145]).

1.4. Conclusions: Summary of key policy ingredients to realise the full potential of primary health care

Table 1.2 summarises the findings of the report. For each chapter, the table highlights the main type of policy levers, which are organised around four categories: regulations to mandate changes in primary health care systems; organisational changes around for example the delivery model, the location or tools available for primary health care systems; economic incentives on the demand and supply sides, and patient empowerment policies including information support, patient's education or counselling. In the second columns of the table, many country examples of good practice are given.

Table 1.2. Summary of findings

Chapter 2. Improving efficiency	
Type of policy levers	**Country examples**
Regulation – Changes in training	**France**: Introduction of a public health rotation for students in the health sector. **Belgium:** Strengthening of initial and ongoing training on health promotion, disease prevention, shared communication.
	Canada, England, Germany and the United States: Strengthening competencies on the use of digital health technology.
Regulation – Develop new support roles for nurses, community pharmacists and other community health workers	**Australia:** Upskilling primary health care nurses in mental health literacy and clinical skills. **Latvia**: Introduction of second practice nurses in primary health care teams to deliver health checks and public health care. **Ireland:** Development of registered nurse prescribers to be able to prescribe a range of medicinal products. **Canada:** Development of nurse navigators to improve co-ordination and continuity of care
	Belgium: Introduction of pharmacist co-ordinators to take the lead in medication reviews. **United Kingdom**: Community Pharmacist Consultation Service is being introduced to develop the role of community pharmacy in primary health care. **Switzerland:** Development of the "No to Colorectal Cancer" campaign in community pharmacies. **Finland:** Diabetes programme for community pharmacists called "Apteenkkien Diabetesohjelma". **Italy**: The first national diabetes prevention campaign in pharmacies was organised in 2017.
	Canada: Development of primary health counsellor to provide mental health services. **United States**: Development of community health educator referral liaison to link patient with community-based services. **Costa Rica**: Introduction of health promotor to increase the focus on health promotion and disease prevention in primary health care settings. **United Kingdom**: Five different primary health care roles are being introduced (clinical pharmacists, social prescribing link workers, physician associates, first contact physiotherapists and first contact community paramedics) to provide clinical services, patient education and link patients with community-based services.
Organisational change – Use of digital technology (teleconsultation, EHR and ePrescription)	**Canada:** The Ontario Telehomecare project provides co-ordinated support from primary health care teams to people with complex chronic diseases. **Estonia**: eConsultation service in primary health care is implemented to allow primary health care physicians to consult with specialists on difficult cases online. **United Kingdom:** Babylon GP at Hand offers digital and face-to-face consultations to registered patients.
	Finland: POTKU model provides primary health care physicians with the locally developed Evidence-Based Medicine electronic Decision Support system, which is matched with EHR. **Spain:** EHR is integrated with a patient portal, an electronic prescription system and tele-monitoring service. **Israel:** Portable EHR in community care supports the sharing of information among physicians, laboratories, diagnostic centres, hospitals and patients.
	Estonia, Sweden, Australia, New Zealand, Lithuania: ePrescription service is well-developed in primary health care settings.

Organisational change – Availing primary and community care (intermediate care facilities and discharge home-based programmes)	**France**: More than 500 local hospitals will act as intermediate care facilities to provide primary health care services, rehabilitation and nursing care. **Norway, Netherlands**: Intermediate care facilities are well established to reduce the number of hospital admissions and emergency department visits. **Costa Rica**: Development of interdisciplinary outpatient units for people with mental health issues and of health hostels for patients with chronic conditions. **Ireland**: Introduction of community intervention teams to provide post-acute and nursing care. **Mexico**: Introduction of Health Centers with Extended Services (called *CESSAS*) as intermediate care facilities.
	Canada, the United Kingdom: Virtual wards provides short-term transitional care at home to high risk patients with complex needs who have recently been discharged from hospitals. **Germany**: Introduction of discharge home-based programmes for patients with mental health care issues.
Economic incentive – Design pay-for prevention, for co-ordination, for performance and other value-based payment	**Canada**: Additional fees are offered to primary health care physicians to compensate for communicating and sharing information with the care team. **Iceland, Italy, Israel**: Additional remuneration for primary health care physicians responsible for patient with chronic conditions. **Australia**: The Practice Incentives Program supports general practice activities that encourage continuing improvement and quality care including improving health outcomes relating to chronic diseases. **France**: *Experimentations de nouveaux modes de remuneration* entailed a lump-sum payment per patient for co-ordinating activities, provision of new services and inter-professional co-operation. **Austria, Denmark, Germany, Sweden, Netherlands**: Implementation of pay for co-ordination schemes. **United States**: The Comprehensive Primary Care Plus model allow providers to bill for care co-ordination and care transition services. **Czech Republic, Denmark, Norway, Sweden, the United Kingdom**: Hospitals or municipalities are fined for excessive delays in discharge from hospital. **Canada**: Primary health care physicians are provided with a financial incentive for a timely primary health care appointment post-hospital discharge.
	England: The Quality and Outcome Framework included 75 indicators in 2017-19. **France**: *Remunération sur Objectifs de Santé Publique* targeted management of chronic conditions, prevention activities and efficiency in 2018. **Estonia**: The Quality Bonus System targets prevention, monitoring of chronic diseases according to national guidelines and enhanced services. **Chile**: The P4P programme has two components: the health goals and the primary health care activity. **Czech Republic**: Each health insurance fund designs its own P4P programme **United States**: P4P programmes designed for community pharmacists to increase their role in the delivery of primary health care services.

Chapter 3 – A. More effective and patient-centred care through disease prevention and care co-ordination

Type of policy levers	Country examples
Organisational change – Develop new models of primary health care delivery based on teams or networks	**United States**: Development of Patient-Centered Medical Homes, and recently the Comprehensive Primary Care Plus. **Australia**: Establishment of 31 Primary Health Networks, and 132 Health Care Homes. **Canada**: Development of the Physician Integrated Framework, which gave an impetus to the development of My Health Team in several provinces. **France**: Development of *Centres de Santé* and *Communautés Professionnelles Territoriales de Santé*. **Austria**: Establishment of primary health care units.
Organisational change – Implementing portable EHR	**Spain**: Use of risk stratification by unifying EHR with various data sources, including demographics, primary health care, hospital care and prescription data. **Israel**: All the health funds have comprehensive EHR in community care to support delivery of care processes. **United States**: HealthConnect, the largest EHR implemented by Kaiser Permanente, has many functionalities to support primary health care teams.

Type of policy levers	Country examples
Economic incentive – Bundled payments, needs-based capitation and population-based payments	**Australia**: Funding for Health Care Homes is bundled into periodic payments (levels of payments linked to patient's level of complexity). **Canada**: Introduction of Comprehensive Care Management (CCM) in Manitoba for patients with chronic conditions (5 tariffs are available according to patient's level of complexity). **France**: Experimentation of bundled payments (*Paiement en Equipe des Professionnels de Santé*) for patients followed by a multi-disciplinary team. **Belgium**: Interprofessional Integrated Needs-based Capitation payment introduced to take into account patient's level of complexity and stimulate collaboration.
	United States: Implementation of several population-based payments with a shared saving approach in ACOs. **Germany**: Gesundes Kinzigtal GmbH is an integrated care model whith a shared saving approach. **France**: Implementation of a five-year pilot programme called *Incitation à une Prise en Charge Partagée*, which is similar to shared savings population-based financing.

Chapter 3 – B. More effective and patient-centred care through patient self-management and greater responsiveness

Type of policy levers	Country examples
Patient empowerment – Collecting primary health care on clinical performance and undertake quality improvement actions	**Israel**: The Quality Indicators in Community Healthcare programme captures more than 35 measures of quality of primary health care. **Sweden**: Primary Care Quality Sweden is a quality improvement system comprising around 150 quality measures and technical methods for collecting data automatically. **Italy**: In the region of Lazio, primary health care quality indicators are systematically used by the Health Plan Directorate to evaluate clinical performance for chronic conditions. **Spain**: Performance indicators help to target strategic areas of improvement in health centres. **United States**: The CAHPS surveys collect PREMs indicators at practice level and for specific health conditions. **England**: The GP Patient Survey assesses patient's experience of health care services provided by GP practices within the NHS.
Patient empowerment – Individual and group-based services to support better self-management	**Netherlands**: Implementation of several Combined Lifestyle Intervention such as the Coaching on Lifestyles intervention and the SLIMMER diabetes prevention lifestyle intervention. **Canada, Czech Republic, Germany**: Implementation of brief alcohol intervention in primary health care settings and the workplace. **Italy, Japan, Estonia**: Implementation of health education and counselling in primary and community settings to improve diets, physical activity and screening uptake. **Australia, New Zealand, the United Kingdom and the United States**: Peer support groups used for mental health care to provide education, emotional support and practical problem-solving assistance. **Canada**: Your Way to Wellness programme in Nova Scotia is a self-management programme for those living with chronic diseases.
Organisational change – Use of digital technology (patient-provider portals, smartphones, internet-based monitoring)	**Finland**: The Oulu Self Care Service is an electronic platform providing self-care services. **Canada**: miHealth application is a secure platform for patients and physicians to communicate. **Estonia**: Patient portal allows access to personal health information, to relevant health information based on their health status and to treatment plans. **Turkey**: E-pulse is the personal health record system where people can share their medical records with their doctor, make medical appointments, and self-monitoring their condition.
	Australia: The Symptom Checker is an online tool to guide consumers to the most appropriate health care and to provide advice. **United Kingdom**: Babylon Health GP at Hand deliver personalised health assessments, treatment advice and face-to-face appointments.
	Denmark: TeleCare North is a telemonitoring programme for chronic conditions involving the North Denmark regional authority, its hospitals, GPs and 11 municipalities. **Austria**: The Health Dialogue Diabetes Mellitus campaign offers telemonitoring programme. **Czech Republic**: Telemonitoring programmes are offered for chronic heart failure and diabetes. **Ireland**: Telemonitoring programme are offered for epilepsy. **Lithuania**: Telemonitoring programme are offered for palliative care.

Type of policy levers	Country examples
Economic incentive – Health care vouchers or coupons, personal health budgets and conditional cash transfers	**United States**: California's Medicaid programme introduced non-health-related incentives (movie tickets or gift certificates) to reward patients who keep up with scheduled well-child. **Germany:** Health care vouchers for accessing primary health care services was introduced for refugees.
	England: Personal health budgets are offered to people with long-term conditions to improve quality of life, well-being and encourage greater choice and control.
	United States: Conditional cash transfers are used to encourage greater use of preventive health services.
Chapter 4 – Less inequalities and more inclusive societies	
Type of policy levers	Country examples
Regulation – Readjust the role of health professionals to improve access to primary health care services in remote and under-served areas	**Australia:** The Allied Health Rural Generalist Program and the Rural Generalist Medical Programme for GPs to address requirements for training, development and ongoing support in rural or remote areas. **United States:** Community health aids provide primary health care services in remote areas (for example Alaskan villages) **France:** A new decree has established the profession of Advanced Nurse Practitioner in 2018, and the role of pharmacists is increasingly growing as part of *Ma Santé 2022*. **Switzerland:** Netcare programme offers opportunities to pharmacists to provide primary triage and non-urgent primary health care.
Organisational change – Use of digital consultation or tele-expertise	**Norway, Sweden, Finland, Costa Rica, Korea**: Video consultations are possible for people living in rural and remote areas. **Czech Republic:** Telemedicine services are possible in cardiology and diabetes care. **Canada (Saskatchewan):** Patients can receive primary health care by visiting the nearest telehealth site and meeting with a professional in a virtual exam room. The Remote Presence Technology pilot allows the primary health care team in the community to have access to expertise on demand. **Lithuania, Portugal:** Tele-expertise between primary health care teams and specialists is possible for dermatology consultation. **Ireland:** Pilot mental telehealth sites have being established. **France, United Kingdom, Germany, Switzerland, Belgium:** Several platforms (such as LIVI, Babylon GP at Hand, or Medlanes) offer fee-charging or non-fee charging video consultations with primary health care teams.
Organisational change – Development of mobile health clinics to reach the most vulnerable populations	**United States**: Mobile primary health care clinics provide screening, preventive care, and management of chronic diseases for deprived population. **Mexico:** Health Windows provide primary health care to localities that do not have access to health services due to their geographic dispersion or characteristics of the population. **Germany, Portugal:** Mobile health clinics are being implemented in some rural areas to guarantee adequate primary health care and to help alleviate workforce shortages. **Latvia:** Mobile primary health care facilities are specifically designed to perform screening, and physical health and dental checks in rural areas. **France:** Mobile health care units (*équipes mobiles psychiatrie précarité*) target mental health care needs for the most vulnerable population. **Greece:** Mobile Mental Health Units provide a range of health care services and educational programmes for the community in rural and remote areas.
Organisational change – Integrate primary health care and social care to address social health determinants	**Canada:** Access Centres and Community Health Centres provide primary health care and health promotion programmes for individuals, and work in close collaboration with the community to address social conditions. **United States:** Development of community partnerships aims at linking patients with community services to address health-related social needs.
Organisational change – Conduct primary health care actions in the workplace	**Sweden:** Rehabilitation coordinators work in primary health care to enhance return to work for patients with common mental disorders. **Belgium:** Prevention advisors give guidance to workplaces on psychological well-being, and support the preparation of risk assessment plans to minimise stress and violence at work. **Germany:** Occupational medical doctors work in collaboration with the primary health care team in order to promote people's health and employability.
Economic incentive – Expanding coverage for primary health care services and reducing out-of-pocket payments	**Greece:** Introduction of universal coverage with primary health care services in 2016. **Belgium:** Introduction of a bill to prevent patients from paying out-of-pocket payments above a certain threshold. **Iceland:** Introduction of a ceiling, and when the upper limit is reached, patients will only pay a low fixed sum every month.

Patient empowerment – Improving the availability of health information and health literacy skills for populations	**Australia:** Healthdirect provides every Australian with access to the trusted information and advice they need to manage their own health **France**: *Santetresfacile* provides information about health professionals to ease access to care, and provide friendly and understandable information to help people monitor their health. **Spain**: The Network of Health Schools for Citizenship offers a wide range of programmes, training tools and evidence-based health information to patients, relatives and caregivers.
	Sweden: Information sessions are organised to encourage discussion among immigrants about common problems with navigating the health care system. **United States**: Kaiser Permanente has telephone-based interpreter services that can be accessed at all times to provide instant translation for foreign-born population.
	Ireland: ENGAGE initiative to equip primary health care providers with the skills and resources to best work with some target population. **Netherlands**: PHAROS offers tools for primary health care providers to optimize the delivery of primary health care services to migrant population.

References

Agency for Healthcare Research and Quality (2018), *Potentially Avoidable Hospitalizations.*, http://www.ahrq.gov/research/findings/nhqrdr/chartbooks/carecoordination/measure3.html (accessed on 9 April 2019). [16]

AHRQ (2016), "Team-Based Primary Care: Convergence of Improving Engagement, Safety, and Enhanced Joy in Practice", *AHRQ Pub. No. 16-0035*, https://micmrc.org/system/files/BEllin%20teambased-1_0.pdf. [108]

AIHW (2019), *Potentially preventable hospitalisations in Australia by small geographic areas*, Web Report, Cat. no. HPF 36. Canberra: AIHW., https://www.aihw.gov.au/reports/primary-health-care/potentially-preventable-hospitalisations/contents/overview (accessed on 5 September 2019). [58]

Aihw (2018), *Emergency department care 2017-18 Australian hospital statistics*, http://www.aihw.gov.au. [24]

Atherton, H. et al. (2018), "Alternatives to the face-to-face consultation in general practice: Focused ethnographic case study", *British Journal of General Practice*, http://dx.doi.org/10.3399/bjgp18X694853. [133]

Auraaen, A., L. Slawomirski and N. Klazinga (2018), "The economics of patient safety in primary and ambulatory care: Flying blind", *OECD Health Working Papers*, No. 106, OECD Publishing, Paris, https://dx.doi.org/10.1787/baf425ad-en. [56]

Bates, D. and A. Bitton (2010), *The future of health information technology in the patient-centered medical home*, http://dx.doi.org/10.1377/hlthaff.2010.0007. [105]

Bell, D., N. Gachuhi and N. Assefi (2018), *Perspective Piece: Dynamic clinical algorithms: Digital technology can transform health care decision-making*, American Society of Tropical Medicine and Hygiene, http://dx.doi.org/10.4269/ajtmh.17-0477. [88]

Berchet, C. (2015), "Emergency Care Services: Trends, Drivers and Interventions to Manage the Demand", *OECD Health Working Papers*, No. 83, OECD Publishing, Paris, https://dx.doi.org/10.1787/5jrts344crns-en. [15]

Bonner, L. (2016), "As pay for performance grows, health plans work with pharmacies", *Pharmacy Today*, http://dx.doi.org/10.1016/j.ptdy.2016.02.024. [97]

Borgermans, L. et al. (2018), "How Leapfrogging in primary care can contribute to upscaling NCD core services", *Eurohealth*, Vol. 24/1. [99]

Bourgueil, Y., F. Jusot and Leleu Henri (2012), "In What Way Can Primary Care Contribute to Reducing Health Inequalities? A Review of Research Literature", *Question d'Economie de la Santé*, http://www.irdes.fr/EspaceAnglais/Publications/IrdesPublications/QES179.pdff. [130]

Buerhaus Peter (2018), *Nurse Practitioners: Nurse Practitioners: A solution to America's primary care crisis*, American Enterprise Institute. [72]

Caffery, L. et al. (2017), *Outcomes of using telehealth for the provision of healthcare to Aboriginal and Torres Strait Islander people: a systematic review*, http://dx.doi.org/10.1111/1753-6405.12600. [132]

Campanella, P. et al. (2016), *The impact of electronic health records on healthcare quality: A systematic review and meta-analysis*, http://dx.doi.org/10.1093/eurpub/ckv122. [78]

Campbell, R. et al. (2003), "Cervical cancer rates and the supply of primary care physicians in Florida", *Family Medicine*. [35]

Carinci, F. (2020), "Covid-19: preparedness, decentralisation, and the hunt for patient zero; Lessons from the Italian outbreak", *BMJ*, Vol. 368, http://dx.doi.org/10.1136/bmj.m799. [117]

Chandrashekar, P. (2018), "Do mental health mobile apps work: evidence and recommendations for designing high-efficacy mental health mobile apps", *mHealth*, http://dx.doi.org/10.21037/mhealth.2018.03.02. [127]

Chaudhry, B. et al. (2006), "Systematic review: impact of health information technology on quality, efficiency, and costs of medical care", *Annals of internal medicine*, http://dx.doi.org/10.7326/0003-4819-144-10-200605160-00125. [77]

Chetty, U. et al. (2016), "The role of primary care in improving health equity: Report of a workshop held by the WONCA Health Equity Special Interest Group at the 2015 WONCA Europe Conference in Istanbul, Turkey", *International Journal for Equity in Health*, http://dx.doi.org/10.1186/s12939-016-0415-8. [38]

Chipman, A. (2019), *Value-Based Healthcare In Sweden: Reaching the next level*, Economist Intelligence Unit Limited, https://eiuperspectives.economist.com/sites/default/files/value-basedhealthcareinswedenreachingthenextlevel.pdf. [116]

Conejo-Cerón, S. et al. (2017), *Effectiveness of psychological and educational interventions to prevent depression in primary care: A systematic review and meta-analysis*, Annals of Family Medicine, Inc, http://dx.doi.org/10.1370/afm.2031. [29]

Cookson, R. et al. (2017), "Primary care and health inequality: Difference-in-difference study comparing England and Ontario", *PLoS ONE*, http://dx.doi.org/10.1371/journal.pone.0188560. [43]

Couturier, B., F. Carrat and G. Hejblum (2016), "A systematic review on the effect of the organisation of hospital discharge on patient health outcomes", http://dx.doi.org/10.1136/bmjopen-2016. [63]

Cravo Oliveira Hashiguchi, T. (2020), "Bringing health care to the patient: An overview of the use of telemedicine in OECD countries", *OECD Health Working Papers*, No. 116, OECD Publishing, Paris, https://dx.doi.org/10.1787/8e56ede7-en. [134]

Cylus, J., I. Papanicolas and P. Smith (2016), *Health System Efficiency. How to make measurement matter for policy and management*, WHO Regional Office for Europe, Copenhagen, Denmark. [25]

Dahl, U., A. Steinsbekk and R. Johnsen (2015), "Effectiveness of an intermediate care hospital on readmissions, mortality, activities of daily living and use of health care services among hospitalized adults aged 60 years and older - A controlled observational study", *BMC Health Services Research*, http://dx.doi.org/10.1186/s12913-015-1022-x. [89]

de Bakker, D. et al. (2012), "Early results from Adoption of bundled payment for diabetes care in the Netherlands show improvement in care coordination", *Health Affairs*, http://dx.doi.org/10.1377/hlthaff.2011.0912. [111]

De Maeseneer, J. and P. Boeckxstaens (2012), *Debate & analysis James Mackenzie lecture 2011: Multimorbidity, goal-oriented care, and equity*, http://dx.doi.org/10.3399/bjgp12X652553. [96]

Declaration of Astana - Global Conference on Primary Health Care (2018), *Declaration of Astana*, https://www.who.int/docs/default-source/primary-health/declaration/gcphc-declaration.pdf. [7]

Deetjen, U. (2016), "European E-Prescriptions: Benefits and Success Factors", *Cyber Studies Programme*, No. 5, Oxford Internet Institute, University of Oxford, http://www.politics.ox.ac.uk/centre/cyber-studies-programme.html (accessed on 18 July 2019). [83]

DeJesus, R. et al. (2018), "Impact of a 12-week wellness coaching on self-care behaviors among primary care adult patients with prediabetes", *Preventive Medicine Reports*, http://dx.doi.org/10.1016/j.pmedr.2018.02.012. [120]

Del Fiol, G., T. Workman and P. Gorman (2014), *Clinical questions raised by clinicians at the point of care a systematic review*, http://dx.doi.org/10.1001/jamainternmed.2014.368. [54]

Duijzer, G. et al. (2017), "Effect and maintenance of the SLIMMER diabetes prevention lifestyle intervention in Dutch primary healthcare: A randomised controlled trial", *Nutrition and Diabetes*, http://dx.doi.org/10.1038/nutd.2017.21. [122]

East Melbourne, V. (ed.) (2018), *General Practice: Health of the Nation 2018*, http://www.racgp.org.au. [46]

Erni, P. et al. (2016), "netCare, a new collaborative primary health care service based in Swiss community pharmacies", *Research in Social and Administrative Pharmacy*, http://dx.doi.org/10.1016/j.sapharm.2015.08.010. [142]

EuroHealthNet (2016), *How the Netherlands and PHAROS are reducing health inequalities and improving health literacy*, http://eurohealthnet-magazine.eu/how-the-netherlands-is-reducing-health-disparities-and-ensuring-heath-and-good-quality-care-for-all-thanks-to-pharos (accessed on 6 June 2019). [145]

Fisher, R. et al. (2017), *GP views on strategies to cope with increasing workload: A qualitative interview study*, http://dx.doi.org/10.3399/bjgp17X688861. [49]

Fleetcroft, R. et al. (2018), "Does practice analysis agree with the ambulatory care sensitive conditions' list of avoidable unplanned admissions?: A cross-sectional study in the East of England", *BMJ Open*, http://dx.doi.org/10.1136/bmjopen-2017-020756. [57]

Frenk, J. et al. (2010), *Health professionals for a new century: Ttransforming education to strengthen health systems in an interdependent world*, http://dx.doi.org/10.1016/S0140-6736(10)61854-5. [50]

Friedberg, M. et al. (2015), "Effects of a medical home and shared savings intervention on quality and utilization of care", *JAMA Internal Medicine*, http://dx.doi.org/10.1001/jamainternmed.2015.2047. [102]

Garåsen, H., R. Windspoll and R. Johnsen (2007), "Intermediate care at a community hospital as an alternative to prolonged general hospital care for elderly patients: A randomised controlled trial", *BMC Public Health*, http://dx.doi.org/10.1186/1471-2458-7-68. [90]

Grava-Gubins, I., A. Safarov and J. Eriksson (2012), *2010 National Physician Survey : Workload patterns of Canadian Family Physicians*. [47]

Green, L., S. Savin and Y. Lu (2013), "Primary care physician shortages could be eliminated through use of teams, nonphysicians, and electronic communication", *Health Affairs*, http://dx.doi.org/10.1377/hlthaff.2012.1086. [64]

Guanais, F. et al. (2019), "Primary Health Care and Determinants of the Perception of the Health System and Quality of Care in 17 Countries in LAC and the OECD", in Guanais, F. et al. (eds.), *From the Patient's Perspective: Experiences with primary health care in Latin America and the Caribbean*, Inter-American Development Bank, Washington, DC. [36]

Guo, Y. and D. Albright (2018), "The effectiveness of telehealth on self-management for older adults with a chronic condition: A comprehensive narrative review of the literature", *Journal of Telemedicine and Telecare*, http://dx.doi.org/10.1177/1357633X17706285. [128]

Haines, A. et al. (2020), "National UK programme of community health workers for COVID-19 response", *The Lancet*, Vol. 395, https://doi.org/10.1016/S0140-6736(20)30735-2. [69]

Hanlon, P. et al. (2017), *Telehealth interventions to support self-management of long-term conditions: A systematic metareview of diabetes, heart failure, asthma, chronic obstructive pulmonary disease, and cancer*, http://dx.doi.org/10.2196/jmir.6688. [129]

Hartley, L. (2002), "Examination of primary care characteristics in a community-based clinic", *Journal of Nursing Scholarship*, Vol. 34/4, pp. 377-382, http://dx.doi.org/10.1111/j.1547-5069.2002.00377.x. [34]

Hernández, C. et al. (2018), "Implementation of Home Hospitalization and Early Discharge as an Integrated Care Service: A Ten Years Pragmatic Assessment", *International Journal of Integrated Care*, http://dx.doi.org/10.5334/ijic.3431. [93]

Hibbard, J. and J. Greene (2013), "What the evidence shows about patient activation: Better health outcomes and care experiences; fewer data on costs", *Health Affairs*, http://dx.doi.org/10.1377/hlthaff.2012.1061. [119]

Hirschhorn, L. et al. (2019), "What kind of evidence do we need to strengthen primary healthcare in the 21st century?", *BMJ Global Health*, Vol. 4/Suppl 8, p. e001668, http://dx.doi.org/10.1136/bmjgh-2019-001668. [8]

Hobbs, F. et al. (2016), "Clinical workload in UK primary care: a retrospective analysis of 100 million consultations in England, 2007–14", *The Lancet*, http://dx.doi.org/10.1016/S0140-6736(16)00620-6. [44]

Hone, T., J. Macinko and C. Millett (2018), "Revisiting Alma-Ata: what is the role of primary health care in achieving the Sustainable Development Goals?", *The Lancet*, Vol. 392/10156, pp. 1461-1472, http://dx.doi.org/10.1016/S0140-6736(18)31829-4. [9]

Hujala Anneli et al. (2016), *The POTKU project (Potilas kuljettajan paikalle, Putting the Patient in the Driver's Seat), Finland*, http://www.icare4eu.org/pdf/POTKU_Case_report.pdf (accessed on 20 May 2019). [79]

Huntley, A. et al. (2014), "Which features of primary care affect unscheduled secondary care use? A systematic review", *BMJ Open*, http://dx.doi.org/10.1136/bmjopen-2013-004746. [13]

Hussey, P. et al. (2012), "Closing the quality gap: revisiting the state of the science (vol. 1: bundled payment: effects on health care spending and quality).", *Evidence report/technology assessment*. [109]

Iankowitz, N. et al. (2012), "The effectiveness of computer system tools on potentially inappropriate medications ordered at discharge for adults older than 65 years of age: a systematic review.", *JBI library of systematic reviews*, Vol. 10/13, pp. 798-831, http://dx.doi.org/10.11124/jbisrir-2012-68. [82]

IQVIA (2017), *The Growing Value of Digital Health. Evidence and Impact on Human Health and the Healthcare System*, IQVIA Institute for Human Data Science, https://www.iqvia.com/-/media/iqvia/pdfs/institute-reports/the-growing-value-of-digital-health.pdf?_=1562314612052 (accessed on 5 July 2019). [87]

Jakab, M. et al. (2018), *Health systems respond to noncommunicable diseases: time for ambition*, WHO Regional Office for Europe, Copenhagen. [144]

James, C., M. Devaux and F. Sassi (2017), "Inclusive growth and health", *OECD Health Working Papers*, No. 103, OECD Publishing, Paris, https://dx.doi.org/10.1787/93d52bcd-en. [138]

Khan, R. and K. Socha-Dietrich (2018), "Investing in medication adherence improves health outcomes and health system efficiency: Adherence to medicines for diabetes, hypertension, and hyperlipidaemia", *OECD Health Working Papers*, No. 105, OECD Publishing, Paris, https://dx.doi.org/10.1787/8178962c-en. [81]

Kirkland, S., A. Soleimani and A. Newton (2018), "The impact of pediatric mental health care provided outpatient, primary care, community and school settings on emergency department use – a systematic review.", *Child Adolesc Ment Health* 23, pp. 4-13. [14]

Kitsiou, S. et al. (2017), "Effectiveness of mHealth interventions for patients with diabetes: An overview of systematic reviews", *PLOS ONE*, Vol. 12/3, p. e0173160, http://dx.doi.org/10.1371/journal.pone.0173160. [85]

Kringos, D. et al. (2010), "The breadth of primary care: a systematic literature review of its core dimensions.", *BMC health services research*, Vol. 10, p. 65, http://dx.doi.org/10.1186/1472-6963-10-65. [40]

Kringos, D. et al. (2013), "Europe's Strong Primary Care Systems Are Linked To Better Population Health But Also To Higher Health Spending", *Health Affairs*, Vol. 32/4, pp. 686-694, http://dx.doi.org/10.1377/hlthaff.2012.1242. [28]

Levine, D., B. Landon and J. Linder (2019), "Quality and Experience of Outpatient Care in the United States for Adults With or Without Primary Care", *JAMA Internal Medicine*, Vol. 179/3, p. 363, http://dx.doi.org/10.1001/jamainternmed.2018.6716. [37]

Liddy, C. et al. (2014), "Health coaching in primary care: A feasibility model for diabetes care", *BMC Family Practice*, http://dx.doi.org/10.1186/1471-2296-15-60. [131]

Lin, I., S. Wu and S. Huang (2015), "Continuity of Care and Avoidable Hospitalizations for Chronic Obstructive Pulmonary Disease (COPD)", *The Journal of the American Board of Family Medicine*, Vol. 28/2, pp. 222-230, http://dx.doi.org/10.3122/jabfm.2015.02.140141. [20]

Lorenzoni, L. et al. (2019), "Health Spending Projections to 2030: New results based on a revised OECD methodology", *OECD Health Working Papers*, No. 110, OECD Publishing, Paris, https://dx.doi.org/10.1787/5667f23d-en. [6]

Macinko, J., B. Starfield and T. Erinosho (2009), "The Impact of Primary Healthcare on Population Health in Low- and Middle-Income Countries", *Journal of Ambulatory Care Management*, Vol. 32/2, pp. 150-171, http://dx.doi.org/10.1097/jac.0b013e3181994221. [27]

Macinko, J., B. Starfield and L. Shi (2003), "The contribution of primary care systems to health outcomes within Organization for Economic Cooperation and Development (OECD) countries, 1970-1998", *Health Services Research*, http://dx.doi.org/10.1111/1475-6773.00149. [26]

Maier, C. and L. Aiken (2016), *Expanding clinical roles for nurses to realign the global health workforce with population needs: A commentary*, http://dx.doi.org/10.1186/s13584-016-0079-2. [73]

Matthys, E., R. Remmen and P. Van Bogaert (2017), "An overview of systematic reviews on the collaboration between physicians and nurses and the impact on patient outcomes: What can we learn in primary care?", *BMC Family Practice*, http://dx.doi.org/10.1186/s12875-017-0698-x. [71]

McHale, P. et al. (2013), "Who uses emergency departments inappropriately and when - a national cross-sectional study using a monitoring data system", *BMC Medicine*, Vol. 11/1, http://dx.doi.org/10.1186/1741-7015-11-258. [23]

Medical Association, C. (2017), *CMA Workforce Survey 2017*, http://www.cma.ca/pdc. [48]

Morton, K. et al. (2017), "Using digital interventions for self-management of chronic physical health conditions: A meta-ethnography review of published studies.", *Patient education and counseling*, http://dx.doi.org/10.1016/j.pec.2016.10.019. [86]

Mousquès, J. (2011), "Le regroupement des professionnels de santé de premiers recours : quelles perspectives économiques en termes de performance ?", *Revue française des affaires sociales*, Vol. 2-3, p. pages 253 à 275. [100]

NAP (2019), *State of the science: a synthesis of interprofessional collaborative practice research*, National Academies of Practice, Lexingtion, https://napractice.org/Portals/0/NAP%20State%20of%20the%20Science%20-%20Final%20for%20publication.pdf. [106]

NCQA (2017), *Patient-Centered Medical Home Recognition*. [103]

NHS (2019), *Investment and evolution: A five-year framework for GP contract reform to implement The NHS Long Term Plan*, NHS England. [70]

NHS (2019), *The Community Pharmacy Contractual Framework for 2019/20 to 2023/24: supporting delivery for the NHS Long Term Plan*, Depatment of Health and social care, NHS and PSNC, https://assets.publishing.service.gov.uk/government/uploads/system/uploads/attachment_data/file/819601/cpcf-2019-to-2024.pdf. [98]

Nicholson, P. and J. Gration (2017), "What occupational medicine offers to primary care", *British Journal of General Practice*, Vol. 67/662, pp. 392-393, http://dx.doi.org/10.3399/bjgp17X692213. [141]

Nuffieldtrust (2019), *Potentially preventable emergency hospital admissions*, https://www.nuffieldtrust.org.uk/resource/potentially-preventable-emergency-hospital-admissions (accessed on 9 April 2019). [18]

Oderkirk, J. (2017), "Readiness of electronic health record systems to contribute to national health information and research", *OECD Health Working Papers*, No. 99, OECD Publishing, Paris, https://dx.doi.org/10.1787/9e296bf3-en. [118]

OECD (2020), *Beyond Containment: Health systems responses to COVID-19 in the OECD*, OECD Publishing, Paris, http://www.oecd.org/coronavirus/policy-responses/beyond-containment-health-systems-responses-to-covid-19-in-the-oecd-6ab740c0/. [68]

OECD (2019), *Health at a Glance 2019: OECD Indicators*, OECD Publishing, Paris, https://doi.org/10.1787/4dd50c09-en. [59]

OECD (2019), *Health for Everyone?: Social Inequalities in Health and Health Systems*, OECD Health Policy Studies, OECD Publishing, Paris, https://dx.doi.org/10.1787/3c8385d0-en. [39]

OECD (2019), *Health in the 21st Century: Putting Data to Work for Stronger Health Systems*, OECD Health Policy Studies, OECD Publishing, Paris, https://dx.doi.org/10.1787/e3b23f8e-en. [2]

OECD (2019), *Risks that Matter: Main Findings from the 2018 OECD Risks that Matter Survey*, OECD, Paris, http://www.oecd.org/social/risks-that-matter.htm. [1]

OECD (2018), "How resilient were OECD health care systems during the "refugee crisis"?", *Migration Policy Debates*, Vol. 17. [143]

OECD (2018), *Policy Survey on the Future of Primary Care*. [65]

OECD (2017), *Caring for Quality in Health: Lessons Learnt from 15 Reviews of Health Care Quality*, OECD Reviews of Health Care Quality, OECD Publishing, Paris, https://dx.doi.org/10.1787/9789264267787-en. [114]

OECD (2017), *OECD Digital Economy Outlook 2017*, OECD Publishing, Paris, https://doi.org/10.1787/9789264276284-en (accessed on 3 July 2019). [123]

OECD (2017), *Preventing Ageing Unequally*, OECD Publishing, Paris, https://dx.doi.org/10.1787/9789264279087-en. [140]

OECD (2017), *Tackling Wasteful Spending on Health*, OECD Publishing, Paris, https://dx.doi.org/10.1787/9789264266414-en. [60]

OECD (2016), *Better Ways to Pay for Health Care*, OECD Health Policy Studies, OECD Publishing, Paris, https://dx.doi.org/10.1787/9789264258211-en. [94]

OECD (2016), *Health System Characteristics Survey*, http://www.oecd.org/els/health-systems/characteristics.htm. [66]

OECD (2016), *Health Workforce Policies in OECD Countries: Right Jobs, Right Skills, Right Places*, OECD Health Policy Studies, OECD Publishing, Paris, https://dx.doi.org/10.1787/9789264239517-en. [51]

OECD/EU (2018), *Health at a Glance: Europe 2018: State of Health in the EU Cycle*, OECD Publishing, Paris/EU, Brussels, https://doi.org/10.1787/health_glance_eur-2018-en. [4]

OECD/IDB (2016), *Broadband Policies for Latin America and the Caribbean: A Digital Economy Toolkit*, OECD Publishing, Paris, https://dx.doi.org/10.1787/9789264251823-en. [74]

Ormel, H. et al. (2018), "Self-monitoring physical activity with a smartphone application in cancer patients: a randomized feasibility study (SMART-trial)", *Supportive Care in Cancer*, http://dx.doi.org/10.1007/s00520-018-4263-5. [125]

OTN (2018), *OTN Annual Report 2017/2018*, Ontario Telemedicine Network, https://otn.ca/wp-content/uploads/2017/11/otn-annual-report.pdf (accessed on 3 July 2019). [135]

PAE - Pain Alliance Europe (2018), *Survey on chronic pain and your work life: A survey in 14 EU countries.*, Pain Alliance Europe. [3]

Payne, J. et al. (2018), "Defining Adherence to Dietary Self-Monitoring Using a Mobile App: A Narrative Review", *Journal of the Academy of Nutrition and Dietetics*, http://dx.doi.org/10.1016/j.jand.2018.05.011. [126]

Pecina, J. and F. North (2016), "Early e-consultation face-to-face conversions", *Journal of Telemedicine and Telecare*, http://dx.doi.org/10.1177/1357633X15602634. [84]

Peritogiannis, V. et al. (2017), "Mental healthcare delivery in rural greece: A 10-year account of a mobile mental health unit", *Journal of Neurosciences in Rural Practice*, http://dx.doi.org/10.4103/jnrp.jnrp_142_17. [136]

PGEU (2020), *PGEU overview of the expansion of community pharmacy services/activities in relation to COVID-19*, PGEU. [67]

Pimperl, A. et al. (2017), "Case Study: Gesundes Kinzigtal, Germany - Accountable care in Practice: Global perspectives", *Research Gate - Technical Report*. [113]

Purdy, S. (2010), *Avoiding hospital admissions*, The King's Fund, London, https://www.kingsfund.org.uk/publications/avoiding-hospital-admissions. [17]

Ranjan, P., A. Kumari and A. Chakrawarty (2015), "How can doctors improve their communication skills?", *Journal of Clinical and Diagnostic Research*, http://dx.doi.org/10.7860/JCDR/2015/12072.5712. [55]

Reynders, D. et al. (2018), *A new drive for primary care in Europe rethinking the assessment tools and methodologies : report of the Expert Group on Health Systems Performance Assessment*, Publications Office of the European Union. [115]

Rosano, A. et al. (2013), "The relationship between avoidable hospitalization and accessibility to primary care: a systematic review.", *European journal of public health*, Vol. 23/3, pp. 356-60, http://dx.doi.org/10.1093/eurpub/cks053. [11]

Ruano, A., J. Furler and L. Shi (2015), "Interventions in Primary Care and their contributions to improving equity in health", *International Journal for Equity in Health*, http://dx.doi.org/10.1186/s12939-015-0284-6. [42]

Ryan, A. et al. (2016), "Long-term evidence for the effect of pay-for-performance in primary care on mortality in the UK: a population study", *The Lancet*, http://dx.doi.org/10.1016/S0140-6736(16)00276-2. [95]

Salmi, L. et al. (2017), "Interventions addressing health inequalities in European regions: the AIR project", http://dx.doi.org/10.1093/heapro/dav101. [41]

Sans-Corrales, M. et al. (2006), *Family medicine attributes related to satisfaction, health and costs.*, http://dx.doi.org/10.1093/fampra/cmi112. [33]

Santana, M. et al. (2019), *Measuring patient-centred system performance: A scoping review of patient-centred care quality indicators*, BMJ Publishing Group, http://dx.doi.org/10.1136/bmjopen-2018-023596. [62]

Saver, B. (2002), "Financing and Organization Findings Brief", *Academy for Research and Health Care Policy*, Vol. 5/1-2. [32]

Schäfer, W. et al. (2016), "Two decades of change in European general practice service profiles: Conditions associated with the developments in 28 countries between 1993 and 2012", *Scandinavian Journal of Primary Health Care*, Vol. 34/1, pp. 97-110, http://dx.doi.org/10.3109/02813432.2015.1132887. [61]

Schuchman, M., M. Fain and T. Cornwell (2018), "The Resurgence of Home-Based Primary Care Models in the United States", *Geriatrics*, http://dx.doi.org/10.3390/geriatrics3030041. [104]

Shaw T, M. Hines and C. Kielly-Carroll (2017), *Impact of Digital Health on the Safety and Quality of Health Care*, ACSQHC, Sydney. [75]

Shi, L. and B. Starfield (2005), "Primary Care, Income Inequality, and Self-Rated Health in the United States: A Mixed-Level Analysis", *International Journal of Health Services*, http://dx.doi.org/10.2190/n4m8-303m-72ua-p1k1. [31]

Shipman, S. and C. Sinsky (2013), "Expanding primary care capacity by reducing waste and improving the efficiency of care", *Health Affairs*, http://dx.doi.org/10.1377/hlthaff.2013.0539. [52]

Sinsky, C. and T. Bodenheimer (2019), "Powering-Up Primary Care Teams: Advanced Team Care With In-Room Support", *Ann Fam Med*, Vol. 17/4, pp. 367-371, http://dx.doi.org/10.1370/afm.2422. [107]

Sinsky, C. et al. (2016), "Allocation of physician time in ambulatory practice: A time and motion study in 4 specialties", *Annals of Internal Medicine*, http://dx.doi.org/10.7326/M16-0961. [53]

Socha-Dietrich, K. (2019), *Interprofessional Teams for Complex Patients in Primary Health Care: Patients' and health professionals' experience. Fast Track Paper presented at the 25th Session of the Health Committee*, OECD, Paris. [101]

Starfield, B., L. Shi and J. Macinko (2005), "Contribution of Primary Care to Health Systems and Health", *The Milbank Quarterly*, Vol. 83/3, pp. 457–502. [19]

Stokes, J. et al. (2018), *Towards incentivising integration: A typology of payments for integrated care*, http://dx.doi.org/10.1016/j.healthpol.2018.07.003. [112]

Struijs, J. and C. Baan (2011), "Integrating Care through Bundled Payments — Lessons from the Netherlands", *New England Journal of Medicine*, http://dx.doi.org/10.1056/nejmp1011849. [110]

Sung, N., Y. Choi and J. Lee (2018), "Primary care comprehensiveness can reduce emergency department visits and hospitalization in people with hypertension in South Korea", *International Journal of Environmental Research and Public Health*, Vol. 15/2, http://dx.doi.org/10.3390/ijerph15020272. [21]

Tanner, C. et al. (2015), "Electronic Health Records and Patient Safety Co-occurrence of early EHR implementation with patient safety practices in primary care settings", *APPLIED CLINICAL INFORMATICS*, http://dx.doi.org/10.4338/ACI-2014-11-RA-0099. [80]

Thompson, M. and F. Walter (2016), "Increases in general practice workload in England", *The Lancet*, http://dx.doi.org/10.1016/s0140-6736(16)00743-1. [45]

Trivedi, D. (2017), *Cochrane Review Summary: Interventions for improving outcomes in patients with multimorbidity in primary care and community settings*, Cambridge University Press, http://dx.doi.org/10.1017/S1463423616000426. [30]

Valverde-Albacete, J. et al. (2019), *Benchmarking deployment of eHealth among general practitioners (2018)*, European Commission, http://dx.doi.org/10.2759/511610. [76]

Van den Berg, M., T. Van Loenen and G. Westert (2016), "Accessible and continuous primary care may help reduce rates of emergency department use. An international survey in 34 countries", *Family Practice*, Vol. 33/1, pp. 42-50, http://dx.doi.org/10.1093/fampra/cmv082. [22]

van der Brug, F. (2017), "Readmission rates: what can we learn from the Netherlands?", *Nuffieldtrust*, https://www.nuffieldtrust.org.uk/news-item/readmission-rates-what-can-we-learn-from-the-netherlands. [91]

van Loenen, T. et al. (2014), "Organizational aspects of primary care related to avoidable hospitalization: a systematic review", *Family Practice*, Vol. 31/5, pp. 502-516, http://dx.doi.org/10.1093/fampra/cmu053. [12]

van Rinsum, C. et al. (2018), "The coaching on lifestyle (CooL) intervention for overweight and obesity: A longitudinal study into participants' lifestyle changes", *International Journal of Environmental Research and Public Health*, http://dx.doi.org/10.3390/ijerph15040680. [121]

Wammes, J., P. van der Wees and M. Tanke (2018), "Systematic review of high-cost patients' characteristics and healthcare utilization", *BMJ Open*, Vol. 8, p. e023113. [5]

Whitehead, L. and P. Seaton (2016), *The effectiveness of self-management mobile phone and tablet apps in long-term condition management: A systematic review*, http://dx.doi.org/10.2196/jmir.4883. [124]

WHO (2017), *Protecting workers' health Fact sheets*, https://www.who.int/news-room/fact-sheets/detail/protecting-workers'-health. [139]

Wolters, R., J. Braspenning and M. Wensing (2017), *Impact of primary care on hospital admission rates for diabetes patients: A systematic review*, Elsevier Ireland Ltd, http://dx.doi.org/10.1016/j.diabres.2017.05.001. [10]

Yu, S. et al. (2017), *The scope and impact of mobile health clinics in the United States: A literature review*, http://dx.doi.org/10.1186/s12939-017-0671-2. [137]

Zhu, Q. et al. (2015), "Effectiveness of nurse-led early discharge planning programmes for hospital inpatients with chronic disease or rehabilitation needs: A systematic review and meta-analysis", *Journal of Clinical Nursing*, http://dx.doi.org/10.1111/jocn.12895. [92]

Notes

[1] Data are taken from the UEMO questionnaire.

[2] Store and forward telemedicine collects clinical information (such as medical history, laboratory reports, images, or videos) and sends this information to another site for evaluation and for health care professionals to access.

[3] A negative incentive is an incentive that require individuals or organisations to perform in order to avoid a loss.

2 Greater efficiency

This chapter analyses the efficiency of primary health care across OECD countries. The chapter starts with a review of published studies which shows that strong primary health care makes health systems more efficient, notably by containing the rate of growth in health spending, and by reducing the use of costly hospital inputs. The chapter then goes on to show that there are unrealised opportunities from better primary health care, and that systems will need to operate differently in order to reap better efficiency from primary health care across OECD countries. The chapter concludes by identifying areas where policy makers need to act so as to realise efficiency gains. Special emphasis is devoted to changes in training and improved matching of skills to tasks, greater use of digital technology, financial incentives that encourage good primary health care processes and good health outcomes, as well as availing primary and community care options.

Key findings

- Good primary health care can make health systems more efficient, notably by reducing rates of avoidable hospitalisations and unnecessary emergency department visits.
- In many OECD countries primary health care is not achieving the expected results, as demonstrated by high rates of avoidable hospitalisations and inappropriate prescribing:
    - Inappropriate use of antibiotics in general practice ranges between 45% and 90% of all systemic antibiotic prescriptions.
    - Hospital admissions for chronic conditions were equivalent to 5.8% of hospital bed days in 2016, many of which could be avoided with good primary health care.
- Shortcomings in primary health care services may partly be attributed to the shortage of required skills and skills mismatches in primary health care practice. Reductions in the share of generalist medical practitioners, coupled with imbalances between skills and tasks, is a source of sub-optimal use of resources in primary health care.
- There are many opportunities to improve technical and allocative efficiency in primary health care practice and it is essential that primary health care teams have the following:
    - Expertise in a wide range of areas, which goes beyond treating infectious diseases and includes, for example, providing information on nutrition, dealing with addiction and mental health issues. Primary health care teams also need soft skills, such as counselling, shared communication, collaboration and the ability to use health technology. France and Belgium have recently developed programmes to expand the skills and knowledge of primary health care teams in areas of health promotion and disease prevention. England, Germany and the United States, have also introduced modules in the medical curricula to build the attitudes and skills necessary for an effective deployment of digital health technology.
    - An appropriate mix of professionals with the right combination of skills. New support roles for nurses, community pharmacists or health workers (e.g. as developed in Canada and the United Kingdom) will help meet patient's clinical needs more effectively and comprehensively, with less use of physician time and at lower costs: this will improve technical efficiency.
    - Access and training to enable the functionalities offered by digital technologies to be fully embraced. Telemedicine, mHealth, electronic health records (EHR) and ePrescribing have been shown to enhance appropriateness of treatment, accuracy of diagnosis and patient experiences with primary health care. In particular, implementing well-structured and portable EHR systems is critical for improving workflow, communication and the clinical practices recommended for safe patient care in primary health care settings (e.g. the system used in Israel).
    - Greater diffusion of payment systems targeting desired activities, including the management of chronic diseases (e.g. Iceland, Italy and Israel), care co-ordination (e.g. Austria, Denmark, Germany and Sweden), early discharge from hospitals (e.g. the Czech Republic, Norway, Sweden and the United Kingdom) or other targets (e.g. Estonia, France and the United States) have great potential to maximise health care outputs through better processes of care, and to reduce the use of expensive inputs by moving care out of the hospital sector. To be effective, such payment systems need to encourage the delivery of appropriate services in primary health care that can be directly influenced by the level of the primary health care team's efforts.

- Developing intermediate care facilities (e.g. Costa Rica, Mexico, the Netherlands and Norway) and home-based programmes (e.g. Canada, Germany and the United Kingdom) are good options to reduce instances where costly hospital inputs are used instead of less expensive alternatives. Such policies consist of ensuring that patients with minor and non-acute conditions are in the right place at the right time.

2.1. Primary health care is associated with reduced use of costly hospital and emergency department inputs

High performing primary health care has been shown to help control health care spending. Not only do studies show that health care systems in which specialist or hospital care is only accessible after referral by a general practitioner (GP) have lower health care costs or are better able to contain the growth of health spending, but others suggest that primary health care also helps reduce the avoidable use of hospitals. Together, these conclusions suggest that when patients can be treated in the primary health care sector, fewer expensive services need to be provided at secondary levels of care, which can contain the growth in health care costs.

Delnoij et. al. (2000[1]), showed that in countries with gatekeeping GPs, ambulatory care expenditure has increased more slowly than in non-gatekeeping systems. Using international health expenditure and OECD data, Gerdtham et al (2011[2]) confirm this result by showing that the use of primary health care "gatekeepers" resulted in lower health expenditure. This relationship can be explained, in part, due to the role of primary health care systems in avoiding unnecessary procedures or avoidable use of costly facilities, such as emergency rooms and hospitals, through better preventive care.

A large number of empirical studies have confirmed the ability of primary health care to avoid unnecessary procedures and reduce the use of costly facilities, such as emergency rooms and hospitals, through better preventive care (World Health Organization, 2018[3]). Indeed, there is strong evidence that associates primary health care with lower rates of hospitalisations (Wolters, Braspenning and Wensing, 2017[4]; Rosano et al., 2013[5]; Van den Berg, Van Loenen and Westert, 2016[6]) and emergency department use (Kirkland, Soleimani and Newton, 2018[7]; Huntley et al., 2014[8]; Berchet, 2015[9])for so-called ambulatory care sensitive conditions (ACSCs).

ACSCs are conditions for which people-centred primary health care can generally prevent the need for hospitalisation, or for which early intervention can reduce the risk of complications or prevent more severe diseases developing (Agency for Healthcare Research and Quality, 2018[10]). Diabetes, chronic obstructive pulmonary disease (COPD), asthma, hypertension and congestive heart failure (CHF) are ACSCs with an established evidence base that much of the recommended treatment can be delivered by outpatient care at the primary or community care level. Treated early and appropriately, acute deterioration in people with these conditions and consequent hospital admissions could be avoided, therefore hospitalisations due to ACSCs are defined as "avoidable hospitalisations" (Purdy, 2010[11]; Nuffieldtrust, 2019[12]; Starfield, Shi and Macinko, 2005[13]).

As demonstrated by Starfield, Shi and Macinko (2005[13]), results suggest that people with primary health care physicians as a regular source of care were relatively better protected against hospitalisation for a preventable complication from chronic conditions. Lower rates of hospitalisations for ACSCs are consistently and strongly associated with the receipt of primary health care. In a similar vein, in a review paper identifying research evidence on the value of primary health care, Shi (2012) confirmed that primary health care is associated with a decrease in hospitalisation and emergency department visits (Shi, 2012[14]).

More recently, international literature and research offer some important insights on the significant contribution of care continuity and accessibility of care to explain the relationship between a strong primary health care system and avoidable hospitalisations for ACSCs. Van Loenon et al (2014[15]; 2016[16]) suggested that there is compelling evidence that adequate physician supply and better longitudinal continuity of care reduced avoidable hospitalisations. The higher the number of primary health care physicians per thousand people, the lower the risk of avoidable hospitalisation for ACSCs. The same negative relationship was found between care continuity and avoidable hospitalisation for ACSCs. The authors concluded that patients with long-term relationships with their primary health care physicians or the primary health care team, are more likely to communicate about changes in their medical conditions, thus reducing the risk of deterioration (van Loenen et al., 2014[15]; 2016[16]).

The negative relationship between care continuity and avoidable hospitalisations has been confirmed for specific conditions including diabetes, COPD and hypertension. Across studies, better care continuity and access to primary health care is associated with a lower likelihood of diabetes-related hospitalisations (Van Loenen et al., 2016[16]; Gibson, Segal and McDermott, 2013[17]; Wolters, Braspenning and Wensing, 2017[18]). Lin, Wu and Huang (2015[19]) show that COPD patients in Taiwan who receive a higher continuity of care have a significantly lower likelihood of avoidable hospitalisations (Lin, Wu and Huang, 2015[19]). Sung, Choi, and Lee (2018[20]), using the nationally representative 2013 Korea Health Panel data, found that adults with hypertension having a primary health care physician as a regular source of care have a lower risk of visiting an emergency department and being hospitalised (Sung, Choi and Lee, 2018[20]).

In addition to generating avoidable hospitalisations, delays in diagnosis and inappropriate therapeutic interventions in primary health care for ACSCs are also key sources of patient harm, and can result in emergency department visits (Lin, Wu and Huang, 2015[19]; Sung, Choi and Lee, 2018[20]; Van den Berg, Van Loenen and Westert, 2016[21]). Such emergency department visits are considered "inappropriate" or "non-urgent" visits, and are characterised by low urgency problems requiring other health services including, for example, telephone-based services and primary or community health care services (McHale et al., 2013[22]). According to national definitions and estimates, "avoidable", "inappropriate" or "non-urgent" visits to emergency departments account for around 9% of emergency department in Australia[1], 12% in the United States, between 11.7% and 15% in England, 20% in Italy, 25% in Canada, 31% in Portugal and 56% in Belgium (Berchet, 2015[9]). Van den Berg et al (2016[21]) suggest that good accessibility to primary health care and a more continuous relationship between patients and the primary health care team helps reduce emergency department visits (Van den Berg, Van Loenen and Westert, 2016[21]).

As unit costs for treating patients with the same condition in primary health care are lower than those observed in emergency departments and hospitals, health systems with strong primary health care may attain higher levels of allocative efficiency, which describes a situation where a different combination of inputs could bring better results. Therefore, avoidable emergency department visits or hospital admissions are indicators of possible misallocation of resources across different types of goods and services or, in this case, levels of care (Cylus, Papanicolas and Smith, 2016[23]).

2.2. Shortcomings in primary health care delivery lead to unnecessary use of more expensive specialised services

Across OECD countries, evidence shows that too many patients do not receive the appropriate primary health care at the appropriate place, leading to unnecessary use of more expensive specialised services. For example, international data, suggest that inappropriate prescribing of medication in general practice is too high: prescriptions for unsuitable antibiotics or opioids are either harmful or do not deliver benefits to patients, costing lives and money for health care systems. Avoidable hospital admissions and inappropriate emergency department visits are also excessive, particularly at a time of great fiscal pressure. Primary health care is thereby not delivering care in the right way, meaning that some health care spending could be eliminated, whilst achieving the same or improved population health outcomes. This means that policy makers could improve both technical efficiency (which describes a situation where a given result is obtained at the lowest possible cost) and allocative efficiency (which describes a situation where a different combination of inputs could bring better results).

These shortcomings may relate to the declining share of primary health care physicians, due in part to the lower attractiveness of general practice relative to specialisation, which means that fewer primary health care physicians are asked to deliver care to a growing number of people with complex care needs.

2.2.1. Too many patients do not receive the right primary health care, at the right place

Inappropriate prescribing in general practice is common in many OECD countries

Inappropriate use of antibiotics

Antibiotics are indispensable for treating bacterial infections, but their effectiveness is threatened by the spread of antibacterial resistance. Antibiotics should only be prescribed where there is an evidence-based need, as overuse will increase the risk of resistant strains.

The amount of all antibiotics prescribed in primary health care in 2017 was 19 defined daily doses per 1 000 inhabitants per day. Total amounts vary more than three-fold across countries, ranging from 10 to 36 defined daily doses, with the Netherlands, Estonia, and Sweden reporting the lowest amounts, and Greece and France reporting volumes much higher than the OECD average. Such discrepancies indicate that a significant share of antibiotic prescription is unnecessary and inappropriate (OECD, 2019[24]).

Recent evidence also shows that general practice services are the areas of most concern, as consistently high levels of inappropriate use are reported, and because the discipline consists of a high volume of patients. The inappropriate use of antibiotics in general practice ranges between 45% and 90% of all systemic antibiotic prescriptions (Figure 2.1). This inappropriate prescribing is likely to have marginal, if any, patient benefit, ignoring the added complications of inappropriate choice of drug, dosage or treatment duration.

Figure 2.1. Inappropriate use of antibiotics in general practice is high

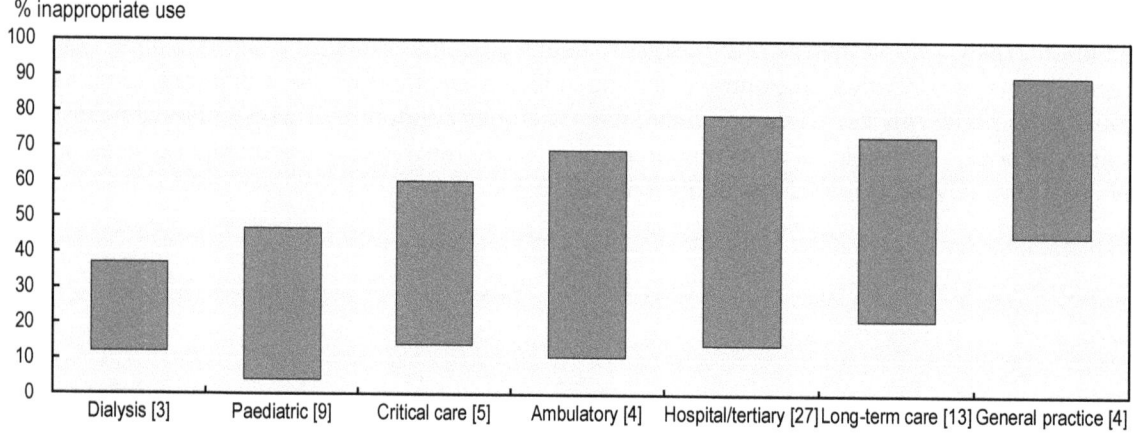

Note: Numbers in brackets indicate the number of studies used to determine the extent of inappropriate use.
Source: OECD (2017[25]), *Tackling Wasteful Spending on Health*, https://doi.org/10.1787/9789264266414-en.

Inappropriate opioid prescribing in general practice

Opioid analgesic prescribing has steadily increased in recent years in OECD countries, and many patients are being treated with opioids for chronic non-malignant pain. While opioid analgesic is beneficial for pain management, the level of usage is now generating significant harm in the community. The number of overdose deaths has mounted to alarming numbers, creating the so-called "opioid crisis" in some OECD countries, such as Canada and the United States (OECD, 2019[26]). Some European countries, are also experiencing a trend of rising opioid consumption and deaths caused by overdoses (OECD, 2019[26]).

Across the OECD, the overall volume of opioids prescribed in 2017 varies almost four-fold across countries, with Iceland leading markedly with the highest volume of opioids prescribed at 40.2 defined daily doses (DDD) per 1 000 inhabitants per day, well above the OECD average, followed by Luxembourg (39.0) and Denmark (23.3) (Figure 2.2). Turkey (0.1) and Korea (0.9) show very modest prescription opioid use with less than 1 DDD per 1 000 inhabitants per day, followed by Estonia and Italy with values of 5.8 and 4.2, respectively.

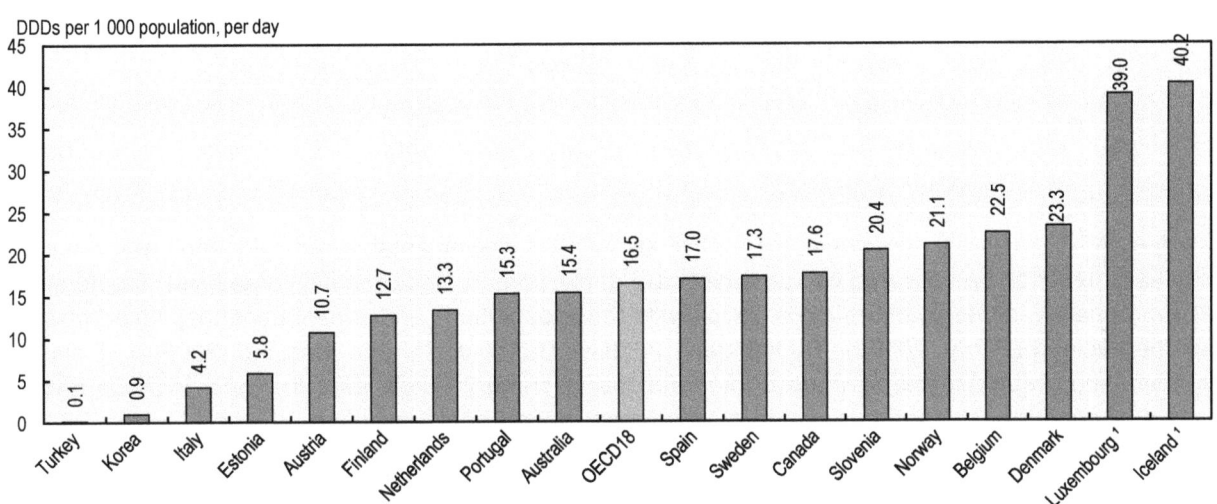

Figure 2.2. The average volume of opioids prescribed in primary health care is more than 16 DDDs per 1 000 population per day, 2017

Note: DDDs = defined daily doses. Exclusion of products used in the treatment of addiction. Some countries cannot split primary health care data from outpatient care or long-term care data. 1. Three-year average.
Source: OECD (2019[24]), *Health at a Glance 2019: OECD Indicators*, https://doi.org/10.1787/4dd50c09-en.

Inappropriate opioid prescribing is associated with non-fatal opioid overdose, fatal opioid overdose and all-cause mortality (Rose et al., 2018[27]). In 25 OECD countries for which data are available, opioid-related deaths have increased by 20% on average in recent years (see Figure 2.3). Among the countries above the average, the United States, Canada, Sweden, Norway, Ireland, and England and Wales have seen particularly worrying trends. The increased mortality rates associated with misuse of opioid prescriptions place a significant cost burden on health systems.

Figure 2.3. Opioid-related deaths in OECD countries have increased by an average of 20% in recent years

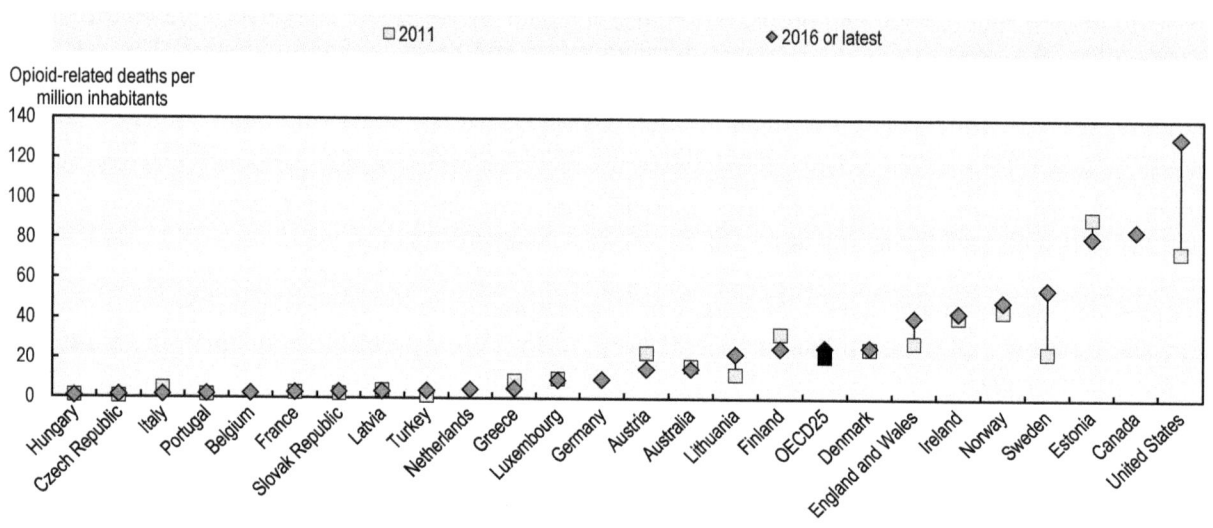

Note: Countries ranked by most recent year with data available.
Source: OECD (2019[26]). *Addressing Problematic Opioid Use in OECD Countries*, https://doi.org/10.1787/a18286f0-en.

Hospital admissions for five chronic conditions are equivalent to 5.8% of total hospital bed days

Diabetes, COPD, asthma, hypertension and CHF are ACSCs with an established evidence base that much of the treatment can be delivered by outpatient care at the primary or community care level. Treated early and appropriately, acute deterioration in people with these conditions and consequent hospital admissions could be avoided (Purdy, 2010[11]; Nuffieldtrust, 2019[12]; Starfield, Shi and Macinko, 2005[13]). Delays in diagnosis and inappropriate therapeutic interventions in primary health care for these ACSCs are key sources of patient harm, and can result in emergency department visits (Lin, Wu and Huang, 2015[19]; Sung, Choi and Lee, 2018[20]; Van den Berg, Van Loenen and Westert, 2016[21]).

Analysis of hospital admission data for five chronic conditions (diabetes mellitus, hypertensive diseases, heart failure, COPD, and asthma) across 30 OECD countries shows that in 2016, just over 5.6 million hospitalisations with a principal diagnosis of one of these five conditions took place (see Box 2.1 for methodology). The average length of stay across all five diagnoses was eight days, ranging from 6.0 days for asthma to 9.7 for heart failure. In total, in 2016, over 47.5 million bed days were consumed by admissions for these five chronic conditions alone across OECD countries, amounting to 5.8% of the total hospital bed day (Figure 2.4). For statistical purposes a bed day is a day during which a person is confined to a bed and in which the patient stays overnight in a hospital.

> **Box 2.1. Estimating the opportunity cost related to avoidable hospitalisation for chronic conditions**
>
> The data on hospital admissions refer to discharges (including deaths in hospital). They include patients in all age groups, but exclude outpatient and day cases (patients who do not stay overnight in hospital). Following the methodology employed by Auraane, Slawomirski and Klazinga (2018[28]), the number of bed days was calculated by multiplying the number of admissions (discharges) by the average length of stay.
>
> The data on cost per hospital bed day refer to the 2011 WHO-CHOICE model, which gives an estimation of cost per bed day for primary, secondary and tertiary public hospitals across 193 countries. The cost is expressed in US dollars. For the purpose of the report, the cost per bed day for secondary hospitals was used as an average value for each country. It is important to note that these estimates represent only the "hotel" component of hospital costs (including costs such as personal, capital and food costs), excluding the cost of drugs, treatment and diagnostic tests. This means that the opportunity cost related to avoidable hospitalisation is grossly underestimated.

Figure 2.4. Share of potentially avoidable hospital admissions due to five chronic conditions as a percentage of total hospital bed days, 2016

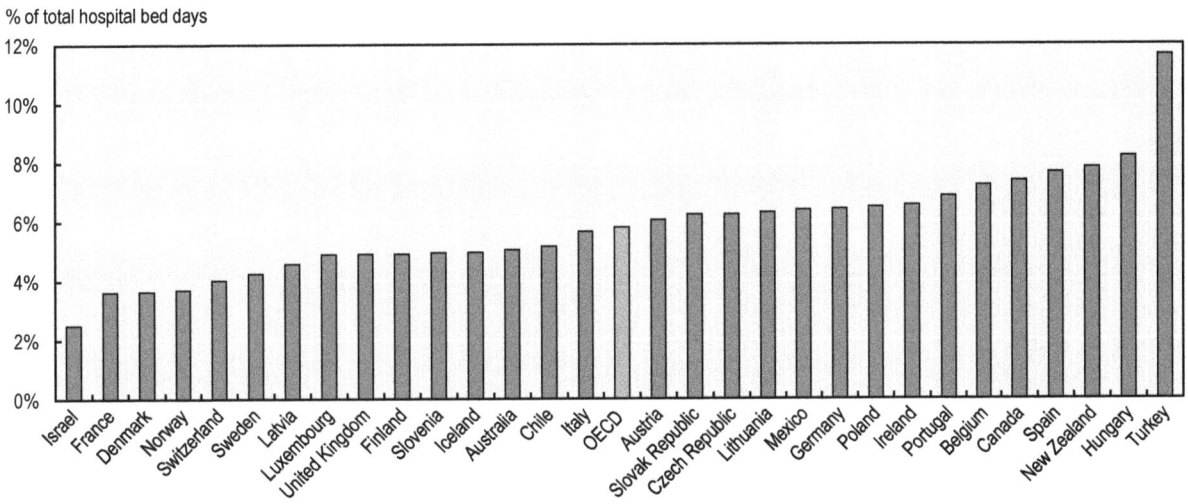

Note: The data includes only admissions with a minimum of one night's hospital stay. Not counted are 'same-day' admissions (e.g. a patient with acute on chronic conditions admitted for observation but discharged a few hours later). These "same-day" admissions consume hospital resources. In addition, the share of avoidable hospital admissions is also largely underestimated as there are more causes of hospitalisations that are potentially preventable. In Australia for example, potentially avoidable hospitalisations for 22 conditions accounted for 9% of all hospital bed days in 2016-17 (AIHW, 2019[29]). Cross-country comparisons of potentially avoidable hospital admissions should also be interpreted with caution, as many other factors, beyond better access to primary health care, can influence the statistics, including data comparability and the prevalence of these chronic conditions. These are crude data and are not age-standardised.
Source: OECD estimates based on OECD Health Statistics 2018, https://doi.org/10.1787/health-data-en.

The use of "cost per hospital bed day", as estimated by the 2011 WHO CHOICE model, gives a rough estimation of the opportunity cost associated with avoidable hospitalisation for ACSCs across OECD countries. On a methodology point, it is important to emphasise that only the "hotel" component of hospital costs (including costs such as personnel, capital and food costs) is considered here. The WHO CHOICE model estimation excludes the cost of drugs, treatment and diagnostic tests, meaning that the cost related to avoidable hospitalisation is largely underestimated. Moreover, there are more causes of hospitalisation that are potentially avoidable than just the five conditions listed in this estimation (including angina, influenza and other vaccine preventable diseases, illnesses resulting from nutritional deficiencies, etc.) (Fleetcroft et al., 2018[30]). The Australian Institute of Health and Welfare for example defined 22 conditions for which hospitalisation is considered potentially preventable across three broad categories (vaccine-preventable conditions, acute conditions and chronic conditions) (AIHW, 2019[29]). The total number of avoidable hospitalisations is also significantly underestimated.

The total cost generated by avoidable hospitalisations for these five chronic conditions in 30 OECD countries is estimated to be USD 21.1 billion in 2016 (Table 2.1). Equipped with the right resources, good primary health care can avoid many of these hospitalisations, increasing efficiency of health systems and improving people's well-being.

Table 2.1. Cost of avoidable hospitalisation for chronic conditions in 30 OECD countries

	Number of hospital bed days	Unit cost of hospital bed days (secondary hospital)	Cost in USD (million)
Australia	1 176 886	660	777
Austria	1 097 267	666	731
Belgium	872 987	625	545
Canada	1 827 485	606	1 108
Chile	516 240	113	58
Czech Republic	1 226 609	255	313
Denmark	162 691	826	134
Finland	390 616	678	265
France	3 994 807	582	2 327
Germany	12 084 564	590	7 128
Hungary	1 522 572	184	280
Iceland	12 088	704	9
Ireland	240 666	821	198
Israel	226 710	347	79
Italy	3 124 832	497	1 552
Latvia	117 965	173	20
Lithuania	319 203	166	53
Luxembourg	32 627	1 852	60
Mexico	1 362 369	113	154
New Zealand	398 323	375	149
Norway	177 011	1 371	243
Poland	3 136 231	160	502
Portugal	458 124	293	134
Slovak Republic	488 094	211	103
Slovenia	126 992	342	43
Spain	2 597 803	452	1 175
Sweden	357 999	707	253
Switzerland	482 199	901	434
Turkey	6 197 769	113	700
United Kingdom	2 800 763	577	1 615
Total	47 530 492	-	21 142
Average	1 584 350	532	843

Note: See Box 2.1 for the methodology. These estimates represent only the "hotel" component of hospital costs (including costs such as personal, capital and food costs), excluding the cost of drugs, treatment and diagnostic tests. Moreover, there are more causes of hospitalisation that are potentially avoidable than just the five conditions listed in this estimation (diabetes mellitus, hypertensive diseases, heart failure, COPD, and asthma). This means that the opportunity cost related to avoidable hospitalisation is grossly underestimated.
Source: OECD estimates based on OECD Health Statistics 2018, https://doi.org/10.1787/health-data-en.

Almost 30% of elderly people visited an emergency department for conditions that could have been treated in primary health care settings

Attendance at emergency departments for low-urgency problems that could be dealt with within the primary health care sector is another source of inefficiency for OECD health care systems.

While injuries are the most common reason for using emergency services, many other emergency department visits are motivated by low-urgency problems that do not require emergency admissions. Drivers of avoidable emergency department visits include, among others, a lack of alternatives to hospital care, misaligned financial incentives with system objectives or patient preference for hospital services over primary health care (notably among the most disadvantaged populations) (Berchet, 2015[9]). Unwarranted use of emergency services is costly and potentially harmful to patients. Indeed, costly hospital inputs are used instead of less expensive ones, with no additional benefit to the patient. Within hospitals, inappropriate emergency department visits lead to overcrowding, which results in delayed diagnosis and treatment (OECD, 2017[25]).

Recent international data show that a significant proportion of elderly patients visited the emergency department for a condition that could have been equally well addressed, or better treated, in primary health care. In 2017, the proportion of inappropriate emergency department visits among elderly people was the highest in France and the United States, with more than 40% of elderly patients visiting an emergency department for a condition that could have been treated by the primary health care team (Figure 2.5). The proportion of inappropriate emergency department visits was also very high in Canada and Switzerland, where 25% and 30% of elderly people inappropriately visited the emergency department, respectively. At the other end of the scale, Australia, Sweden and New Zealand had fewer inappropriate emergency department visits, at around 20% of elderly patients. Recent data from the Australian Institute of Health and Welfare show that after-hours lower urgency emergency department visits fell by 3.4% over 2015-16 to 2017-18 (Aihw, 2018[31]).

Figure 2.5. On average almost 30% of elderly patients visited an emergency department for a condition that could have been treated in primary health care, 2017

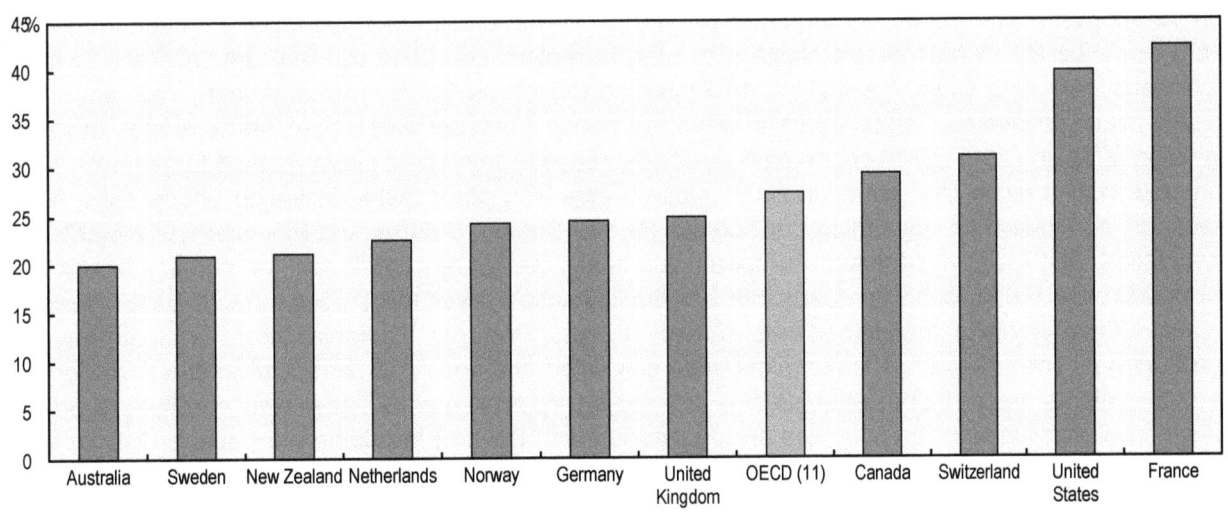

Note: Respondents were asked: "The last time you went to the hospital emergency department, was it for a condition that you thought could have been treated by the doctors or staff at the place where you usually get medical care if they had been available?" Results show the proportion of people responding "yes" to the question. In Australia, recent data from the Australian Institute of Health and Welfare show that in 2017-18, 37% of all ED presentations were for lower urgency care (Aihw, 2018[31]).
Source: The Commonwealth Fund, 2017, International Health Policy Survey of Older Adults (65+).

REALISING THE POTENTIAL OF PRIMARY HEALTH CARE © OECD 2020

The opportunity cost associated with avoidable emergency department visits can be large (OECD, 2017[25]). In the United States, a recent cost estimates study showed that around one-fifth of emergency department visits could be avoided, with an annual estimated expense of greater than USD 60 billion (Galarraga and Pines, 2016[32]).

2.2.2. The declining share of primary health care physicians and skills mismatches in primary health care make it increasingly difficult to meet complex care needs

A shortage and mismatch of skills in primary health care practice is an important factor causing shortcomings in primary health care systems. Indeed, international figures demonstrate a reduction in the share of primary health care physicians, while at the same time there are imbalances between skills and tasks. Together, this might adversely affect the quality of patient care, and lead to sub-optimal use of resources in primary health care.

Reduction in the share of generalist medical practitioners and new burdens in workload increase the need for more technical efficiency in primary health care

The number of doctors and nurses has never been greater in OECD countries. In 2017, there was on average 3.5 doctors and 8.8 nurses per 1 000 inhabitants in OECD countries, up from 2.7 doctors and 7.4 nurses per 1 000 inhabitants in 2000 (OECD, 2019[33]). However, while the overall number of doctors and nurses has largely increased, the share of generalist medical practitioners dropped between 2000 and 2017 in the majority of countries (see Figure 2.6). On average across OECD countries, generalists made up about 29% of all physicians in 2017. Between 2000 and 2017, the share of generalist medical practitioners decreased by more than 20% in Australia, the United Kingdom, Israel, Denmark, Estonia and Ireland (Figure 2.6).

While there are proportionally fewer doctors, the upward trend in both the clinical and administrative workload of general practice is putting strain on primary health care services, and this trend is likely to continue to grow especially in view of population ageing and the rising burden of chronic conditions across OECD countries. In the United Kingdom, for example, the number of consultations per patient per year rose by roughly 12% between 2007-08 and 2013-14, which is equivalent to a 16% rise in clinical workload (Hobbs et al., 2016[34]; Thompson and Walter, 2016[35]). In Australia, 40% of GPs stated that their workload can be excessive and more than a quarter of GPs (27%) have seen their workload increase in the past two years (The Royal Australian College of General Practitioners, 2018[36]). Similarly, in Canada family physicians work long hours: the 2017 CMA Physician Workforce Survey indicates that family physicians or GPs work on average 48.69 hours a week, 14 hours more per week than the average Canadian. Between 2004 and 2017, CMA observed a steady decrease in time spent directly caring for patients, which contrasts with a rising time commitment to indirect care and other tasks, including phone calls, family meetings, administration, managing practice etc. (Grava-Gubins, Safarov and Eriksson, 2012[37]; Medical Association, 2017[38]). In 14 other European countries, the current workload for primary health care physicians was found to be unreasonable and unsustainable over the longer term (Croatia, Hungary, Ireland, Lithuania, Malta, the Netherlands, Norway, Poland, Portugal, Romania, Slovenia, Spain, Sweden and Turkey)[2]. The growing workload might adversely affect the quality of patient care, and is inadequate to meet patients' need (Fisher et al., 2017[39]). A recent study also shows that over one-third of primary health care physicians in ten countries are dissatisfied with the time available per patient (Osborn et al., 2015[40]), which can in turn compromises the care provided and adversely affects physician stress and workload (Irving et al., 2017[41]).

Figure 2.6. The share of generalist medical practitioners continues to drop across the majority of OECD countries

% changes between 2000 and 2017

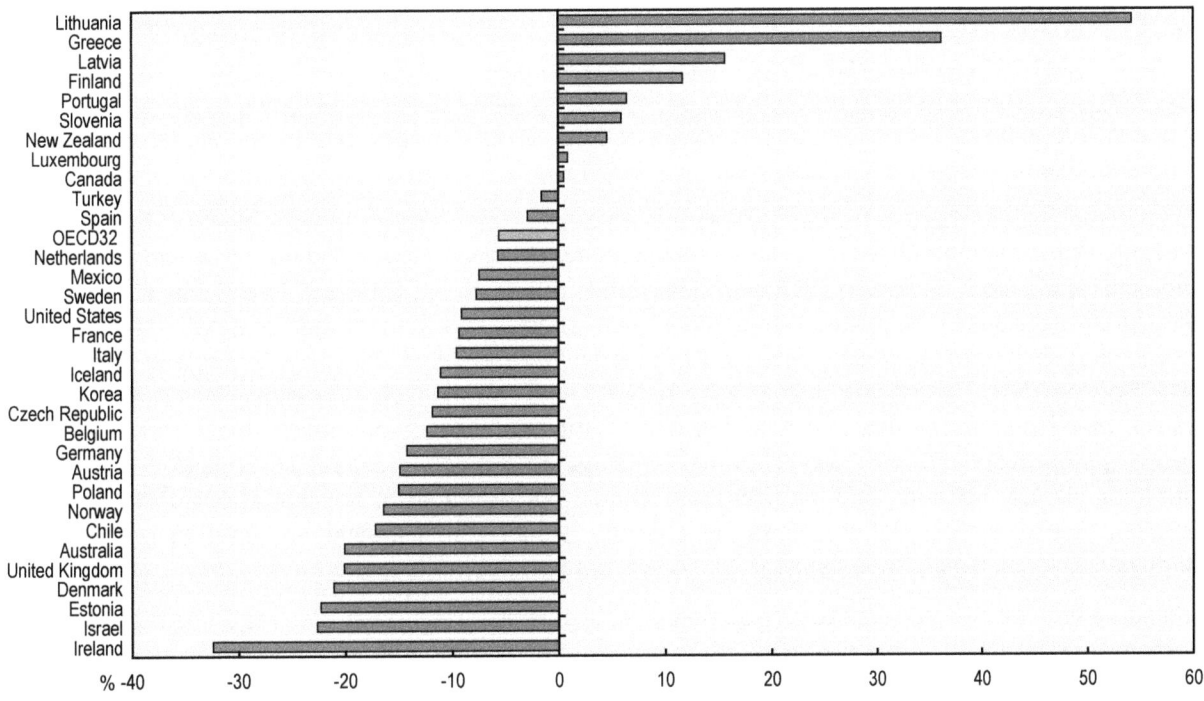

Note: The category of generalist medical practitioners includes general practitioners, district medical doctors, family medical practitioners, primary health care physicians, general medical doctors, general medical officers, medical interns or residents specialising in general practice or without any area of specialisation yet. Generalist medical practitioners do not limit their practice to certain disease categories or methods of treatment, and may assume responsibility for the provision of continuing and comprehensive medical care to individuals, families and communities. There are many breaks in the series for Australia, Estonia, and Ireland over the period. In some countries (Ireland, Israel, Korea and Poland), the share of general practitioners among all doctors has increased over the same period.
Source: OECD Health Statistics 2019, https://doi.org/10.1787/health-data-en.

On the issue of the supply of primary health care physicians, several factors explain the growing imbalance away from general practice in favour of greater specialisation, including: the retirement of GPs, lower remuneration in general medicine compared with specialised medicine and high workload in primary health care (OECD, 2016[42]). In most OECD countries, specialists earn significantly more than the GPs (OECD, 2017[43]). In 2015, the income gap between specialists and GPs was particularly high in Australia, Belgium and Luxemburg, where the self-employed specialists earned over twice the remuneration earned by GPs. The income gap between GPs and specialists continues to widen, reducing the financial attractiveness of general practice. Since 2005, the remuneration of specialists has risen faster than that of generalists in Canada, Finland, France, Hungary, Iceland, Israel, Luxembourg and Mexico.

However, budgetary constraints make it very unlikely that remuneration of primary health care physicians will increase, unless gains in productivity can be achieved simultaneously. Therefore, increases in technical efficiency in primary health care are central to addressing the potential shortage in primary health care workforce (Shipman and Sinsky, 2013[44]).

A better match of skills to tasks is more important than ever, especially given the challenges and opportunities offered by digital technologies

Beyond pressures coming from a reduction in the share of GPs and increasing workload, there is evidence that the distribution of skills and tasks among primary health care teams is inefficient (OECD, 2016[42]). On the one hand, 76% of doctors and 79% of nurses reported being overskilled for some of the tasks they have to do in their day-to-day work. For nurses, those who have a postgraduate degree (master's level or equivalent) are twice as likely to report being overskilled for some of the work they do, compared to those with qualifications up to and including a bachelor's degree. Given the significant length of training of doctors and nurses, this represents a dramatic waste in human capital.

In the United States, there is evidence that the amount of administrative work doctors have to do is increasing. For every hour physicians were seeing patients, they were spending nearly two additional hours on administrative work (including EHR and deskwork) (Sinsky et al., 2016[45]). In another study, primary health care physicians in the United States have been found to spend more than one-half of their workday (equivalent to six hours) interacting with the EHR (Brian G. Arndt et al., 2017[46]). In England, the National Health Service (NHS) estimates that 11% of a GP's time is taken up by paperwork (The Economist, 2019[47]). Many primary health care systems aim to improve care co-ordination and it may be that the increase in paperwork and other administrative tasks relates to these increased responsibilities. This is not a bad thing per se, but such non-medical tasks should be delegated to appropriately qualified, but also less expensive workforce. Not only does this strategy reduce administrative workload for primary health care physicians, but it also improves time for patient care and communication.

At the same time as being overskilled for some tasks, physicians and nurses also report being underskilled for others. Across OECD countries, 51% of doctors and 43% of nurses, reported being underskilled for some of the tasks they have to do. Rapid progress in medical research, demographic and epidemiological transition, combined with increased expectations for the management of complex cases in primary health care practices, may be drivers for reports of underskilling. A systematic review found that, on average, clinicians have more than one question about patient care for every two clinical encounters, and 49% of these questions are never pursued (Del Fiol, Workman and Gorman, 2014[48]). Of the total questions raised, 34% were related to drug treatment and 24% to causes of a symptom or diagnostic test result. In addition, medical doctors might not have the required soft skills, including shared communication, collaboration and partnership, to deliver people-centred care (Ranjan, Kumari and Chakrawarty, 2015[49]). The need for change in the training and development of primary health care teams is thereby evident (see also Section 3.1).

2.3. Policy options to enable the workforce to deliver more efficient primary health care

There are many opportunities to improve technical and allocative efficiency in primary health care practice. Policy options having most potential range from changes in training and improved matching of skills to tasks, greater use of digital technology (notably of EHR), financial incentives that encourage good primary health care processes and good health outcomes, as well as availing primary and community care options to avoid unnecessary use of hospitals.

2.3.1. New mechanisms for workforce recruitment and training are needed to ensure the right mix of skills and competences throughout primary health care teams

Changes in training are required, especially with technological progress and new ways of delivering services

Professional education in primary health care may not be aligned with changes related to technological progress and new ways of delivering services. Furthermore, it may not match increasing citizen expectations, and there is a mismatch of competences to patient needs (Frenk et al., 2010[50]). Available evidence for example show that primary health care practices still deliver reactive care that predominantly focuses on disease treatment and do not engage sufficiently in preventive care (Schäfer et al., 2016[51]) (see also Chapter 3).

Changes in training are required to ensure that the primary health care teams have expertise in a wide range of areas, which go beyond treating infectious diseases and include nutrition, addiction, mental health and healthy ageing. In addition, "soft" and transversal skills (including behaviour counselling, shared communication, collaboration, or partnership) are also needed to deliver people-centred and proactive care (Ranjan, Kumari and Chakrawarty, 2015[49]).

Providing initial and continuing training programmes in all these areas is critical to improve technical efficiency. Initial and continuing education should, in particular, prepare primary health care teams to better understand the signs and symptoms of chronic diseases and associated risk factors, to recognise the importance of environmental determinants of unhealthy behaviour and the factors that impact behavioural change. Ideally, health promotion and disease prevention should be integrated into initial and continuing training for all members of the primary health care team (primary health care physicians, but also nurses, pharmacists, auxiliaries and community health workers). Screening assessment tools, individual counselling, behavioural change programmes and multidisciplinary collaboration in primary health care should be the main priority of training programmes, at least to the same extent as diagnosis and treatment of diseases. The need to learn about technology-enabled consultation, data-coding and analytics is also important at a time when digital health and new technologies show promise in improving care processes.

Achieving skills for person-centred communication will also be vital to expand attention to patients' personal and social situations. This is a prerequisite to improve diagnosis and tailor care plans, but also to practice shared decision making and consider patients' goals and values. Lastly, to break down professional silos and foster effective working with other health and social care professionals, primary health care teams should achieve skills for effective teamwork and interprofessional collaboration.

A few health care systems are working toward these goals. In France, the Ministry of Health, jointly with the Ministry of Education, recently announced that primary health care workforces will have to perform a public health rotation (see Box 2.2). In Belgium, the Flemish Coalition Agreement 2014-19 includes a simplification of primary health care structures and a strengthening of primary health care. In the area of education, the ongoing plan is to ensure that initial and ongoing training for primary health care professionals follows an integrated care approach, in which the patient takes the central position, whilst also promoting interdisciplinary partnership. The plan assumes that primary health care professionals will be trained following a broad definition of care, not only including treatment of disease and monitoring recovery, but also continued care through health promotion, disease prevention and shared communication and collaboration.

Another good example is the NHS in England, which created the NHS Digital Academy, which aims at strengthening providers' competencies in IT-based quality improvement tools. Canada, Germany, and the United States, have also introduced modules in the medical curricula to build the attitudes and skills necessary for an effective deployment of digital health technology. The courses address the skills needed for data-driven quality development and digital literacy, but also for interprofessional collaboration.

> **Box 2.2. The public health rotation in France**
>
> The Ministry of Health, jointly with the Ministry of Education, recently announced that students in the health sector will have to perform a public health rotation (called "*service sanitaire*"). The new curricula for medical doctor, nurse, pharmacist and physiotherapist students consists of going to public places, such as universities and high schools, to undertake prevention activities on four priority areas: diet, physical activity, addictions, and sexual health.
>
> This rotation will last 6 weeks with three phases:
>
> 1. a theoretical phase of training to give students the appropriate tools and knowledge
> 2. a practical phase where students are expected to implement a preventive strategy
> 3. a final phase where students will have to demonstrate the effectiveness of the prevention strategy.
>
> In the longer term, the public health rotation will be expanded to workplaces, elderly care facilities, social care facilities and prisons, and will also target rural and remote areas where health care supply is scarce.
>
> Source: OECD (2018[52]), Policy Survey on the Future of Primary Care.

The use of community-based teams has been found to improve the efficiency of primary health care providers

To meet local health needs and realise efficiency gains, the primary health care workforce needs to have sufficient professionals with the right mix of skills. Nurses, community pharmacists and health agents can have important "soft skills" and relevant knowledge about their communities, and have thereby the potential to reduce the workload of primary health care physicians without undermining the quality of care and patient satisfaction (Green, Savin and Lu, 2013[53]). With appropriate training and adequate legislation, OECD health care systems could develop new support roles for nurses, community pharmacists and other community health agents. This could consist of introducing new roles of care co-ordinators, care planners, and patient navigators to provide continuous care across different specialist areas while promoting healthy living, and preventing and managing some diseases. These functions often extend beyond traditional health care boundaries, and include close working relationships with social services and long-term care teams. Primary health care physicians will remain leaders of health care teams, notably by guiding other members of the team with their diagnostic and management skills and by taking care of patients' medical needs.

Only a few health care systems have moved toward this goal. In 2016, the majority of nurses or assistants independently provided immunisation, health promotion and routine checks for chronically ill patients in less than half of OECD countries (Table 2.2). In 2018, 19 out of 27 OECD countries had implemented concrete policy measures in the last five years to develop the primary health care workforce (Figure 2.7).

Table 2.2. Involvement of nurses and assistants in health promotion and prevention

	At least 75% of nurses or assistants independently provide immunisations	At least 75% of nurses or assistants independently provide health education	At least 75% of nurses or assistants independently provide routine checks of chronically ill patients
Austria	No	No	No
Belgium	No	No	No
Canada	No	Yes	Yes
Chile	Yes	Yes	Yes
Czech Republic	Yes	No	No
Denmark	No	Yes	No
Estonia	Yes	Yes	Yes
Finland	Yes	Yes	Yes
France	No	Yes	No
Greece	No	Yes	Yes
Iceland	Yes	No	No
Ireland	Yes	Yes	Yes
Israel	Yes	Yes	Yes
Italy	No	No	No
Latvia	Yes	Yes	Yes
Luxembourg	No	No	No
Netherlands	Yes	Yes	Yes
Norway	No	No	No
Poland	Yes	Yes	Yes
Portugal	Yes	Yes	Yes
Slovenia	No	No	No
Spain	Yes	Yes	Yes
Sweden	Yes	Yes	Yes
Switzerland	No	Yes	No
Turkey	Yes	NR	NR
United Kingdom	Yes	Yes	Yes
Total "yes" responses (out of 26 countries)	15	17	14

Source: OECD (2016[54]), Health System Characteristics Survey, http://www.oecd.org/els/health-systems/characteristics.htm.

Figure 2.7. Strategies to develop the primary health care workforce have been implemented in 19 OECD countries in the last five years

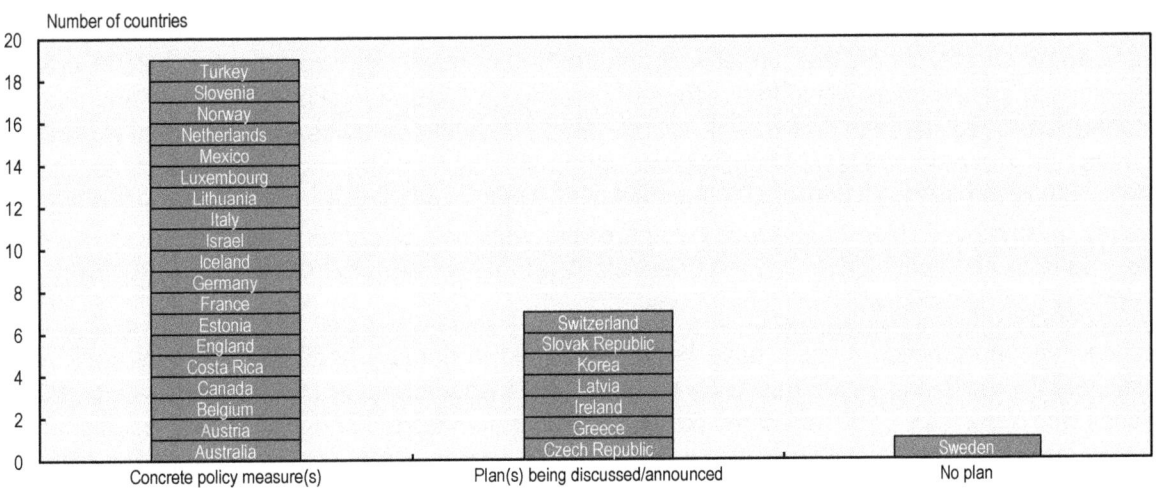

Source: OECD (2018[52]), Policy Survey on the Future of Primary Care.

Research confirms that expanding professional roles or delegating tasks to some primary health care professionals improves efficiency. Nurses or community pharmacists can, for example, help meet patients' clinical needs more effectively and comprehensively, with less use of physician time, and at lower costs. Some estimations show that up to 77% of preventive care and 47% of chronic care could be effectively delegated to non-physician team members (Shipman and Sinsky, 2013[44]). In England, the NHS estimates that 30% of GP time is spent on musculoskeletal problems which could be handled by a physiotherapist, while the latter costs around half as much as a GP (The Economist, 2019[47]). Experiences from the United States also show that care co-ordinators, flow managers or an empowered community based workforce helping with clerical duties can markedly improve physicians' efficiency (Shipman and Sinsky, 2013[44]). Such initiatives are found to increase the number of patients a GP can manage on their list, at the same time as reducing after-hours work for physicians, and resulting in less overtime for the primary health care team. Physician assistants in the United States who are licensed to diagnose, treat, and prescribe medicines, have helped to decrease hospital readmission rates, length of hospital stays and infection rates. In a similar vein, Green, Saving and Lu (2013[53]) show that the use non-physician providers expands manageable patient numbers for GPs, and offsets, to some extent, the primary health care physician shortage (Green, Savin and Lu, 2013[53]). Matthys, Remmen and Bogaert (2017[55]), in their systematic review of more than 60 studies, provide a firm evidence base for greater engagement of nurses in general practice by providing patient education, co-ordination, prevention advice or drug prescriptions and by working in collaboration with primary health care physicians (Matthys, Remmen and Van Bogaert, 2017[55]). The review shows that primary health care teams that include nurses with an advanced role lead to better patient outcomes, greater patient satisfaction and reduced hospitalisation.

The following section presents country specific examples relating to expanding roles for nurses, community pharmacists and community health workers.

Expanding nurses' roles

In Canada, registered nurses and nurse navigators have an important role in improving co-ordination and continuity of care in the MyHealthTeam model of primary health care. Nurses with a navigator role ensure that patients move appropriately through the health care system, and that they receive the appropriate care in the appropriate place. Evidence shows that nurses with a co-ordination role offer value in the care of cancer, cardiovascular illnesses and for patients with other chronic conditions, by supporting patients in managing their symptoms. These measures have been shown to reduce the need to seek additional medical attention such as expensive hospital care (Martin-Misener and Bryant-Lukosius, 2014[56]).

In other OECD countries, such as Estonia, Ireland, Mexico, Sweden and the United Kingdom[3], registered nurses are also allowed to prescribe medication. In Ireland, for example, a 6-month education programme has been established to enhance the skills of nurses and midwifes to become registered nurse prescribers. Registered nurse prescribers are, under authority from their health service provider, able to prescribe a range of medicinal products within their scope of practice. In 2016, a total of 894 nurses and midwives in the country were registered to prescribe medicinal products. Available evidence shows that expanding role of nurses has improved the level of appropriate referrals to specialists, and increased the satisfaction of patients, carers and nurses. At the same time, extending the power to prescribe medications to nurses and midwives in advanced roles has reduced some of the workload of primary health care physicians, and decreased both non-compliance with treatment plans and polypharmacy[4] (Adam et al., 2017[57]). Overall, the strategy has demonstrated efficiency gains.

In Latvia, "second practice nurses" have been introduced in primary health care teams, their role is to deliver health checks and public health care. Employing a second nurse became mandatory in 2014 for practices with more than 1 800 registered patients or 800 patients aged under 18. These additional general practice nurses focus on health promotion and disease prevention. They are expected to deal with lifestyle risk factors such as smoking and harmful alcohol consumption and to carry out behavioural counselling (OECD, 2016[58]).

Finally, in Australia, there is a specific project aimed at upskilling primary health care nurses in mental health literacy and clinical skills. The objective is also to develop a flexible and sustainable model of care that will deliver effective mental health care across a range of health settings. The programme will enable a mental health nurse to transition between acute and primary health care settings. The overarching objective is to improve continuity of care, but also streamline workflow to realise efficiency gains.

Expanding community pharmacists' role

The role of community pharmacists could also evolve to better meet patients' needs. Beyond dispensing medications, community pharmacists have a role to play as medical counsellors and educators, and in performing preventive care screenings. Pharmacists with advanced roles contribute to health improvement, help patients to make the best use of their medicines and help prevent harm that may arise from taking medicines incorrectly (International Pharmaceutical Federation, 2016[59]).

In some OECD countries community pharmacists are engaged in health promotion activities, screening programmes, vaccination and counselling activities. They are allowed to monitor particular clinical parameters and screen for undiagnosed conditions including, for example, cardiovascular risk assessment, colon cancer screening, and some infectious diseases such as HIV and tuberculosis. In Switzerland, for example, the "No to Colorectal Cancer" campaign was recently developed by the Swiss Pharmacy Association. The programme offers a screening service in collaboration with doctors. Pharmacists have to screen patients aged between 50 and 75 who have not had a colonoscopy within ten years. The pharmacist uses a questionnaire to determine a patient's risk of colon cancer. Then either a stool test is performed by the pharmacist, or the pharmacist will refer the patient to a primary health care physician. The pharmacist discusses the results of the stool test and those patients with negative results are scheduled for follow-up screening in two years. Evidence from the Swiss Pharmacy Association shows that within six weeks, the programme detected an estimated 58 cases of cancer and 368 cases of advanced adenoma. Overall, the programme was found cost-neutral, compared to the cost of preventive treatments. Through the campaign, pharmacists are starting to be recognised as advocates of health promotion, which is a positive step towards better using pharmacists' skills for preventive care.

The involvement of community pharmacists in care management for patients suffering from chronic conditions is also a valuable initiative that other OECD countries should consider. Evidence is somewhat conclusive that when community pharmacists provide patient education and behavioural counselling this can improve medication adherence and therapeutic outcomes in patients with chronic conditions (Mossialos et al., 2015[60]). Unfortunately, community pharmacists are given these roles in a disappointingly small number of OECD countries at present.

In the England, the announcement of new Community Pharmacy Contractual Framework (CPCF) arrangements for 2019/24 outlines an important future for community pharmacy in delivering clinical services as a fully integrated partner within local Primary Care Networks (NHS, 2019[61]). The five year agreement will expand the role of pharmacists in a multi-faceted approach, encompassing urgent care, medicines optimisation and prevention to better utilise the skills and reach of community pharmacies. An expanded range of services will be commissioned from community pharmacies alongside legislative reforms designed to free up capacity to enable pharmacists to spend more time delivering face to face services with patients. These new services will see more people triaged to community pharmacies for a wide range of support and advice. The CPCF for 2019/24 will introduce a Community Pharmacist Consultation Service which will develop the role of community pharmacy to support urgent care. It will allow people to be referred direct to a community pharmacy from NHS 111 to receive advice for minor illnesses, including self-care advice and wellbeing support, and treatment as necessary, as well as the supply of urgent medicines. If further testing is successful, this will be expanded over the next five years to include referrals from GPs, Urgent Treatment Centres and NHS 111 online. This will deliver faster access to a clinical consultation for patients with minor illness whilst also helping reduce pressure elsewhere in the health and care system. These new arrangements will continue the New Medicines Service that has been established to improve adherence of patients receiving medication for diabetes, hypertension, asthma and anticoagulant medication. As part of the New Medicines Service, community pharmacists are allowed to carry out either face-to-face or telephone consultations in order to identify any problems, side-effects, concerns or non-adherence to the medication. Recent evaluation of the service provides evidence that the New Medicines Service delivered better patient outcomes through better adherence to treatment (Elliott et al., 2016[62]).

In Finland, the "*Apteenkkien Diabetesohjelma*" is a diabetes programme for community pharmacists which aims at promoting successful diabetes care and prevention. The success factors rely on collaboration between pharmacies or other health care professionals. A diabetes contact is nominated within the pharmacy to be responsible for the implementation of the pharmacy programme at local level. According to the International Pharmaceutical Federation, the programme is now offered in over 650 Finnish community pharmacies (International Pharmaceutical Federation, 2016[59]).

Italy launched its first national diabetes prevention campaign in pharmacies in 2017. More than 5 600 community pharmacies co-operated throughout the national territory and a total of 160 313 patients were examined under the scheme. Among the patients examined, around 3% were found to be diabetic and 9% had a previous diagnosis of diabetes. In addition, 36% of patients were diagnosed with prediabetes, with high risk of developing diabetes within the next ten years.

Belgium introduced the concept of "pharmacist co-ordinators" in 2017. Patients with chronic diseases can choose a pharmacist co-ordinator to take the lead in medication reviews. The pharmacist is expected to have a global view of all of the patient's medications, to co-ordinate with the primary health care team and assess potential gaps in medication use. The aim is to allow patients with chronic illnesses to better manage their health and to stay autonomous as much as possible, but also to reduce the workload of primary health care physicians.

Such initiatives enable pharmacists to provide preventive care and early interventions to reduce the risk of complications or prevent more severe diseases, which could lead to the use of more costly interventions. Increasing the role for community pharmacists can also improve access to primary health care services in remote or underserved areas where there is a shortage of primary health care physicians (see Chapter 4).

Developing community health workers' roles

Beyond expanding the role of nurse practitioners and community pharmacists, some health care systems are working towards the development of community health workers within the primary health care team. Community health workers most often are responsible for delivering person-centred, support team-based care, addressing social determinants of health, and promoting improved access to health care for vulnerable and hard to reach populations (see also Chapter 4) (Hartzler et al., 2018[63]; Malcarney et al., 2017[64]). As shown by a systematic studies review, community health workers perform three main functions: providing clinical services, such as assessment of vital signs, lifestyle advice, and routine examinations aided by remote communication with physicians; linking patients with community-based services, such as referrals for transportation or food assistance; and providing health education and coaching, to help patients achieve health goals and increase self-efficacy (Hartzler et al., 2018[63]).

In the United States, Community Health Aides provide primary health care services in remote Alaskan villages, whose population would otherwise have no access to appropriate health care delivery (Golnick et al., 2012[65]). They are the first point of contact with the health care system for the population living in these very remote villages. They work under the supervision of Community Health Practitioners, and there is an integrated referral system that includes physicians, regional hospitals and a tertiary hospital (Golnick et al., 2012[65]). The range of primary health care services delivered by Community Health Aides mostly includes care for chronic illnesses and disease prevention, plus emergency visits for respiratory distress and chest pain.

Canada has recently introduced the new professional role of "primary health counsellors" to provide mental health care services. Their role is to provide early screening and brief interventions for mental health and addiction (Box 2.3). In the Province of Nova Scotia, community paramedics treat and release patients in the community to avoiding unnecessary emergency department visits and advanced paramedics assist in long-term care settings and within palliative patients in their homes.

In the area of health education and linking patients with community-based services, the community health educator referral liaison (CHERL) is a primary health care role that has been introduced in the United States (Holtrop et al., 2008[66]). Their objective is to reduce unhealthy behaviour such as tobacco use, unhealthy diet, lack of physical activity and risky alcohol use. CHERL assesses health risks, provides health and behaviour change counselling and co-ordinates care with practices, patients, and community resources. Evaluation results show that after six months improvements were reported for BMI, dietary patterns, alcohol use, tobacco use, health status, and days of limited activity in the past month (Holtrop et al., 2008[66]). In a similar vein, Costa Rica has established "health promotors" to specifically increase the focus on health promotion and disease prevention in primary health care settings. This new group of primary health care workforce are encouraged to prescribe physical activity for at-risk population groups with follow-up programmes supervised by other primary health care providers.

In the United Kingdom, the GP contract five year framework provides funding to contribute towards an extra 20 000 non-GP roles in general practice including clinical pharmacists, social prescribing link workers, physician associates, first contact physiotherapists and first contact community paramedics. These roles will provide clinical services, patient education and link patients with community-based services. These roles have been chosen to meet the strong practice demand, and because the tasks they perform can help reduce GP workload, improve practice efficiency and better meet health system objectives (NHS, 2019[67]). According to NHS England, the five roles will enrich the skills mix of general practice teams nationwide and enable all GPs to concentrate their time on tasks specifically requiring physician input. It is expected that the new roles will use data analysis to intervene early to help prevent illness.

Overall, health care systems need to ensure that their community-based workforce is able to take on different roles for the benefit of patients, such as prevention activities, co-ordination roles or person-centred communication. A greater use of a community-based workforce has all the potential to increase efficiency in primary health care practice, notably by increasing the panel size of primary health care physicians, reducing after-hours work for physicians, and by meeting patient's clinical needs more effectively and comprehensively. Health care systems will need to ensure that laws and regulations in OECD countries do not restrict the scope of practice of primary health care staff. It is vital to allow nurse practitioners and other primary health care staff to practice to the fullest extent of their training and ability, and remove restrictions that limit their scope of practice (Buerhaus Peter, 2018[68]; Maier and Aiken, 2016[69]; Shipman and Sinsky, 2013[44]).

> ### Box 2.3. Introduction of community health workers in Costa Rica and Canada to target specific health needs
>
> **Health promotors in Costa Rica**
>
> Costa Rica has recently established a new health profession called "health promotors" to specifically increase the focus on health promotion and disease prevention in primary health care settings.
>
> Health promotors will participate in the diagnosis of community health issues and in the design of indicators and registration systems to help identify health determinants in order to prioritise areas of intervention.
>
> They are expected to participate in interdisciplinary teams and to co-ordinate with primary health care teams. They will conduct counselling, training and guidance in health promotion and prevention of disease, and will also participate to inter-sectoral projects to address social determinants of health.
>
> **Mental health counsellors in Canada**
>
> The primary role of mental health counsellors is to provide early screening and brief interventions for mental health and addiction as part of the shared care services offered in primary health care settings. The mental health counsellor will work in partnership with the patient to identify the support and assistance they need to achieve their health goals.
>
> Where possible, the mental health counsellor and the family physician (and even the psychiatrist) work in the same office or clinic, so all services can be offered from the same location. The mental health counsellor will provide individual, family or group counselling depending on the needs of the individual. Services are short term and time limited. The psychiatrist will provide assessment and consultation with the family physician around treatment for those who need specialised mental health care.
>
> Source: OECD (2018[52]), Policy Survey on the Future of Primary Care.

2.3.2. The vast growth in digital technologies for health has brought both benefits and new challenges for primary health care

Digital health is closely related to the concept of eHealth, which can be defined as the use of information and communication technology in support of health and health-related fields (WHO, 2016[70]). Digital health covers this term and includes emerging areas, such as the use of advanced computer sciences in genomics, "big data", and artificial intelligence (WHO, 2019[71]). Health sectors across countries are undergoing a profound transformation as they capitalise on the opportunities provided by information and communication technologies. Key objectives shaping this transformation process include improved efficiency, productivity and quality of care (OECD/IDB, 2016[72]).

Patients and providers are more aware than ever about advances in technology and that these can be used in health-related issues. Health systems are responding and adapting in different ways to this trend. In Europe, a recent report found that in all the 27 countries surveyed, eHealth adoption in primary health care has increased between 2013 to 2018, with the highest levels of implementation in Denmark, Estonia, Finland, Spain, Sweden and the United Kingdom, while in Greece, Luxembourg and the Slovak Republic uptake remains relatively low (Valverde-Albacete et al., 2019[73]). Figure 2.8 shows the proportion of Internet users in OECD countries utilising common digital technologies or engaged in selected online activities. Notably, health-related searches are the second most common use of the Internet, with almost 57% of people using the Internet in this way, only surpassed by online purchases with 59% (OECD, 2017[74]).

Figure 2.8. Seeking health information ranks second in the utilisation of digital technologies

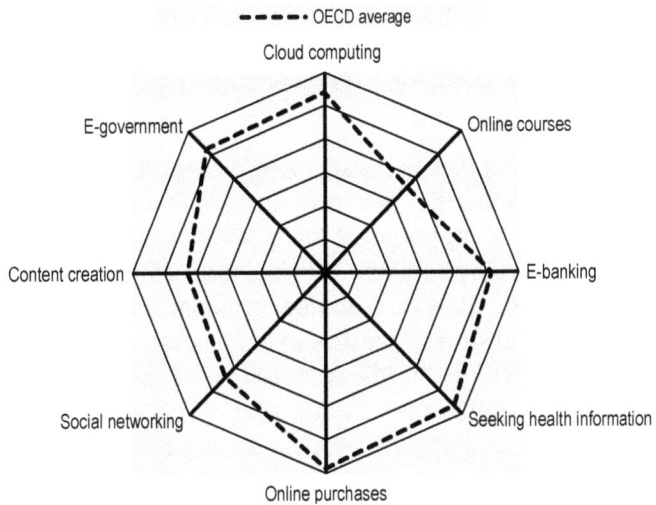

Note: All indicators have been standardised with a range between 0 and 1.
Source: Adapted Figure 1.4, from OECD (2017[74]), *OECD Digital Economy Outlook 2017*, https://doi.org/10.1787/9789264276284-en.

Likewise, a survey of almost 5 000 people in the United States, found that among the respondents who indicated that they are open to using digital tools: the majority said they would prefer to receive them from their primary health care provider; 58% said they would prefer to receive appointment reminders by email, text or phone; 53% would prefer to use EHR; 53% would choose to have email and online communication; and 50% favoured having video or online doctor's appointments (Cordina, Qian and Sanfilippo, 2019[75]).

The following section is focused on three of the most relevant and developed digital technologies used in primary health care: telemedicine, mobile health, and electronic medical support systems.

Telemedicine can result in a better use of resources to improve health care processes and is cost-effective in the majority of studies

Telemedicine can be classified into three categories (Flodgren et al., 2015[76]): telemonitoring, store and forward and interactive telemedicine. Telemonitoring is the use of mobile devices and platforms to conduct routine medical tests, communicate the results to health care workers in real time, and potentially launch pre-programmed automated responses. Store and forward is similar, but is used for clinical data that are less time-sensitive and for which a delay between transmission and response is acceptable. Interactive or real-time telemedicine involves direct and synchronous communication between providers and patients, also called digital consultations (e.g. direct-to-patient or in health care facilities).

Telemedicine may contribute to providing care in the right place at the right time

Telemedicine may contribute to providing care in the right place at the right time in several different ways, notably by improving the process of care and appropriateness of referrals. Teleconsultations, which are one of the most utilised telemedicine interventions in primary health care, may also lead to GPs feeling less isolated from their peers and being better able to triage and treat patients. Indeed, primary health care professionals aided with telemedicine can contact specialists to get specific medical expertise for a consultation. This is associated with continuous learning between peers and with a reduction of unnecessary referrals to secondary care. A review found that face-to-face visits with specialists are reduced between 22% and 68% with the use of teleconsultations (Liddy et al., 2019[77]). Importantly, the same review found that patients were highly satisfied with teleconsultation (median ratings of five on a five-point Likert scale) in terms of expectations being met and confidence in the service, and patients rated the service high for quality of care, timeliness, improved access and safety.

In Colombia, the development of telemedicine is a priority objective to improve quality and access to primary health care to the population. Efforts are being made to develop the regulation and guidelines for a safe use of telemedicine, and to ensure sustainable financing and payment mechanisms of telemedicine services.

In Canada the Ontario Telehomecare project provides co-ordinated support from primary health care teams to people with complex chronic diseases in their own homes. The overarching objective is to provide people with chronic conditions access to appropriate care when needed and decrease the need for emergency department visits and acute hospital admissions, thereby increasing efficiency. The programme focuses on people with CHF, COPD, diabetes, patients transitioning from hospital to home and patients requiring remote monitoring in a shared post-acute care model. Recent evaluations show positive results: patients with CHF and/or COPD reported increased confidence in self-managing symptoms, while hospital emergency department visits and hospital admissions decreased (OTN, 2016[78]).

In Estonia, telemedicine and tele-expertise support interactions among professionals, save time and make care more efficient. The eConsultation service in primary health care has been implemented to allow primary health care physicians to consult with specialists on difficult cases online. The use of the eConsultation service has increased among primary health care physicians and has great potential to reduce unnecessary referrals to specialist care. In 2018, 882 primary health care physicians used the eConsultation service compared to 670 in 2017 (Eesti Haigekassa, 2019[79]).

In the United Kingdom, Babylon GP at Hand offers digital and face-to-face consultations to registered patients. Although there are several questions around the financial sustainability of the GP at Hand practice and other nearby practices (notably because telemedicine services attract younger and healthier patients than other GP practices) (Burki, 2019[80]; Cravo Oliveira Hashiguchi, 2020[81]), a recent evaluation shows that patients were positive about the quality of care they received, the level of antibiotics prescribing was lower among GP at Hand patients than among patients in other traditional practices, and GPs working at the practice reported high levels of satisfaction in terms of work-life balance (Iacobucci, 2019[82]; Burki, 2019[80]; Quigley, Hex and Aznar, 2019[83]). Additional evaluation must however be performed to guarantee the benefits of such digital services are maximised, notably with regards to the use of specialised health care services.

Telemedicine has been found to be cost-effective in the majority of analysis, but important cost savings are missing from many economic assessments

An OECD umbrella review of systematic reviews, found that of 19 systematic reviews on cost-effectiveness, 13 concluded that telemedicine interventions were either cost-effective or had the potential to be cost-effective (Cravo Oliveira Hashiguchi, 2020[81]). For instance, cost-minimisation studies show that the cost of teleconsultations can range between USD 5 and USD 298 per session, compared with face-to-face specialist visits that range between USD 56 and USD 338 (Liddy et al., 2019[77]).

However, there are examples that place a cautionary note. A review including studies conducted in primary health care centres and hospitals in Austria, Italy and the United Kingdom, found that tele-dermatology accounts for more time (7.54 minutes extra on average) than conventional consultations and this difference represents an opportunity cost of EUR 29.25 for each remote consultation, with a unitary factor cost of EUR 3.88 per minute (Fuertes-Guiró and Girabent-Farrés, 2017[84]). Moreover, teleconsultation services in primary health care may lead to difficulties in patient pathways when providers have dissimilar objectives and incentives, or are defectively integrated. This problem has been noted in the United States and the United Kingdom, where there is a risk that providers might prioritise easy-to-access, quick and convenient teleconsultations to younger and healthier patients under fee-for-service payment schemes. This risk can be exacerbated when the primary health care provider is not the patient's usual physician, and continuity of care is limited, which creates an inefficient use of resources (Cravo Oliveira Hashiguchi, 2020[81]). In addition, it is important to ensure a strong quality control for telemedicine so that these digital services offer safe and high-quality care to populations across OECD countries (see also Chapter 4).

Despite the growing number of economic assessments of telemedicine in recent years, the comprehensive and methodological approach used in these studies has generated some questions. A review found that most of the economic studies regarding telemedicine have a sufficiently broad sample and use well-defined cost items and outcome variables, but the perspective of analysis remains an unsolved issue (Fusco, Trieste and Turchetti, 2014[85]). Because economic analyses of telemedicine interventions usually take a relatively narrow health system perspective and fail to introduce a social perspective, they tend to miss important cost categories that would make the economic case for telemedicine more favourable. For instance, in 2017, patients in the Canadian Ontario Telemedicine Network avoided travelling 270 million kilometres and the network saved CAD 71.9 million in travel grants (OTN, 2018[86]). While provider savings associated with travel subsidies would be included in a cost-effectiveness analysis with a health system perspective, the significant costs of unsubsidised patient travelling would not. These costs would include not only direct costs (e.g. gas, bus fare, etc.), but also indirect costs in time away from work or leisure, as well as pollutant emissions (Oliveira et al., 2013[87]). While the costs of avoidable and unplanned admissions are frequently considered in cost-effectiveness analyses of telemonitoring interventions, again the potential costs to family members meeting their relatives at the hospital and the productivity loss for the patient and their families are not (Fusco, Trieste and Turchetti, 2014[85]). These are all quantifiable costs that can improve economic evaluations of telemedicine (Cravo Oliveira Hashiguchi, 2020[81]).

Mobile health apps as a tool to embrace technology and bring patients closer to primary health care practices

The use of smartphones and mobile devices has increased at a fast pace in most countries and mobile health (mHealth) has been one of the fastest growing sectors of information and communication technologies in health. Mobile technologies offer a wide range of smart modalities by which patients can interact with health professionals or systems, ranging from prevention, diagnosis, treatment and monitoring (OECD, 2017[74]). Health-related mobile applications available to consumers surpassed 318 500 in 2017, nearly double the number available in 2015, with approximately 200 new apps added to the market each day. Nonetheless, 85% of all health apps have fewer than 5 000 downloads and only 41 apps have registered at least ten million downloads, together representing nearly half of all app download activity (IQVIA, 2017[88]).

In 2015, the World Health Organization surveyed over 125 countries on eHealth and mHealth activities at the national level (WHO, 2016[89]). Over 80% of these countries reported government-sponsored mHealth programmes, many of which are directly related to primary health care, such as call centres, appointment reminders, community mobilisation, mobile telehealth, patient records, patient monitoring, health surveys, treatment adherence and decision support systems. mHealth projects primarily extend existing health programmes and services at the national or local level (Figure 2.9).

Figure 2.9. Adoption of mHealth programmes by type in 125 countries worldwide, 2015

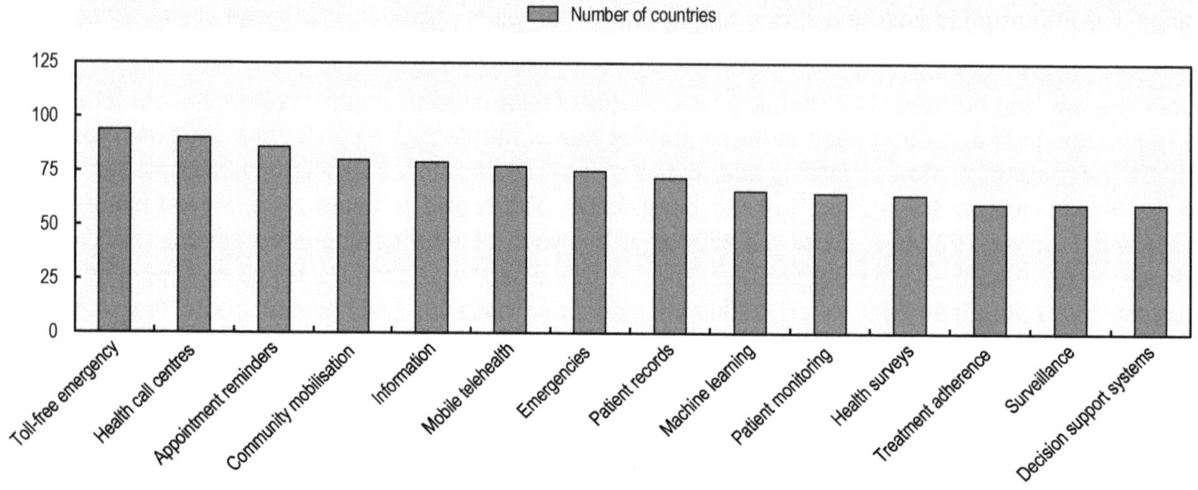

Note: The results include responses from over 600 eHealth experts in 125 countries worldwide.
Source: OECD (2017[74]), *OECD Digital Economy Outlook 2017*, https://doi.org/10.1787/9789264276284-en, based on WHO (2016[89]), *Atlas of eHealth Country Profiles*.

There is an increasing body of evidence about the effectiveness and economic assessments of mHealth interventions, most of which apply for primary health care

mHealth is widely recognised as especially valuable for the management of non-communicable diseases, such as diabetes and cardiac disease, and other health conditions where primary health care has a crucial role. A study by IQVIA (2017) found that there is a growing body of evidence analysing the effectiveness of mobile apps to improve patients' health, with published studies increasing substantially in recent years. In this context, several mobile health apps have achieved significant levels of substantiated clinical evidence supporting them. In particular, three digital apps in the areas of diabetes, depression and anxiety were considered by the report to be candidates for inclusion in clinical guidelines because of favourable scientific evidence supporting them. As an example, an overview of systematic reviews about mHealth for managing diabetes, found that on average mHealth interventions improve glycaemic control (HbA1c), compared to standard care or other non-mHealth approaches, by as much as 0.8% for patients with type 2 diabetes and 0.3% for patients with type 1 diabetes, at least in the short-term (≤12 months) (Kitsiou et al., 2017[90]).

Similarly, there has been a growing number of economic assessments of mHealth. A review that included 39 studies spanning 19 countries (most of which were upper and upper-middle income countries) found economic evaluations about primary mHealth interventions, behaviour change communication (e.g. attendance rates, medication adherence) and use of mHealth short messaging system (SMS) (e.g. used to send reminders, information, provide support, conduct surveys or collect data). In 29 studies (74.3%), researchers reported that the mHealth intervention was cost-effective, economically beneficial, or cost saving at base case (Iribarren et al., 2017[91]). From a health system perspective, this can be explained because of a better use of resources when utilising mHealth. For instance, attendance rates to health care appointments can be improved by using mobile text messages. A review found moderate quality evidence from seven studies that mobile text message reminders improved the rate of attendance at health care appointments compared to no reminders. There was also moderate evidence from three studies that mobile text message reminders had a similar impact to phone call reminders, which require more resources than mobile texts (Gurol-Urganci et al., 2013[92]). At country level, a study which took a health system and social perspective, reported that in the United States using digital health apps in just five patient populations where apps have already been proven to reduce acute care utilisation (diabetes prevention, diabetes, asthma, cardiac rehabilitation and pulmonary rehabilitation) would save the country's health care system USD 7 billion per year and provide tangible improvements (IQVIA, 2017[88]).

A comparative advantage of smartphone or mobile apps is their efficient model due to negligible marginal cost and scalability. Once programming is completed and the app tested and verified, the number of times it can be downloaded and used is virtually unlimited. There is no need for hardware as users will generally not purchase a smartphone only to use health and wellness apps. Any improvements or corrections to the software are automatically updated on the user's smartphone via the Internet. More importantly, an app can be used over and over, incurring only a one-off expense to the consumer. However, successful integration of mHealth in health care systems requires a number of adaptations: the performance and clinical utility of mobile applications must be assessed for reliable and efficient use in health care, and incentives are needed to encourage take-up of mobile applications that are both effective and cost-effective. In addition, exchanges of information must be protected by appropriate levels of cybersecurity (OECD, 2017[93]).

Beyond digital apps, the development of web-based patient portals shows promise for improving self-efficacy, health behaviours and clinical outcomes (Whitehead and Seaton, 2016[94]; Bender et al., 2011[95]). In Finland, the Oulu Self Care Service was launched in 2010 in the City of Oulu. The eService platform provides self-care services, including secure communication with health care professionals, booking appointments, checking laboratory results, accessing personal information, a self-care library (with content for self-care for diabetes, asthma and blood pressure), electronic health-checks and digital coaching (e.g. sleep, stress, weight and exercise) (Lupiañez-Villanueva, Sachinopoulou and Theben, 2015[96]). The platform is integrated with a person's EHR. The Oulu Self Care Service has been recognised as a key enabler of the chronic care model to improve health outcomes, and make care more efficient through a shared use of data among health and social care providers. Similar services are also available in Canada, Estonia and Turkey (see Chapter 3).

Electronic health records and electronic prescription systems can improve clinical decision making in primary health care

Electronic clinical support systems store and analyse data to help health care providers make decisions and improve patient care. They can also issue risk alerts, reminders and provide information about interaction between medicines. They are usually based on EHR and electronic medication prescription systems, which provide the foundation for more complex functionalities that promise greater care co-ordination and improved clinical management (OECD, 2017[74]; Santos et al., 2019[97]).

EHR have expanded in OECD countries and can improve primary health care clinical practice

In 2016, an OECD survey of 30 OECD countries revealed that most countries are investing in the development of EHR (Oderkirk, 2017[98]). Twenty-three countries reported that they are implementing EHR systems at a national level, but only 18 reported comprehensive record sharing within one countrywide system designed to support each patient having only one EHR, aiming to cover primary health care and hospitals. Moreover, six countries indicated that they are not aiming to implement an EHR system at the national level at this time (Chile, Czech Republic, Japan, Mexico and the United States).

In relation to primary health care, 15 countries reported that at least 90% of primary health care physician offices are capturing patient diagnosis and treatment information in EHR. Conversely, Mexico and Poland reported that less than one-third of primary health care physician offices are using EHR (see Figure 2.10). Comparing with data collected in 2012 (OECD, 2013[99]), some countries have substantially increased their EHR coverage in primary health care, for instance, Poland from 15% to 30%, Mexico from 15% to 30.3%, Japan from 15.2% to 35.6%, Switzerland from 20% to 40%, Canada from 41.3% to 77.2%, the United States from 57% to 83%, and Denmark from 51% to 100%. In Lithuania, the coverage of EHR also substantially increased during the past year.

Figure 2.10. Percentage of primary health care physician offices using electronic health records in OECD countries, 2016

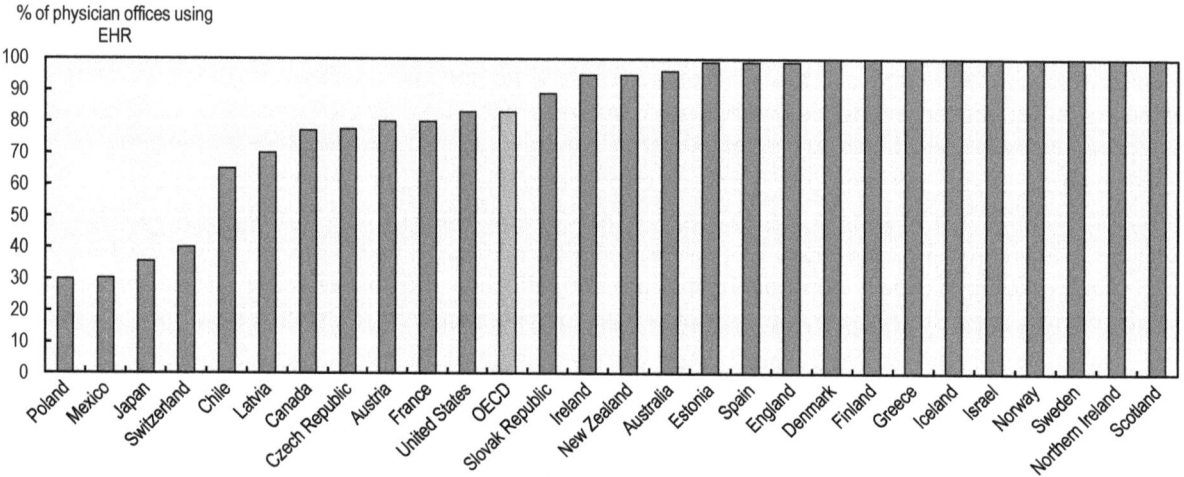

Note: The data for Canada refer to the percentage of physicians, as opposed to physician offices.
Source: Oderkirk (2017[98]), "Readiness of electronic health record systems to contribute to national health information and research", https://dx.doi.org/10.1787/9e296bf3-en.

There is mounting evidence today to demonstrate that the introduction of EHR can contribute to better health care. A systematic review that conducted several meta-analyses found that EHR resulted in 33% higher adherence to guidelines and 54% reduction in medication errors, and 34% reduction in adverse drug effects. However, no association with mortality rates was found (Campanella et al., 2016[100]).

In Finland, the POTKU model has the potential to increase adherence to guidelines and to reduce medication errors. The model provides primary health care physicians with the locally developed Evidence-Based Medicine electronic Decision Support (EBMeDS) system, which is matched with patient records to provide personalised care guidance, and generate automated reminders and warnings (Hujala Anneli et al., 2016[101]).

EHR can also be accessed online by patients, allowing for a relatively new type of relationship between the primary health care system and the patient. A systematic review found that patients reported improved satisfaction with online access and services compared with standard provision, improved self-care, and better communication and engagement with clinicians. For instance, safety improvements were patient-led, for example, by identifying medication errors and facilitating more use of preventive services. Use of EHR also resulted in a moderate increase of email exchanges, no change on telephone contact, with variable effects on face-to-face contact. However, other tasks were necessary to sustain these services, which impacted on clinician time (Mold et al., 2015[102]).

Regarding economic evaluations, there seems to be a salient lack of recently published economic evaluations about EHR in primary health care. A 2003 study (Wang et al., 2003[103]), found that the implementation of an EHR system in primary health care can result in a positive financial return on investment to the health care organisation, estimating a net benefit for a 5-year period of USD 86 400 per provider. Sensitivity analysis showed results ranging from a USD 2 300 net cost to a USD 330 900 net benefit. Benefits accrue primarily from savings in drug expenditure, improved utilisation of radiology tests, better capture of charges, and decreased billing errors. More recent discussion is focused on how the data coming from EHR can help develop economic evaluations of other interventions (Hazra, Rudisill and Gulliford, 2019[104]).

Spain, for example, as part of its "Chronicity Strategy" to provide integrated care to frail elderly adults and patients with multi-morbidity in the Basque country, integrates EHR with a patient portal, an electronic prescription system and tele-monitoring service. Based on a predictive model, risk stratification and case finding are used to unify various data sources, including demographics, primary health care, hospital care and prescription data. Risk stratification and case finding allow the alignment of the delivery of preventive services for groups at higher risk of worse health outcomes and to elaborate needs-based care plans. A recent evaluation of the project shows that the integrated care model was associated with a reduced number of hospital admissions and visits to emergency departments, and with higher satisfaction from patients and health care professionals. Overall, the analysis show that this intervention is cost effective (de Manuel Keenoy, 2018[105]; Scirocco, 2017[106]).

In Israel, all the health funds have comprehensive EHR in community care, which supports the sharing of information among physicians, laboratories, diagnostic centres, hospitals and patients. EHRs are used across the community care setting and they capture detailed patient level information, including demographics, diagnostic and testing information, and drug utilisation data (see also Chapter 3).

In Colombia, the National Government is currently working to improve the interoperability of EHR through defining the legal framework, the sources of financing and training needs.

ePrescription programmes can reduce medication errors and bring financial gains to primary health care

Electronic prescription (ePrescription) allows prescribers to write prescriptions that can be retrieved by a pharmacy electronically, to assess a patient's medication regimen at the point of care and to identify non-adherence. It may also be possible to notify a prescriber or pharmacist about refills, which can help trigger an intervention to avoid a potential gap in medication use and can improve the accuracy and efficiency of pharmaceutical drug dispensing (Khan and Socha-Dietrich, 2018[107]).

The rate of ePrescribing has been increasing in OECD countries. For instance, by 2014 the adoption of ePrescribing in primary health care was approximately 32% of European GPs. National ePrescribing services were established in 11 countries, with pilot projects underway in most others. The highest adoption rates were observed in countries with national health service models, concentrated in the Nordic area and the United Kingdom (Brennan, McElligott and Power, 2015[108]). Other OECD countries, for example Australia and New Zealand, also have ePrescribing infrastructures in place. In New Zealand, as of March 2019, the ePrescription service was used by 160 GP practices, up from 87 in March 2018 (84% increase) and prescribers generated 251 542 ePrescriptions compared to 148 450 the year before (Ministry of Health, 2019[109]). In Australia, by 2015, 95.7% of GPs had implemented Electronic Transfer of Prescription and the Australian Department of Human Services also mandated that all pharmacies have to move to online claiming (HIQA, 2018[110]). In Sweden, all pharmacies use the eHealth data base to get the information they need to dispense a prescription. In Lithuania, electronic medical records, including electronic prescriptions, has grown significantly since 2017. 100% of pharmacies are connected to central eHealth system and can issue medicines by electronic prescriptions. Health care institutions can use the central eHealth portal for free or they can use their own Information system to send medical documents including for example referrals, descriptions of consultations or ePrescription.

Published economic evaluations of ePrescription systems in primary health care settings are relatively scarce. Among the economic benefits described for ePrescribing (Deetjen, 2016[111]), there are efficiency gains for prescribers, mainly by reducing the time devoted to writing prescriptions and in obtaining information on patients' co-morbidities and other medications. Similarly, efficiency gains for dispensers arise from lower workload, better stock management, reduced volumes of paper to be sorted out for reimbursement, and the possibility of preparing orders before patients arrive. In addition, ePrescriptions can enable transparency, by making doctors more accountable for what they prescribe (e.g. allowing the evaluation of adherence to clinical guidelines), and making pharmacies more accountable for what they dispense and in what timescales. Fraud reduction has been signalled as an economic benefit too, by facilitating detection and audit trials. Finally, printing costs are immensely reduced as well. A systematic review found that cost savings due to improved patient outcomes and decreased patient visits are estimated to be between USD 140 billion and USD 240 billion over ten years for practices that implement ePrescribing (Porterfield, Engelbert and Coustasse, 2014[112]).

In Estonia, the direct cost of implementing the service was almost EUR 500 000, including the set up costs, annual running costs for servers and maintenance, but this does not include the cost of auxiliary registries, project management and system integration for pharmacists and health care service providers (Parv et al., 2014[113]). Savings in printing materials were calculated to exceed the EUR 63 668 saved in 2009 to savings of around EUR 100 000 in 2010 (Deetjen, 2016[111]). In Sweden, by 2008 the cumulative investment costs, including operating expenditure over the eight years since nationwide implementation, were estimated at EUR 155 million, while the estimated cumulative benefits were estimated to be EUR 330 million (European Commission, 2008[114]).

Since ePrescribing is usually part of a wider health information system, a study (Dobrev et al., 2009[115]) evaluated the development of ePrescription systems attached to EHR in 11 different health care settings, including primary health care, specialist ambulatory care and hospital care. The experiences considered were from Bulgaria, the Czech Republic, France, Israel, Italy, Spain, Sweden, Switzerland, the United Kingdom and the United States. The study found that the average cumulative socio-economic returns on investment of interoperable EHR and ePrescribing systems was 78%, on average, over the evaluation timescales of between nine and 13 years. It took at least four and up to nine years, before initiatives produced their first positive annual socio-economic return, and 6-11 years, to realise a cumulative net benefit. These findings highlight the importance of long-term investments in EHR and ePrescribing systems to obtain both health and economic benefits.

2.3.3. New payment structures can help teams deliver primary health care more effectively

There are several forms of payment structure that encourage certain desirable behaviours at specific points of the care continuum, including providing additional payments to remunerate specific activities and pay-for-performance (P4P) programmes. Providing additional payments can support the management of chronic diseases, care co-ordination or early discharge from hospitals, while P4P targets quality or performance outcomes. Overall, such forms of payment are keys to incentivise primary health care teams to operate differently. Such economic incentives are designed to maximise health care output through better care processes, and to reduce the use of expensive inputs by moving care out of the hospital sector. Overall, this can help to improve technical and allocative efficiency.

To be effective, paying for specific activities or P4P needs to encourage the delivery of appropriate services in primary health care that can be directly influenced by the level of the primary health care team's efforts.

Paying for disease prevention, care co-ordination and for early discharge from hospitals signals how services should be delivered to improve care processes

Paying for disease prevention and for care co-ordination is a way of targeting specific dimensions of the care provision in order to improve health outcomes, notably through the establishment of care plans, collaborative care meetings or the provision of patient education, particularly for those suffering from multi-morbidity. The 2018 OECD Policy Survey on the Future of Primary Care shows that 11 OECD countries use this type of payment to incentivise care co-ordination or disease prevention (Figure 2.11).

In Canada, for example, the funding model encourages collaboration and communication among providers. Additional fees are offered to physicians to compensate for time spent communicating with other health care providers involved in the patient's care and for sharing information with other providers to better manage complex needs. In Iceland and some regions of Italy, physicians have additional remuneration when they are responsible for patients with chronic disorders or with special care needs. They are expected to collaborate with specialists, nurses and social workers. In Israel, additional payments have been introduced to stimulate state-mandated health service organisations to improve quality and access to primary health care. The programme, for example, rewards providers for taking care of chronic patients in multi-disciplinary teams.

Australia has invested in the Practice Incentives Program, which supports general practice activities that encourage continuing improvement, quality care, enhance capacity and improve upon access and health outcomes for patients, including improving health outcomes relating to chronic disease. Components of the Practice Incentives Program include the use of outcomes payments to general practices. As of 1 August 2019, a new Practice Incentives Program Quality Improvement was introduced to provide funding to general practice to undertake continuous quality improvement activities through the collection and review of practice data in partnership with their local Primary Health Network (PHN). The Practice Incentives Program Quality Improvement will support work already underway where practices share data and work closely with their PHN to improve patient care. In addition, practice nurses can receive additional payments for co-ordinating activities. In 2011, the "working with others" programme was introduced as an annual payment for community pharmacists who collaborate with other health professionals.

In France, the *Experimentations de nouveaux modes de rémunération* (ENMR) entailed a lump-sum payment per patient for three types of activities: i) co-ordinating activities; ii) provision of new services, such as patient education; and iii) inter-professional co-operation. Pay-for-co-ordination schemes also exist in Austria, Denmark, Germany and Sweden (Suzuki, 2018[116]). In Austria and Germany, pay-for-co-ordination emerged out of disease management programmes for chronic diseases. In Sweden, municipalities can provide bonuses to primary health care physicians for care co-ordination. In Denmark, general practitioners get pay-for-coordination, notably when they have more responsibility for treatment of chronically ill patients (e.g. diabetes).

In the United States, the Comprehensive Primary Care Plus model (mentioned further in Chapter 3) is a unique public-private partnership, in which practices receive additional financial resources and flexibility to make investments, improve quality of care, and reduce the number of unnecessary services their patients receive. In addition, within the Medicare programme, new billing codes have been recently implemented so that providers can bill for care co-ordination and care transition services.

Other health care systems employ economic incentives to encourage reductions in delayed hospital discharge and to improve care transitions out of hospital. These often take the form of negative incentives, whereby an organisation is required to perform a certain way in order to avoid incurring a loss. In this case, hospitals or municipalities are fined for excessive delays in discharge from hospital, as seen in the Czech Republic, Denmark, Norway, Sweden and the United Kingdom. In Canada, by contrast, the primary health care physicians are provided with a financial incentive for a timely primary health care appointment post-hospital discharge (within seven days).

Experience from OECD countries also shows that financial incentives may be a useful way to compensate primary health care teams for the costs of transition associated with the introduction of digital technologies. In the United States, for example, the Medicare and Medicaid Promoting Interoperability Programs (previously called "meaningful use") are incentive schemes aimed at encouraging the adoption of certified EHR which, as mentioned in Section 2.3.2, has been found to improve efficiency in primary health care (Shipman and Sinsky, 2013[44]; Green, Savin and Lu, 2013[53]). The adoption of EHR should follow three stages:

- Stage 1: focus on promoting the adoption of certified technologies. The first stage establishes requirements for the electronic capture of clinical data and giving patients access to electronic copies of their own health information.

- Stage 2: emphasise care co-ordination and the exchange of patient information. This increases the thresholds of criteria compliance and introduces more clinical decision support, care co-ordination requirements and patient engagement rules.
- Stage 3: aim at improving health outcomes by implementing protected health information, ePrescribing, clinical decision support, computerised provider order entry, patient provider access, co-ordinated care through patient engagement, health information exchange, clinical data registry and case reporting.

Previous studies show that paying for specific activities is simple to implement and does not require large IT investment (OECD, 2016[117]). In France, available evidence suggests the ENMRs showed beneficial impact on both the quality of care and health care costs. The multidisciplinary structures signed up to the ENMR achieved better results than traditional practices for nearly all care indicators (diabetes care processes, disease prevention and efficient prescribing of medications). The organisation of care was also found to be more effective through greater collaboration and greater care co-ordination between health professionals (Mousquès and Bourgueil, 2014[118]). In Norway, the financial sanctions imposed on local authorities between 2012 and 2015 for delays in discharging patients from hospital was followed by a significant reduction in delayed discharges (OECD, 2017[25]). It is important to note that despite positive evaluation, it is always difficult to disentangle the contribution of economic incentives or sanctions from the influence of other factors.

Figure 2.11. Number of OECD countries using paying for prevention/co-ordination vs pay for performance incentives, 2018

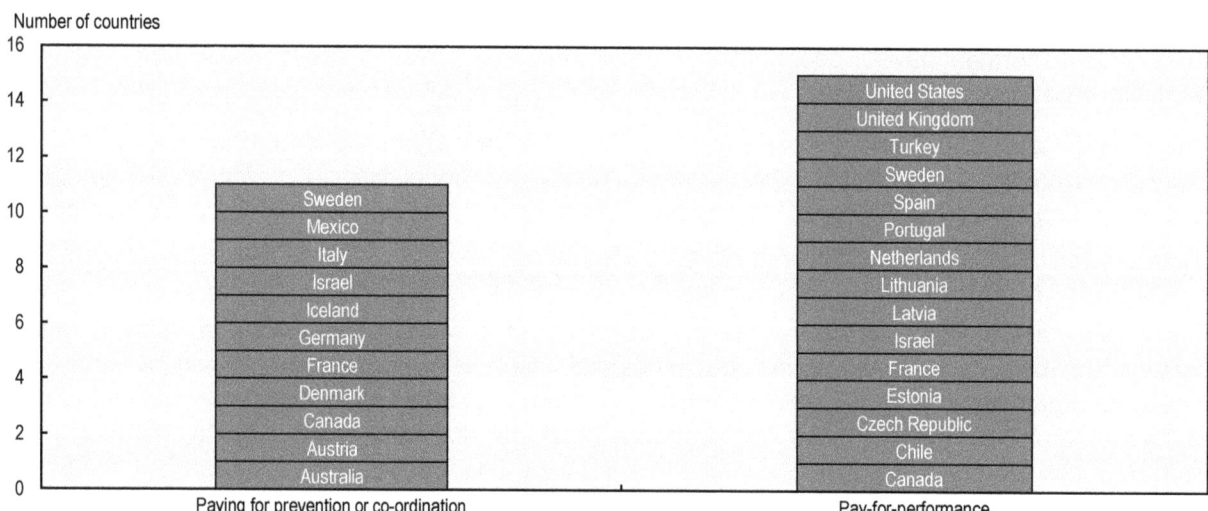

Source: OECD (2018[52]), Policy Survey on the Future of Primary Care, and OECD (2016[54]), Health System Characteristics Survey, http://www.oecd.org/els/health-systems/characteristics.htm.

When properly designed and implemented, P4P programmes have the potential to encourage clinical excellence in primary health care

There are some P4P programmes in primary health care across OECD countries. The payment most often depends on quality or performance targets, and relates to the degree of achievement of certain objectives. Providers have to report the required indicators and outcomes, and have to demonstrate they have met the targets to receive payments. By contrast, if providers do not meet the required targets, the payment is withheld.

The latest evidence indicates that 15 OECD countries have introduced P4P schemes in primary health care. These schemes typically use process indicators to reward clinical excellence (such as blood pressure checks for patients with hypertension or tests for HgbA1c for diabetic patients) or better intermediate outcomes (such as cholesterol control in people with diabetes or controlled blood pressure for patients with hypertension).

In England, for example, these indicators are included in the Quality and Outcome Framework (QOF), a voluntary annual reward and incentive programme for all GP surgeries. In 2017-19, the QOF included 75 indicators, consisting of three domains. The three domains are clinical (e.g. heart failure, hypertension and chronic diseases), public health (e.g. blood pressure, prevention of cardiovascular disease, obesity and smoking) and public health additional services (e.g. cervical screening and contraception). As demonstrated by Roland and Guthrie (2016[119]), the successes of QOF included more systematic management of chronic conditions by multi-disciplinary teams and the widespread introduction of EHR. The QOF has been found to slightly improve care quality and to reduce socio-economic inequalities in care delivery (Roland and Guthrie, 2016[119]). Findings from Dusheiko et al (2011[120]) show that the QOF improves intermediate outcomes for stroke care, which was associated with reduced hospital costs (Dusheiko et al., 2011[120]). Harrison et al (2014[121]) confirmed these findings by suggesting that the introduction of the QOF in England was associated with a decrease in emergency admissions for conditions incentivised under the scheme, compared with conditions that were not incentivised (Harrison et al., 2014[121]). Rates of emergency admissions decreased by 10.9% in 2010/11. However, other studies show that the QOF had no positive impact on health outcomes. Using population-level mortality statistics between 1994 and 2010 for the United Kingdom and other high-income countries not implementing P4P schemes, Ryan et al (2016[122]) have shown that the QOF was not associated with changes in population mortality. Results are therefore highly inconsistent across studies (Ryan et al., 2016[122]).

Table 2.3. Indicators used as part of the Estonian pay-for-performance programme

	Indicators of the P4P programme
Part 1 – Prevention	
Immunisations	Pertussis, diphtheria, tetanus, poliomyelitis, measles, mumps, rubella, hepatitis B, haemophilus influenza type b according to immunisation plan
Children's health check	1, 3, 6, and 12-month checks, 2-year check, preschool health check
Cardio-vascular disease prevention programme	For the population aged 40-60 years, blood pressure, glucose, cholesterol with fractions SCORE calculation
Part 2 – Chronic diseases	
Diabetes mellitus type 2	Register of patients with type 2 diabetes, measuring glucose and HbA1c, cholesterol with fractions, serum creatinine testing, urine tests to detect microalbuminuria, blood pressure measurement, nurse counselling
Hypertension	Register of patients with hypertension, divided into 3 stages, measuring glucose, cholesterol with fractions, serum creatinine testing, urine tests to detect microalbuminuria, blood pressure, ECG, nurse counselling, treatment with ACE inhibitors
Myocardial infarction	Register of patients with myocardial infarction, measuring cholesterol with fractions, ECG, blood pressure, nurse counselling
Hypothyroidism	Register of patients with hypothyreosis, TSH testing
Part 3- Enhanced services	Observation of pregnancy, pap smear tests, minor surgery procedures, participation in CME courses

Source: Merilind et al (2016[123]), "Pay for performance of Estonian family doctors and impact of different practice- and patient-related characteristics on a good outcome: A quantitative assessment", https://doi.org/10.1016/j.medici.2016.04.003.

In France, the P4P programme is called the *Remunération sur Objectifs de Santé Publique* (ROSP). In 2018, the ROSP targeted management of chronic conditions (including diabetes, hypertension and cardiovascular diseases), prevention activities (such as for influenza, cancer screening and addiction) and efficiency (such as rate of antibiotic prescriptions). In Estonia, the Quality Bonus System also contains three major parts: prevention, monitoring of chronic diseases according to national guidelines and enhanced services (see Table 2.3).

In Chile, the P4P scheme has two components. The first one is called the "Health Goals", which defines eight goals with ten indicators. It targets frontline workers in primary health care, who have the opportunity to receive bonus wages every three months, which can add up to two months of potential extra bonus salary per year. The goals were developed to target the main burdens of disease in the country and areas with low-compliance to set standards. The second component is called the Primary care Activity Indicators, which determine the monthly capitation payment from the Ministry of Health to municipalities. Three categories of activity are included: general activity (such as coverage of preventive medical examinations), continuity of care (such as around the clock availability) and compliance with care standards. Evaluations are conducted quarterly, and if the annually set goals for each of the indicators are not met, monthly capitation rates are lowered accordingly.

In the Czech Republic, each health insurance fund designs its own P4P programme for its contractual primary health care providers. Most of the programmes share some core features, albeit with different weights, targets and benefits. Primary health care providers will, for example, receive bonus payments according to the share of registered patients who receive annual preventive treatments, the share of patients (aged 40+) who receive colorectal cancer screening, the share of elderly patients inoculated against influenza or the share of generic medication among prescribed drugs.

There are also interesting P4P programmes outside of GP practices to encourage the expansion of the role of community pharmacies in the delivery of primary health care services, as seen in the United Kingdom or the United States (see Box 2.4).

All of these different schemes in different countries have a common aim of targeting important clinical areas and encouraging the delivery of appropriate services in a primary health care setting and that can be directly influenced by the level of provider's efforts. This is an important prerequisite for successful implementation.

However, and as mentioned previously, evidence on the impact of P4P on health outcomes and performance remains inconclusive (OECD, 2016[117]), and some researchers argue that P4P schemes go in the opposite direction of goal-oriented care (De Maeseneer and Boeckxstaens, 2012[124]). P4P programmes and related quality and performance targets should thereby incentivise outcomes that matter the most to patients (such as improving quality of life or improving daily life activities through better management of chronic conditions) and on patient-centred care processes (such as care co-ordination). P4P programmes, and value-based payments more generally, need to be properly designed and blended with other payment schemes. Appropriate information systems is also required to monitor and follow up process- and outcome-indicators.

> **Box 2.4. Pay-for-performance programmes outside of GP practice**
>
> The Community Pharmacy Quality Payments Scheme in the **United Kingdom** was established in 2016. The scheme rewards community pharmacies for delivering quality criteria in all three of the quality dimensions: clinical effectiveness, patient safety and patient experience. Among the defined criteria to be met are public health, clinical efficacy for certain chronic conditions, and workforce development. For example, the scheme aims at:
>
> - more effective treatment for asthma, by referring asthma patients who have been dispensed too many short-acting reliever inhalers without any preventer inhaler for an asthma review
> - better care for people with dementia, by ensuring that 80% of all pharmacy staff working in patient-facing roles take part in the Alzheimer's Society's Dementia Friends Scheme
> - increased support for healthy living, by ensuring there is a Royal Society of Public Health trained health champion in every one of the healthy living pharmacies across England.
>
> Since April 2017, over 90% of pharmacies have taken part in the Pharmacy Quality Scheme. As part of the new Community Pharmacy Contractual Framework for 2019/2024, the Quality Payment Scheme continues under a new name, the Pharmacy Quality Scheme.
>
> In the **United States**, a P4P programme for pharmacists is run by the Inland Empire Health Plan (IEHP), a non-profit Medicare and Medicaid health plan in Southern California. The quality measures that pharmacies must meet include: proportion of days covered (PDC) for diabetes, PDC for hypertension, PDC for statins, statin use in people with diabetes, absence of controller therapy in patients with asthma, sub-optimal control in patients with asthma, use of high-risk medications in older people and the generic dispensing rate. The programme also entails close follow-up with patients. For those suffering from diabetes for example, pharmacists check the medication history and associated past adverse events and follow-up with the patient's physician if necessary (Bonner, 2016[125]).
>
> Source: Based on OECD (2018[52]), Policy Survey on the Future of Primary Care, Bonner (2016[125]) "As pay for performance grows, health plans work with pharmacies", https://doi.org/10.1016/j.ptdy.2016.02.024 and NHS (2019[61]), "The Community Pharmacy Contractual Framework for 2019/20 to 2023/24: supporting delivery for the NHS Long Term Plan", https://assets.publishing.service.gov.uk/government/uploads/system/uploads/attachment_data/file/819601/cpcf-2019-to-2024.pdf.

2.3.4. Availing primary and community care is essential to reduce inappropriate use of costly hospital inputs

To reduce instances where costly hospital inputs are used instead of less expensive options, it is important to avail less costly options at primary health care and community level. Intermediate care facilities and home-based programmes have opportunities to offer effective treatment at the primary health care level. Making full use of primary and community care helps to replace a substantial share of the workload in emergency departments and to prevent hospitalisations for chronic conditions. Such policies ensure that patients with minor and non-acute conditions are treated in the appropriate place at the appropriate time. This can increase allocative and technical efficiency due to the lower cost of primary health care alternatives compared with hospital care.

Developing intermediate care facilities

Intermediate care facilities (also called primary health care centres, community hospitals or local hospitals) provide non-urgent care and a mix of post-acute, rehabilitation and nursing care 24 hours a day, seven days a week. Intermediate care facilities are therefore available at times that suit the population and for emergencies outside of normal working hours. Intermediate care facilities can also deliver short-term care for patients who no longer require acute hospital care, but require a level of support that they could not obtain if they were discharged directly home. The overarching objective of intermediate care facilities is to strengthen the role of the primary and community care systems, to improve experiences for patients, while moving care out of the hospital sector to reduce health care costs.

There is already a large body of evidence confirming that using intermediate care following a hospital admission may reduce the need for further hospital admissions, and reduces the number of emergency department visits. In Norway, for example, studies have shown that intermediate facilities significantly reduce the number of hospital readmissions for the same disease, increase the quality of life for patients, and did not result in an increased risk of mortality (Dahl, Steinsbekk and Johnsen, 2015[126]; Garåsen, Windspoll and Johnsen, 2007[127]). In the Netherlands, van der Brug (2017[128]) found that the use intermediate care facilities was associated with reduced hospital readmission rates (van der Brug, 2017[128]). More recently, intermediate care facilities have been established in three countries: Costa Rica (interdisciplinary outpatient units for people with mental health issues and health hostels for patients with chronic conditions), Ireland (Community Intervention Teams) and Mexico (CESSAS).

In France, the National Plan "*Ma Santé 2022*" envisages the establishment of more than 500 local hospitals to act as intermediate care facilities. Local hospitals will provide primary health care services, rehabilitation, nursing care for the population and will ensure access to technical imaging and medical biology. Local hospitals will help care for frail elderly people in their own homes by providing higher levels of support than GP practices, and by offering prevention activities. The objective is to bridge primary health care services with secondary care services in order to ensure more consistent patient pathways.

Providing post-discharge care at home

Early discharge home-based programmes allow patients to return home when they might previously have stayed longer in the hospital or been referred to a nursing home. This goes in line with the preference of patients for treatment at home. For policy makers, the objective is to curb hospital costs and to mitigate delays that are driven by insufficient availability of community care, while improving patient experience and health outcomes. Home-based early discharge programmes generally consist of providing post-discharge care at home, telephone support, counselling and education to improve self-management, care co-ordination with other community support, including social support and remote monitoring of vital signs (Zhu et al., 2015[129]).

A handful of studies provide evidence that patients receiving home interventions experience reduced length of hospital stays and lower risk of readmission (Zhu et al., 2015[129]). More recently, Hernandez el al (2018[130]) have shown that providing home hospitalisation and post-discharge care at home, results in good clinical outcomes and reduced length of stay in hospital (Hernández et al., 2018[130]). The benefit of early discharge home-based programmes is mostly evidenced among patients aged 60 years old and over, and those having chronic diseases, both groups of which are high users of emergency departments.

Some health care systems are increasingly providing post-discharge care at home as an alternative to hospital-based care. In Canada and the United Kingdom, virtual wards have been developed to reduce hospital readmissions, by providing short-term transitional care to high-risk patients with complex needs who have recently been discharged from hospital. Patients are referred to a virtual ward based on the use of an algorithm that predicts the risk of readmission, and they are provided with home-based care by a primary health care team. In the New Brunswick Region, a new extra-mural programme has been recently introduced to help patients and their families. The team provides home health care services, ranging from health education to more complex medical needs such as rehabilitative care, medication management, dementia, and end of life care. In Nova Scotia, the INSPIRED programme (Implementing a Novel and Supportive Program of Individualised care for patients and families living with a Respiratory Disease) aimed at decreasing inpatient hospitalisations due to ambulatory care sensitive conditions through supported self-management of COPD, reduced emergency department visits and improved patient outcomes. The programme allowed more patients to be treated in their homes and prevented (or better managed) the disease exacerbations that are common with advanced COPD. In Germany, since 2017, mental health care following discharge from psychiatric hospitals can be delivered within the patient's home. In such cases, the responsibility for the treatment process remains with the hospital, but the primary health care team will have a key role in delivering care co-ordination, counselling and education.

Digital technologies, including Internet-enabled home monitors, apps for mobile health, and digital consultations, are key levers for bringing care into patient's homes (see Section 2.3.2). Digital technologies will play a central role in expanding opportunities for accessing routine monitoring and counselling by primary health care teams, and for patients to receive support to manage health conditions at home. Of course, this will only be relevant for non-intensive medical conditions with no requirement for around the clock attention or human monitoring.

2.4. Conclusions

A high performing primary health care service offers opportunities to make health care systems more efficient. The literature suggests that when patients can be treated in a strong primary health care sector, fewer expensive services need to be provided at secondary levels of care, which can contain growth in health care costs. However, international figures demonstrate that there are several shortcomings across OECD countries. High rates of avoidable hospitalisations for chronic conditions and inappropriate prescribing in general practice are important sources of unnecessary use of more expensive resources for OECD health care systems. These shortcomings suggest that there is scope to improve both technical and allocative efficiency in primary health care.

Country experiences demonstrate that a number of policy solutions have great potential to improve efficiency in primary health care. These include: changes in training and improved matching of skills to meet patients' needs more effectively and at lower costs; a greater use of digital technology, notably of EHR to improve workflow, communication and clinical practices; and availing primary and community care options to make sure patients with minor and non-acute conditions are treated in the appropriate place at the appropriate time. To support these changes, the use of payments linked to outcomes or desired activities, such as those encouraging the management of chronic diseases, care co-ordination or discharge from hospitals, will help to improve technical and allocative efficiency.

References

Adam, E. et al. (2017), *Advancing the role of nurses and midwives in ireland: Pioneering transformation of the health workforce for non-communicable diseases in Europe*, http://www.euro.who.int/en/health-topics/Health-systems/health-systems-response-to-ncds/publications/2017/advancing-the-role-of-nurses-and-midwives-in-ireland-pioneering-transformation-of-the-health-workforce-for-noncommunicable-diseases-in-europe-2017. [57]

Agency for Healthcare Research and Quality (2018), *Potentially Avoidable Hospitalizations.*, http://www.ahrq.gov/research/findings/nhqrdr/chartbooks/carecoordination/measure3.html (accessed on 9 April 2019). [10]

AIHW (2019), *Potentially preventable hospitalisations in Australia by small geographic areas*, Web Report, Cat. no. HPF 36. Canberra: AIHW., https://www.aihw.gov.au/reports/primary-health-care/potentially-preventable-hospitalisations/contents/overview (accessed on 5 September 2019). [29]

Aihw (2018), *Emergency department care 2017-18 Australian hospital statistics*, http://www.aihw.gov.au. [31]

Auraaen, A., L. Slawomirski and N. Klazinga (2018), "The economics of patient safety in primary and ambulatory care: Flying blind", *OECD Health Working Papers*, No. 106, OECD Publishing, Paris, https://dx.doi.org/10.1787/baf425ad-en. [28]

Bender, J. et al. (2011), "Can pain be managed through the Internet? A systematic review of randomized controlled trials", *Pain*, http://dx.doi.org/10.1016/j.pain.2011.02.012. [95]

Berchet, C. (2015), "Emergency Care Services: Trends, Drivers and Interventions to Manage the Demand", *OECD Health Working Papers*, No. 83, OECD Publishing, Paris, https://dx.doi.org/10.1787/5jrts344crns-en. [9]

Bonner, L. (2016), "As pay for performance grows, health plans work with pharmacies", *Pharmacy Today*, http://dx.doi.org/10.1016/j.ptdy.2016.02.024. [125]

Brennan, J., A. McElligott and N. Power (2015), "National Health Models and the Adoption of E-Health and E-Prescribing in Primary Care – New Evidence from Europe", *Journal of Innovation in Health Informatics*, Vol. 22/4, pp. 399-408, http://dx.doi.org/10.14236/jhi.v22i4.97. [108]

Brian G. Arndt, M. et al. (2017), "Tethered to the EHR: Primary Care Physician Work- load Assessment Using EHR Event Log Data and Time- Motion Observations", *Annals of Family Medicine*, http://dx.doi.org/10.1370/afm.2121. [46]

Buerhaus Peter (2018), *Nurse Practitioners: Nurse Practitioners: A solution to America's primary care crisis*, American Enterprise Institute. [68]

Burki, T. (2019), "GP at hand: a digital revolution for health care provision?", *The Lancet*, Vol. 394, https://doi.org/10.1016/S0140-6736(19)31802-1. [80]

Campanella, P. et al. (2016), "The impact of electronic health records on healthcare quality: a systematic review and meta-analysis", *The European Journal of Public Health*, Vol. 26/1, pp. 60-64, http://dx.doi.org/10.1093/eurpub/ckv122. [100]

Cordina, J., M. Qian and L. Sanfilippo (2019), *Healthcare consumerism today: Accelerating the consumer experience*, Consumer Health Insights Survey 2018. McKinsey & Company, https://www.mckinsey.com/industries/healthcare-systems-and-services/our-insights/healthcare-consumerism-today-accelerating-the-consumer-experience?utm_content=buffere2156&utm_medium=social&utm_source=twitter.com&utm_campaign=buffer (accessed on 3 July 2019). [75]

Cravo Oliveira Hashiguchi, T. (2020), "Bringing health care to the patient: An overview of the use of telemedicine in OECD countries", No. 116, OECD, Paris, https://dx.doi.org/10.1787/8e56ede7-en. [81]

Cylus, J., I. Papanicolas and P. Smith (2016), *Health System Efficiency. How to make measurement matter for policy and management*, WHO Regional Office for Europe, Copenhagen, Denmark. [23]

Dahl, U., A. Steinsbekk and R. Johnsen (2015), "Effectiveness of an intermediate care hospital on readmissions, mortality, activities of daily living and use of health care services among hospitalized adults aged 60 years and older - A controlled observational study", *BMC Health Services Research*, http://dx.doi.org/10.1186/s12913-015-1022-x. [126]

De Maeseneer, J. and P. Boeckxstaens (2012), *Debate & analysis James Mackenzie lecture 2011: Multimorbidity, goal-oriented care, and equity*, http://dx.doi.org/10.3399/bjgp12X652553. [124]

de Manuel Keenoy, E. (2018), *Good Practice on digitally-enabled, integrated, personcentred care in the Basque Country*, https://ec.europa.eu/health/sites/health/files/non_communicable_diseases/docs/ev_20181212_co01_en.pdf (accessed on 24 July 2019). [105]

Deetjen, U. (2016), "European E-Prescriptions: Benefits and Success Factors", *Cyber Studies Programme*, No. 5, Oxford Internet Institute, University of Oxford, http://www.politics.ox.ac.uk/centre/cyber-studies-programme.html (accessed on 18 July 2019). [111]

Del Fiol, G., T. Workman and P. Gorman (2014), *Clinical questions raised by clinicians at the point of care a systematic review*, http://dx.doi.org/10.1001/jamainternmed.2014.368. [48]

Delnoij, D. et al. (2000), "Does general practitioner gatekeeping curb health care expenditure?", *Journal of Health Services Research and Policy*, http://dx.doi.org/10.1177/135581960000500107. [1]

Dobrev, A. et al. (2009), *The socio-economic impact of interoperable electronic health record (EHR) and ePrescribing systems in Europe and beyond*, European Commission, DG INFSO & Media, http://www.ehr-impact.eu (accessed on 18 July 2019). [115]

Dusheiko, M. et al. (2011), "Does better disease management in primary care reduce hospital costs? Evidence from English primary care", *Journal of Health Economics*, http://dx.doi.org/10.1016/j.jhealeco.2011.08.001. [120]

East Melbourne, V. (ed.) (2018), *General Practice: Health of the Nation 2018*, http://www.racgp.org.au. [36]

Eesti Haigekassa (2019), *An increasing number of family physicians use e-consultation*, https://www.haigekassa.ee/en/uudised/increasing-number-family-physicians-use-e-consultation (accessed on 24 July 2019). [79]

Elliott, R. et al. (2016), "Supporting adherence for people starting a new medication for a long-term condition through community pharmacies: A pragmatic randomised controlled trial of the New Medicine Service", *BMJ Quality and Safety*, http://dx.doi.org/10.1136/bmjqs-2015-004400. [62]

European Commission (2008), *E-Prescriptions: Apoteket and Stockholm County Council, Sweden-eRecept, an E-Prescribing Application*, http://ehealth-impact.eu/fileadmin/ehealth_impact/documents/ehealth-impact-7-2.pdf (accessed on 17 July 2019). [114]

Fisher, R. et al. (2017), *GP views on strategies to cope with increasing workload: A qualitative interview study*, http://dx.doi.org/10.3399/bjgp17X688861. [39]

Fleetcroft, R. et al. (2018), "Does practice analysis agree with the ambulatory care sensitive conditions' list of avoidable unplanned admissions?: A cross-sectional study in the East of England", *BMJ Open*, http://dx.doi.org/10.1136/bmjopen-2017-020756. [30]

Flodgren, G. et al. (2015), "Interactive telemedicine: effects on professional practice and health care outcomes", *Cochrane Database of Systematic Reviews* 9, http://dx.doi.org/10.1002/14651858.CD002098.pub2. [76]

Frenk, J. et al. (2010), *Health professionals for a new century: Ttransforming education to strengthen health systems in an interdependent world*, http://dx.doi.org/10.1016/S0140-6736(10)61854-5. [50]

Fuertes-Guiró, F. and M. Girabent-Farrés (2017), "Opportunity cost of the dermatologist's consulting time in the economic evaluation of teledermatology", *Journal of Telemedicine and Telecare*, Vol. 23/7, pp. 657-664, http://dx.doi.org/10.1177/1357633X16660876. [84]

Fusco, F., L. Trieste and G. Turchetti (2014), *Approaching 2014: Is Telemedicine Assessed from The Social Perspective*, IARIA, Barcelona, https://www.thinkmind.org/index.php?view=article&articleid=etelemed_2014_13_40_40158 (accessed on 7 July 2019). [85]

Galarraga, J. and J. Pines (2016), "Costs of ED episodes of care in the United States", *American Journal of Emergency Medicine*, http://dx.doi.org/10.1016/j.ajem.2015.06.001. [32]

Garåsen, H., R. Windspoll and R. Johnsen (2007), "Intermediate care at a community hospital as an alternative to prolonged general hospital care for elderly patients: A randomised controlled trial", *BMC Public Health*, http://dx.doi.org/10.1186/1471-2458-7-68. [127]

Gerdtham, U. et al. (2011), "The Determinants of Health Expenditure in the OECD Countries: A Pooled data Analysis", http://dx.doi.org/10.1007/978-1-4615-5681-7_6. [2]

Gibson, O., L. Segal and R. McDermott (2013), "A systematic review of evidence on the association between hospitalisation for chronic disease related ambulatory care sensitive conditions and primary health care resourcing", *BMC Health Services Research*, http://dx.doi.org/10.1186/1472-6963-13-336. [17]

Golnick, C. et al. (2012), *Innovative primary care delivery in rural Alaska: A review of patient encounters seen by community health aides*, http://dx.doi.org/10.3402/ijch.v71i0.18543. [65]

Grava-Gubins, I., A. Safarov and J. Eriksson (2012), *2010 National Physician Survey : Workload patterns of Canadian Family Physicians*. [37]

Green, L., S. Savin and Y. Lu (2013), "Primary care physician shortages could be eliminated through use of teams, nonphysicians, and electronic communication", *Health Affairs*, http://dx.doi.org/10.1377/hlthaff.2012.1086. [53]

Gurol-Urganci, I. et al. (2013), "Mobile phone messaging reminders for attendance at healthcare appointments", *Cochrane Database of Systematic Reviews* 12, http://dx.doi.org/10.1002/14651858.CD007458.pub3. [92]

Harrison, M. et al. (2014), "Effect of a national primary care pay for performance scheme on emergency hospital admissions for ambulatory care sensitive conditions: Controlled longitudinal study", *BMJ (Online)*, http://dx.doi.org/10.1136/bmj.g6423. [121]

Hartzler, A. et al. (2018), "Roles and functions of community health workers in primary care", *Annals of Family Medicine*, http://dx.doi.org/10.1370/afm.2208. [63]

Hazra, N., C. Rudisill and M. Gulliford (2019), "Developing the role of electronic health records in economic evaluation", *The European Journal of Health Economics*, pp. 1-5, http://dx.doi.org/10.1007/s10198-019-01042-5. [104]

Hernández, C. et al. (2018), "Implementation of Home Hospitalization and Early Discharge as an Integrated Care Service: A Ten Years Pragmatic Assessment", *International Journal of Integrated Care*, http://dx.doi.org/10.5334/ijic.3431. [130]

HIQA (2018), *ePrescribing: An International Review*, Health Information and Quality Authority, Ireland, https://www.hiqa.ie/sites/default/files/2018-05/ePrescribing-An-Intl-Review.pdf (accessed on 17 July 2019). [110]

Hobbs, F. et al. (2016), "Clinical workload in UK primary care: a retrospective analysis of 100 million consultations in England, 2007–14", *The Lancet*, http://dx.doi.org/10.1016/S0140-6736(16)00620-6. [34]

Holtrop, J. et al. (2008), *The Community Health Educator Referral Liaison (CHERL). A Primary Care Practice Role for Promoting Healthy Behaviors*, http://dx.doi.org/10.1016/j.amepre.2008.08.012. [66]

Hujala Anneli et al. (2016), *The POTKU project (Potilas kuljettajan paikalle, Putting the Patient in the Driver's Seat), Finland*, http://www.icare4eu.org/pdf/POTKU_Case_report.pdf (accessed on 20 May 2019). [101]

Huntley, A. et al. (2014), "Which features of primary care affect unscheduled secondary care use? A systematic review", *BMJ Open*, http://dx.doi.org/10.1136/bmjopen-2013-004746. [8]

Iacobucci, G. (2019), "GP at Hand: patients are less sick than others but use services more, evaluation finds", *BMJ (Clinical research ed.)*, http://dx.doi.org/10.1136/bmj.l2333. [82]

International Pharmaceutical Federation (2016), *Advanced roles of pharmacists: Written contribution to OECD workshop "Towards a more efficient use of human resources for health*, International Pharmaceutical Federation. [59]

IQVIA (2017), *The Growing Value of Digital Health. Evidence and Impact on Human Health and the Healthcare System*, IQVIA Institute for Human Data Science, https://www.iqvia.com/-/media/iqvia/pdfs/institute-reports/the-growing-value-of-digital-health.pdf?_=1562314612052 (accessed on 5 July 2019). [88]

Iribarren, S. et al. (2017), "What is the economic evidence for mHealth? A systematic review of economic evaluations of mHealth solutions.", *PloS one*, Vol. 12/2, p. e0170581, http://dx.doi.org/10.1371/journal.pone.0170581. [91]

Irving, G. et al. (2017), *International variations in primary care physician consultation time: A systematic review of 67 countries*, http://dx.doi.org/10.1136/bmjopen-2017-017902. [41]

Khan, R. and K. Socha-Dietrich (2018), "Investing in medication adherence improves health outcomes and health system efficiency: Adherence to medicines for diabetes, hypertension, and hyperlipidaemia", *OECD Health Working Papers*, No. 105, OECD Publishing, Paris, https://dx.doi.org/10.1787/8178962c-en. [107]

Kirkland, S., A. Soleimani and A. Newton (2018), "The impact of pediatric mental health care provided outpatient, primary care, community and school settings on emergency department use – a systematic review.", *Child Adolesc Ment Health* 23, pp. 4-13. [7]

Kitsiou, S. et al. (2017), "Effectiveness of mHealth interventions for patients with diabetes: An overview of systematic reviews", *PLOS ONE*, Vol. 12/3, p. e0173160, http://dx.doi.org/10.1371/journal.pone.0173160. [90]

Kringos, D. et al. (2013), "Europe's Strong Primary Care Systems Are Linked To Better Population Health But Also To Higher Health Spending.", *Health affairs (Project Hope)*, Vol. 32/4, pp. 686-94, http://dx.doi.org/10.1377/hlthaff.2012.1242. [131]

Liddy, C. et al. (2019), "A Systematic Review of Asynchronous, Provider-to-Provider, Electronic Consultation Services to Improve Access to Specialty Care Available Worldwide", *Telemedicine and e-Health*, Vol. 25/3, pp. 184-198, http://dx.doi.org/10.1089/tmj.2018.0005. [77]

Lin, I., S. Wu and S. Huang (2015), "Continuity of Care and Avoidable Hospitalizations for Chronic Obstructive Pulmonary Disease (COPD)", *The Journal of the American Board of Family Medicine*, Vol. 28/2, pp. 222-230, http://dx.doi.org/10.3122/jabfm.2015.02.140141. [19]

Lupiañez-Villanueva, F., A. Sachinopoulou and A. Theben (2015), *Oulu Self-Care (Finland) Case Study Report*, European Commission Joint Research Centre, Luxembourg, http://dx.doi.org/10.2791/692203. [96]

Maier, C. and L. Aiken (2016), *Expanding clinical roles for nurses to realign the global health workforce with population needs: A commentary*, http://dx.doi.org/10.1186/s13584-016-0079-2. [69]

Malcarney, M. et al. (2017), "The Changing Roles of Community Health Workers", *Health Services Research*, http://dx.doi.org/10.1111/1475-6773.12657. [64]

Martin-Misener, R. and D. Bryant-Lukosius (2014), *Optimizing the Role of Nurses in Primary Care in Canada*, Canadian Nurses Association. [56]

Matthys, E., R. Remmen and P. Van Bogaert (2017), "An overview of systematic reviews on the collaboration between physicians and nurses and the impact on patient outcomes: What can we learn in primary care?", *BMC Family Practice*, http://dx.doi.org/10.1186/s12875-017-0698-x. [55]

McHale, P. et al. (2013), "Who uses emergency departments inappropriately and when - a national cross-sectional study using a monitoring data system", *BMC Medicine*, Vol. 11/1, http://dx.doi.org/10.1186/1741-7015-11-258. [22]

Medical Association, C. (2017), *CMA Workforce Survey 2017*, http://www.cma.ca/pdc. [38]

Merilind, E. et al. (2016), "Pay for performance of Estonian family doctors and impact of different practice- and patient-related characteristics on a good outcome: A quantitative assessment", *Medicina (Lithuania)*, http://dx.doi.org/10.1016/j.medici.2016.04.003. [123]

Ministry of Health, N. (2019), *New Zealand ePrescription Service*, https://www.health.govt.nz/our-work/ehealth/other-ehealth-initiatives/emedicines/new-zealand-eprescription-service (accessed on 17 July 2019). [109]

Mold, F. et al. (2015), "Patients' online access to their electronic health records and linked online services: a systematic review in primary care.", *The British journal of general practice : the journal of the Royal College of General Practitioners*, Vol. 65/632, pp. e141-51, http://dx.doi.org/10.3399/bjgp15X683941. [102]

Mossialos, E. et al. (2015), "From "retailers" to health care providers: Transforming the role of community pharmacists in chronic disease management", *Health Policy*, http://dx.doi.org/10.1016/j.healthpol.2015.02.007. [60]

Mousquès, J. and Y. Bourgueil (2014), *L'évaluation de la performance des maisons, pôles et centres de santé dans le cadre des Expérimentations des nouveaux modes de rémunération*, Les Rapports de l'IRDES n°559, Paris. [118]

NHS (2019), *Investment and evolution: A five-year framework for GP contract reform to implement The NHS Long Term Plan*, NHS England. [67]

NHS (2019), *The Community Pharmacy Contractual Framework for 2019/20 to 2023/24: supporting delivery for the NHS Long Term Plan*, Depatment of Health and social care, NHS and PSNC, https://assets.publishing.service.gov.uk/government/uploads/system/uploads/attachment_data/file/819601/cpcf-2019-to-2024.pdf. [61]

Nuffieldtrust (2019), *Potentially preventable emergency hospital admissions*, https://www.nuffieldtrust.org.uk/resource/potentially-preventable-emergency-hospital-admissions (accessed on 9 April 2019). [12]

Oderkirk, J. (2017), "Readiness of electronic health record systems to contribute to national health information and research", *OECD Health Working Papers*, No. 99, OECD Publishing, Paris, https://dx.doi.org/10.1787/9e296bf3-en. [98]

OECD (2019), *Addressing Problematic Opioid Use in OECD Countries*, OECD Health Policy Studies, OECD Publishing, Paris, https://dx.doi.org/10.1787/a18286f0-en. [26]

OECD (2019), *Health at a Glance 2019: OECD Indicators*, OECD Publishing, Paris, https://doi.org/10.1787/4dd50c09-en. [24]

OECD (2019), *OECD Health Statistics*, OECD Publishing, Paris, https://doi.org/10.1787/health-data-en. [33]

OECD (2018), *Policy Survey on the Future of Primary Care*. [52]

OECD (2017), *Health at a Glance 2017: OECD Indicators*, OECD Publishing, Paris, https://dx.doi.org/10.1787/health_glance-2017-en. [43]

OECD (2017), *New Health Technologies: Managing Access, Value and Sustainability*, OECD Publishing, Paris, https://dx.doi.org/10.1787/9789264266438-en. [93]

OECD (2017), *OECD Digital Economy Outlook 2017*, OECD Publishing, Paris, https://doi.org/10.1787/9789264276284-en (accessed on 3 July 2019). [74]

OECD (2017), *Tackling Wasteful Spending on Health*, OECD Publishing, Paris, https://dx.doi.org/10.1787/9789264266414-en. [25]

OECD (2016), *Better Ways to Pay for Health Care*, OECD Health Policy Studies, OECD Publishing, Paris, https://dx.doi.org/10.1787/9789264258211-en. [117]

OECD (2016), *Health System Characteristics Survey*, http://www.oecd.org/els/health-systems/characteristics.htm. [54]

OECD (2016), *Health Workforce Policies in OECD Countries: Right Jobs, Right Skills, Right Places*, OECD Health Policy Studies, OECD Publishing, Paris, https://dx.doi.org/10.1787/9789264239517-en. [42]

OECD (2016), *OECD Reviews of Health Systems: Latvia 2016*, OECD Reviews of Health Systems, OECD Publishing, Paris, https://dx.doi.org/10.1787/9789264262782-en. [58]

OECD (2013), *Strengthening Health Information Infrastructure for Health Care Quality Governance: Good Practices, New Opportunities and Data Privacy Protection Challenges*, OECD Health Policy Studies, OECD Publishing, Paris, https://dx.doi.org/10.1787/9789264193505-en. [99]

OECD/IDB (2016), *Broadband Policies for Latin America and the Caribbean: A Digital Economy Toolkit*, OECD Publishing, Paris, https://dx.doi.org/10.1787/9789264251823-en. [72]

Oliveira, T. et al. (2013), "Teleconsultations reduce greenhouse gas emissions", *Journal of Health Services Research & Policy*, Vol. 18/4, pp. 209-214, http://dx.doi.org/10.1177/1355819613492717. [87]

Osborn, R. et al. (2015), "Primary care physicians in ten countries report challenges caring for patients with complex health needs", *Health Affairs*, http://dx.doi.org/10.1377/hlthaff.2015.1018. [40]

OTN (2018), *OTN Annual Report 2017/2018*, Ontario Telemedicine Network, https://otn.ca/wp-content/uploads/2017/11/otn-annual-report.pdf (accessed on 3 July 2019). [86]

OTN (2016), *Telehomecare Deployment Project: Phase 2-Remote Patient Monitoring RPM-05B-Benefits Evaluation Report*, Ontario Telemedicine Network. [78]

Parv, L. et al. (2014), "An evaluation of e-prescribing at a national level", *Inform Health Soc Care*, pp. 1-18, http://dx.doi.org/10.3109/17538157.2014.948170. [113]

Porterfield, A., K. Engelbert and A. Coustasse (2014), "Electronic prescribing: improving the efficiency and accuracy of prescribing in the ambulatory care setting.", *Perspectives in health information management*, Vol. 11/Spring, p. 1g, http://www.ncbi.nlm.nih.gov/pubmed/24808808 (accessed on 18 July 2019). [112]

Purdy, S. (2010), *Avoiding hospital admissions*, The King's Fund, London, https://www.kingsfund.org.uk/publications/avoiding-hospital-admissions. [11]

Quigley, A., N. Hex and C. Aznar (2019), *Evaluation of Babylon GP at hand : Final evaluation report*, Ipsos MORI/York Health Economics Consortium, London, https://www.hammersmithfulhamccg.nhs.uk/media/156123/Evaluation-of-Babylon-GP-at-Hand-Final-Report.pdf. [83]

Ranjan, P., A. Kumari and A. Chakrawarty (2015), "How can doctors improve their communication skills?", *Journal of Clinical and Diagnostic Research*, http://dx.doi.org/10.7860/JCDR/2015/12072.5712. [49]

Roland, M. and B. Guthrie (2016), "Quality and Outcomes Framework: What have we learnt?", *BMJ (Online)*, http://dx.doi.org/10.1136/bmj.i4060. [119]

Rosano, A. et al. (2013), "The relationship between avoidable hospitalization and accessibility to primary care: A systematic review", *European Journal of Public Health*, Vol. 23/3, pp. 356-360, http://dx.doi.org/10.1093/eurpub/cks053. [5]

Rose, A. et al. (2018), "Potentially Inappropriate Opioid Prescribing, Overdose, and Mortality in Massachusetts, 2011–2015", *Journal of General Internal Medicine*, http://dx.doi.org/10.1007/s11606-018-4532-5. [27]

Ryan, A. et al. (2016), "Long-term evidence for the effect of pay-for-performance in primary care on mortality in the UK: a population study", *The Lancet*, http://dx.doi.org/10.1016/S0140-6736(16)00276-2. [122]

Santos, N. et al. (2019), "Interventions to reduce the prescription of inappropriate medicines in older patients", *Revista de Saúde Pública*, Vol. 53, p. 7, http://dx.doi.org/10.11606/S1518-8787.2019053000781. [97]

Schäfer, W. et al. (2016), "Two decades of change in European general practice service profiles: Conditions associated with the developments in 28 countries between 1993 and 2012", *Scandinavian Journal of Primary Health Care*, Vol. 34/1, pp. 97-110, http://dx.doi.org/10.3109/02813432.2015.1132887. [51]

Scirocco (2017), *Basque Country: Care plan for elderly. Overview of SCIROCCO Good Practices*, Scirocco. [106]

Shi, L. (2012), "The Impact of Primary Care: A Focused Review", *Scientifica*, Vol. 2012, pp. 1-22, http://dx.doi.org/10.6064/2012/432892. [14]

Shipman, S. and C. Sinsky (2013), "Expanding primary care capacity by reducing waste and improving the efficiency of care", *Health Affairs*, http://dx.doi.org/10.1377/hlthaff.2013.0539. [44]

Sinsky, C. et al. (2016), "Allocation of physician time in ambulatory practice: A time and motion study in 4 specialties", *Annals of Internal Medicine*, http://dx.doi.org/10.7326/M16-0961. [45]

Starfield, B., L. Shi and J. Macinko (2005), "Contribution of Primary Care to Health Systems and Health", *The Milbank Quarterly*, Vol. 83/3, pp. 457–502. [13]

Sung, N., Y. Choi and J. Lee (2018), "Primary care comprehensiveness can reduce emergency department visits and hospitalization in people with hypertension in South Korea", *International Journal of Environmental Research and Public Health*, Vol. 15/2, http://dx.doi.org/10.3390/ijerph15020272. [20]

Suzuki, E. (2018), *Delayed Discharge From Hospital. Fast track paper for the 23rd Session of the Health Committee, to be held on Wednesday 27 and Thursday 28 June 2018*. [116]

The Economist (2019), *The front line of England's NHS is being reinvented: A shortage of family doctors leaves little choice but to try something new*, https://www.economist.com/britain/2019/06/27/the-front-line-of-englands-nhs-is-being-reinvented. [47]

Thompson, M. and F. Walter (2016), "Increases in general practice workload in England", *The Lancet*, http://dx.doi.org/10.1016/s0140-6736(16)00743-1. [35]

Valverde-Albacete, J. et al. (2019), *Benchmarking deployment of eHealth among general practitioners (2018)*, European Commission, http://dx.doi.org/10.2759/511610. [73]

Van den Berg, M., T. Van Loenen and G. Westert (2016), "Accessible and continuous primary care may help reduce rates of emergency department use. An international survey in 34 countries", *Family Practice*, Vol. 33/1, pp. 42-50, http://dx.doi.org/10.1093/fampra/cmv082. [21]

Van den Berg, M., T. Van Loenen and G. Westert (2016), "Accessible and continuous primary care may help reduce rates of emergency department use. An international survey in 34 countries", *Family Practice*, Vol. 33/1, pp. 42-50, http://dx.doi.org/10.1093/fampra/cmv082. [6]

van der Brug, F. (2017), "Readmission rates: what can we learn from the Netherlands?", *Nuffieldtrust*, https://www.nuffieldtrust.org.uk/news-item/readmission-rates-what-can-we-learn-from-the-netherlands. [128]

Van Loenen, T. et al. (2016), "The impact of primary care organization on avoidable hospital admissions for diabetes in 23 countries", *Scandinavian Journal of Primary Health Care*, http://dx.doi.org/10.3109/02813432.2015.1132883. [16]

van Loenen, T. et al. (2014), "Organizational aspects of primary care related to avoidable hospitalization: A systematic review", *Family Practice*, http://dx.doi.org/10.1093/fampra/cmu053. [15]

Wang, S. et al. (2003), "A cost-benefit analysis of electronic medical records in primary care", *The American Journal of Medicine*, Vol. 114/5, pp. 397-403, http://dx.doi.org/10.1016/S0002-9343(03)00057-3. [103]

Whitehead, L. and P. Seaton (2016), *The effectiveness of self-management mobile phone and tablet apps in long-term condition management: A systematic review*, http://dx.doi.org/10.2196/jmir.4883. [94]

WHO (2019), *WHO guideline: recommendations on digital interventions for health system strengthening*, https://apps.who.int/iris/bitstream/handle/10665/311941/9789241550505-eng.pdf?ua=1 (accessed on 3 June 2019). [71]

WHO (2016), *Atlas of eHealth Country Profiles: The Use of eHealth in Support of Universal Health Coverage: Based on the Findings of the Third Global Survey on eHealth 2015*, World Health Organisation, Geneva, http://www.who.int/ (accessed on 5 July 2019). [89]

WHO (2016), *Global diffusion of eHealth: Making universal health coverage achievable. Report of the third global survey on eHealth*, World Health Organisation, Geneva. [70]

Wolters, R., J. Braspenning and M. Wensing (2017), *Impact of primary care on hospital admission rates for diabetes patients: A systematic review*, http://dx.doi.org/10.1016/j.diabres.2017.05.001. [18]

Wolters, R., J. Braspenning and M. Wensing (2017), *Impact of primary care on hospital admission rates for diabetes patients: A systematic review*, Elsevier Ireland Ltd, http://dx.doi.org/10.1016/j.diabres.2017.05.001. [4]

World Health Organization (2018), *Building the economic case for primary health care: a scoping review*, WHO, Geneva. [3]

Zhu, Q. et al. (2015), "Effectiveness of nurse-led early discharge planning programmes for hospital inpatients with chronic disease or rehabilitation needs: A systematic review and meta-analysis", *Journal of Clinical Nursing*, http://dx.doi.org/10.1111/jocn.12895. [129]

Notes

[1] The Australian Institute of Health and Welfare estimates that 8.8% of emergency department presentations in 2017-18 were assigned to the non-urgent triage category (Aihw, 2018[31]).

[2] Data are taken from the UEMO questionnaire.

[3] In England, only certain nurses are able to prescribe – nurse independent prescribers.

[4] Polypharmacy is defined as the administration of many drugs at the same time (more than five medications concurrently).

3 More effective and patient-centred care

This chapter turns to the question of whether primary health care is delivering effective and responsive care. The chapter shows that as the first point of contact with the health care system, primary health care teams are in a unique position to advise patients on health behaviour, to administer preventive care, and to control the progress of chronic conditions. This is ever more needed as citizen expectations about services are high, societies are ageing and complex cases are costly. The chapter then shows that strong evidence suggests preventive care is inefficient across OECD countries and there are break-downs in communication between primary health care and other sectors of the health care system. The chapter concludes by describing the policy levers needed to encourage both the effectiveness and responsiveness of primary health care. These range from new models of organising services based on a team or network of providers, changes to the incentives that determine clinical practice, better measurements of quality and outcomes of primary health care, to implementing health coaching and counselling.

Key Findings

- Primary health care has great potential to improve population health and responsiveness of care. As shown earlier, the main functions of primary health care – to be the first point of contact, person and community focused, comprehensive, and co-ordinated – make it ideally placed to seek out patients for preventive treatment before they get sick and to better manage chronic conditions over time.
- Recent data show that currently preventive care is not delivered effectively and too many people experience problems of care co-ordination between primary health care, specialists and hospitals:
    - in 2014, one in four patients suffering from certain chronic conditions did not receive any of the recommended preventive tests in the previous 12 months
    - the involvement of general practice in preventive activities has decreased by 13% over the past two decades, while participation in treatment has increased
    - in 11 OECD countries surveyed in 2016, between 29% and 51% of people reported having experienced problems of care co-ordination in the health service.
- Developing new models of primary health care delivery based on teams and networks, backed by portable electronic health records (EHR) and embracing new ways of communicating, can reap the greatest gains for population health outcomes. Multi-disciplinary team practices, providing comprehensive health services and steering population health management, enable preventive work to be more proactive. Such models allow for a co-ordinated approach spanning primary health care, community services, hospital care and social care. Australia, Canada and the United States are at the leading edge of these practices.
- Implementing team-based delivery of primary health care is not a simple undertaking given the traditional divisions of professional silos, and the fact that across many OECD countries, primary health care practices are owned by physicians themselves and operate as small enterprises. Physicians who want to create or migrate into group practices may need effective support, including assistance with the preparation of business plans and access to loans, the selection and training of support staff, drafting of employment contracts, and the implementation of technological solutions. In Austria, the strong focus on practical implementation is the guiding element in the current reform process that aims to establish primary health care units.
- Introducing new forms of remuneration in combination with the existing more traditional payment mechanisms can provide incentives for providers to increase care co-ordination and disease prevention activities. Bundled payments for chronic conditions (as seen in Australia, Canada and the Netherlands), and population-based financing with a shared saving approach (as seen in Germany and the United States) are promising initiatives.
- Collecting patient-reported indicators in primary health care can help evaluate improvements in the quality and responsiveness of that care, as seen with the United States' Consumer Assessment of Health Care Providers and Systems surveys and England's GP Patient survey, which are both used for regulating, monitoring and improving primary health care.
- Enabling patients and primary health care staff to co-design primary health care services through, for example, in-depth interviewing, focus groups or group discussions involving both patients and staff, is an effective option to improve quality and responsiveness, as seen in Australia in the case of mental health services.
- Individual or group-based counselling in primary health care has the potential to support patient self-management of chronic conditions and to manage the wider social and lifestyle aspects of

their health in the long term. Experience of counselling in Dutch primary health care has been effective in achieving and maintaining healthier lifestyle behaviours.
- Online self-management services – for example, patient-provider portals, smartphone applications or Internet-based monitoring – have been found to increase patient-provider communication, improve adherence to treatment regimens and lifestyle changes, and improve self-monitoring practices. Finland's e-service platform can guide other OECD countries as it successfully integrates health information into a common hub of personal health service information, results and advice.
- Health care vouchers, personal health budgets and conditional cash transfers could also be applied to increase patient choice over their health and health care and to change patient's behaviour. In the United States, conditional cash transfers led to positive improvement in the health of poorer families, notably through greater use of preventive health services.

3.1. Good quality primary health care improves health system responsiveness, makes health care more patient-centred and can improve health outcomes for the population

From a population health perspective there is a convincing body of evidence supporting the advantages of a well-developed primary health care system. Strong primary health care systems (see Chapter 1 for a full definition) have been associated with better health outcomes. The underlying hypothesis is that the main functions of primary health care – first point of contact with the health service, to be patient and community focused, offer a comprehensive and co-ordinated service – make the primary health care system better placed to provide preventive activities (both primary and secondary prevention) and to better manage chronic conditions over time (tertiary prevention). Primary health care is in a unique position to understand a patient's medical history and current needs in order to identify patients who are at risk of disease and to seek out patients for preventive treatment before they get sick.

3.1.1. Primary health care improves population health outcomes, health system responsiveness and patient centredness

At an international level, Macinko, Starfield, and Shi (2003) first explored the positive contribution of primary health care on health in 18 OECD countries. The findings from the quantitative analysis show that the stronger a country's primary health care orientation, the higher the population health outcomes. A positive relationship was confirmed for several health outcomes (including all-cause mortality rates, premature mortality, and cause-specific premature mortality from asthma and bronchitis, emphysema and pneumonia, cardiovascular disease, and heart disease) (Macinko, Starfield and Shi, 2003[1]). This held true even after controlling for various system and population characteristics (such as GDP per capita, total physicians per 1 000 population, percentage of elderly people, average number of ambulatory care visits, per capita income, and lifestyle factors). Macinko, Starfield and Erinosho (2009), in their review of 36 studies looking at the impact of primary health care on health outcomes, confirmed this positive relationship in the case of low- and middle-income countries. Greater availability and improved access to primary health care, was particularly associated with reduced infant and child mortality (MacInko, Starfield and Erinosho, 2009[2]).

In line with these findings, Kringos et. al. (2013) have shown more recently that the structure, co-ordination and comprehensiveness of primary health care were positively associated with the health of people with ischemic heart diseases, cerebrovascular diseases and other chronic conditions, including asthma, bronchitis and emphysema (Kringos et al., 2013[3]). In particular, a strong primary health care structure (as measured by the national governance, the economic conditions underpinning primary health care and workforce development) was associated with fewer potential deaths due to ischemic heart disease and cerebrovascular diseases, while better care co-ordination was associated with fewer potential deaths due to chronic asthma, bronchitis, and emphysema.

Several other studies have shown that countries with strong primary health care performed better on other major aspects of health, including patients with complex care needs. Hansen et al (2015) found that subjective assessments of patient health are better for people living in countries with a strong primary health care structure and good care co-ordination. In addition, good accessibility to primary health care helps reduce the risk of having untreated medical conditions (Hansen et al., 2015[4]). A positive relationship between strong primary health care and health outcomes was also confirmed among people with multiple morbidities. These people have a higher chance of having good or very good health if they live in a country with a strong primary health care structure, high continuity of care and a comprehensive primary health care system. Among all primary health care characteristics, comprehensiveness of care was the most influential: people with multiple morbidities were more likely to report having good health, less likely to have limitations in daily functioning and to have undergone long-term medical treatment, if they live in a country with a more comprehensive system of care. This result suggests that offering a broad set of services is especially beneficial for the needs of patients with complex health problems. Continuity of primary health care also appeared beneficial for the health of people with conditions particularly sensitive to management in primary health care. This latter result indicates the importance of the relationship between patients and primary health care teams, managing and communicating health information, and providing care management. The review by Sans-Corrales et al (2006) also supports this conclusion: continuity of care is consistently associated with better health outcomes, such as less back pain, fewer infarcts, liver pathologies, and stomach ulcers (Sans-Corrales et al., 2006[5]). There is also strong evidence that primary health care interventions have a positive impact on measures of mental health indicators, including depression and anxiety (Conejo-Cerón et al., 2017[6]; Trivedi, 2017[7]).

In addition to better population outcomes, there is evidence that strong primary health care also improves health system responsiveness and patient-centredness. A study that included 12 OECD countries and 5 other countries in Latin America and the Caribbean found that, on average, patients that had a regular place of care, where care providers were familiar with their medical history and it was easy to communicate, and help was given to co-ordinate care, were 12.1% less likely to say that their health system needs major changes, and 29.2% more likely to perceive their usual provider as providing high quality care[1] (Guanais et al., 2019[8]). Moreover, patients who had a physician that explained things in a way that was easy to understand and that spent enough time with them during consultations were 8.6% less likely to agree that their health system needs major changes and 69.6% more likely to perceive their usual provider as providing high quality care.

Very recently, Levine, Landon and Linder (2019) have quantified the potential benefit of primary health care with respect to receipt of high-value care and experience with care delivery in the United States. Compared to adults without primary health care, adults with primary health care were more likely to have routine preventive care and to receive high value-care, including high-value cancer screening, recommended diagnostic and preventive testing, and high-value counselling. In addition, adults with primary health care were also more likely to report better access to care and experience with care delivery (Levine, Landon and Linder, 2019[9]). It makes no doubt that primary health care can offer high value, responsive and patient-centred care.

3.1.2. Primary health care is best placed to seek out patients for preventive treatment before they get sick

The role of primary health care in playing an informative, supportive and facilitating function in the uptake of preventive activities is not to be underestimated. A handful of studies provide evidence that primary health care is best placed to carry out preventive interventions given that their focus is on the entire person and not limited to any specific disease or organ system. This conclusion has been especially confirmed for health counselling regarding smoking cessation, immunisations and screening (Shi and Starfield, 2005[10]; Saver, 2002[11]; Sans-Corrales et al., 2006[5]; Hartley, 2002[12]).

In the United States, several studies have suggested a positive relationship between the supply of primary health care physicians and the uptake of preventive care. Shi (2005) and Shi and Starfield (2005) have shown that those states with higher primary health care physician to population ratios, report significantly lower smoking and obesity rates than states with lower ratios of primary health care physicians to population (Shi, 2005[13]; Shi and Starfield, 2005[10]). This suggests that states with larger primary health care system structures have more effective approaches to disease prevention. This is also confirmed by Saver (2002) who showed a positive association between strong primary health care and smoking cessation and immunisation. In particular, care continuity with primary health care physicians was significantly associated with an increased likelihood of smoking cessation and of influenza immunisation. Hartley (2002) also found that care continuity is associated with more effective implementation of preventive activities. Strong primary health care was associated with having a better diet, smoking cessation, vaccination uptake and reduced alcohol consumption. Sans Corrales et al (2006), in their review of 20 studies, concluded that people receiving care from primary health care physicians are more likely to receive effective preventive services and more generic approaches to prevention, which can result in a reduction in morbidity and mortality. The review by Starfield, Shi, Macinko (2005) supports this conclusion: people receiving care from primary health care physicians are more likely to receive recommended preventive services, including pap smears and being up to date on screening and immunisations (Starfield, Shi and Macinko, 2005[14]). Strong primary health care might make the difference by informing the population about preventive care and facilitating access to these services.

The positive relationship between the supply of primary health care and preventive activities was also confirmed for early detection of breast cancer, colon cancer and melanoma (Campbell et al., 2003[15]; Ferrante, Gonzalez and Roetzheim, 2000[16]; Roetzhiem, RG; Pal, N; Gonzalez, EC; Ferrante, JM; Van Durme, 1999[17]). These findings suggest that primary health care physicians (or the broader primary health care team) can have an important impact on the stage at which a disease is diagnosed by performing clinical examinations and by recommending screening programmes to their patients. Although primary health care physicians do not perform screening in many European countries because of the introduction of population-based programmes, the role of the primary health care team can be significant in having a supportive, informative and facilitating role (Yano et al., 2007[18]; Triantafillidis et al., 2017[19]).

3.1.3. Greater investment in primary health care increases the uptake of prevention activities across OECD countries

As shown by previous research, being first point of contact, offering person and community focus with comprehensive and co-ordinated care, are important characteristics of primary health care systems which offer value to population health. Consistent with previous work (Sans-Corrales et al., 2006[5]; Starfield, Shi and Macinko, 2005[14]), new OECD analysis shows that investment in primary health care is associated with more effective implementation of preventive activities (see Box 3.1 for the data and methodology).

In this section, the average relationship between primary health care resources and primary health care performance is estimated. The hypothesis is that, on average, investment in the primary health care sector leads to greater primary health care performance through greater uptake of preventive interventions. Additional investment may, for example, enable more health professionals to be recruited which, in turn, may lead to better patient access. Additional investment may also improve the quality of care through, for example, new training opportunities in communication, prevention activities or through a greater use of new technologies and information infrastructure (Triantafillidis et al., 2017[19])

Analysis of data across OECD countries for the period 2005 to 2015 shows that a 1% increase in primary health care expenditure is associated with a 0.34% increase in cervical screening participation and a 0.52% increase in breast cancer screening participation (see Table 3.1).

These findings confirm results from previous studies. They suggest that investment in the primary health care sector leads to greater uptake of preventive interventions through, for example, increased recruitment, new training opportunities or greater use of new technologies. With such opportunities, the role of the primary health care team leads to greater uptake of preventive activities, which in turn is expected to improve population health outcomes.

Table 3.1. Impact of primary health care spending on cervical and breast cancer screening uptake in the OECD, 2005-15

	Cervical cancer screening	Breast cancer screening
Primary health care expenditure (USD PPP, per capita, log)	0.3373*** (0.0847)	0.5183*** (0.1176)

Note: *** signifies a p value <0.01. The analysis is based on multi-level modelling econometric techniques. Full models control for risk factors, demographic factors, hospital resources and time trends. Standard errors are in brackets. Full results are available upon request.
Source: OECD estimates based OECD Health Statistics 2005-15, https://doi.org/10.1787/health-data-en.

Box 3.1. Data and methodology used to estimate the relationship between primary health care resources and primary health care performance

Data

The analysis combines data from the following sources: (i) OECD Health Statistics and (ii) the Quality and Costs of Primary Care (QALICOPC) study.

OECD Health Statistics

OECD Health Statistics 2017 offers the most comprehensive source of comparable international statistics on health and health systems across OECD countries. It provides rich, national level data for a range of variables that were utilised in this analysis, including primary health care expenditure, primary health care quality outcomes, as well as a range of control variables, such as risk factors and demographic information (see table below).

The QUALICOPC study

The QUALICOPC study collected data on primary health care systems in 34 countries between October 2011 and December 2013. In Europe, 26 EU Member States were included in the project, as well as Iceland, Norway, Turkey, Switzerland and the Republic of North Macedonia. Research institutes from Australia, Canada and New Zealand participated in the collection of data in these countries. The study conducted surveys in each country among samples of general practitioners (GPs) and their patients. The data provide insights into the professional behaviour of GPs and their patients' expectations and experiences. The limitation of using the QUALICOPC data relates to the time difference compared with OECD Health Statistics.

Dependant and independent variables used

	Dependant variables	Key explanatory variables (OECD Health Statistics)	Time varying control variables	Non-time varying variables (health system characteristics[1])
Sources	OECD Health Statistics	OECD Health Statistics	OECD Health Statistics	QUALICOPC data
Name of variables	Breast cancer screening rate	Primary health care expenditure (per capita, USD PPP)	Number of generalist medical practitioners (per 1 000 population)	Health promotion scale
	Cervical cancer screening rate		Per capita GDP	Continuity of care scale
			Gini Coefficient	Collaboration of care scale
			Percentage of the population aged over 65 years	Responsiveness scale
			The number of hospital beds	
			Lifestyle variables (smoking rates, obesity rates and average alcohol consumption)	
			Year	

1. Four country-level characteristics (health promotion, continuity of care, collaboration of care and responsiveness) are used in the analysis to explain why the relationship between primary health care expenditures and screening varies across OECD countries. These characteristics are time invariant in the estimation, while they are not in reality. This is a recognised limitation of the work.

Method

The analysis is based on multi-level modelling econometric techniques. Such models are commonly used in quantitative analysis, particularly when the data involve units at different "levels" of observation. Multi-level modelling can be used when there are repeated observations over time for multiple countries. Analysis of this type of data can help disentangle "within effects" (variations over time) and "between effects" (variation between countries). This is the nature of the data used in the current analysis. The approach is based on previous work (Or, Wang and Jamison, 2005[20]; OECD, 2015[21]). The analysis utilises the longitudinal nature of the data, and in doing so, estimates the OECD average relationship between primary health care resources and performance, as well as individual country trends.

Presented here are only the results of the first stage analysis, which examines the relationship between health care resources and performance, after controlling for a range of health and non-health factors. The model can be characterised as follows:

$$y_{it} = \beta_{0i} + \beta_{1i} I_{it} + \alpha_p x_{pit} + e_{it}$$

$$\beta_{0i} = \tau_0 + \mu_{0i}$$

$$\beta_{1i} = \tau_1 + \mu_{1i}$$

where y_{it} represents cervical or breast cancer screening for country i at time period t. The variable I_{it} represents primary health care expenditure that varies by country and over time. The vector x is a set of p control variables that can vary over time. Both the intercept β_{0i} and the slope coefficients β_{1i} vary by country. e_{it} is the residual error term for the ith country in year t and is assumed to be normally distributed with a mean of zero. Results presented in Table 3.1 focus on the estimates of β_{1i}.

3.2. Disease prevention and care co-ordination are insufficient in a context of rising health care needs

Despite evidence demonstrating the contribution of primary health care to population health outcomes and health system responsiveness, the current organisation of primary health care is not achieving the expected results.

In recent decades, an epidemiological transition has taken place worldwide. In most countries, chronic conditions are now the leading cause of disability-adjusted life years lost and infectious diseases continue to pose a threat to populations across OECD countries. As the first point of contact with the health care system, and as a trusted source of information, primary health care teams are in a unique position to advise patients on lifestyles and health behaviour, to administer preventive care, and to manage and control the progress of chronic conditions. However, recent international data show that too many patients with chronic conditions do not receive the recommended preventive care and that there are significant problems with co-ordination of care between primary health care teams, specialists, and hospitals.

3.2.1. Chronic conditions are on the rise and the risk of infectious diseases continues to pose a threat to populations

Disease prevention and management is becoming increasingly important in ageing societies with a growing number of people living with one or more chronic diseases, such as cardiovascular disease, musculoskeletal disorders, cancer or diabetes. The share of the population aged 65 years and over is expected to grow by more than 60% across OECD countries, from 17.3% in 2017 to 28% by 2050. While it is a remarkable sign of progress that life expectancy for people at age 65 continues to steadily increase, for many people, most of the remaining years of life after that age are lived with health problems and disabilities which decrease quality of life and generate costs to health systems. An elderly population can be expected to have more complex health care needs, more chronic conditions and often multiple chronic conditions.

In addition to ageing, the rise of chronic diseases is also associated with persistent exposure to behavioural risk factors in some OECD countries, such as smoking, alcohol consumption, unhealthy diets and physical inactivity. Obesity rates have, for example, been on the rise in recent decades. In 2015, on average, nearly one in every five adults was obese in OECD countries, up from around one in seven in 2000. OECD countries with historically high rates of obesity are Canada, Chile, Mexico, the United Kingdom and the United States (OECD, 2017[22]).

OECD projections also show a steady increase in obesity rates until at least 2030 (Figure 3.1). Obesity levels are expected to be particularly high in the United States, Mexico and England, where 47%, 39% and 35% of the population, respectively, are projected to be obese in 2030. The level of obesity in France is projected to nearly match that of Spain, at 21% in 2030. Obesity rates are projected to increase at a faster pace in Korea and Switzerland, where rates have been historically low.

Figure 3.1. Evolution and projection of obesity rates in selected OECD countries, 1990-2030

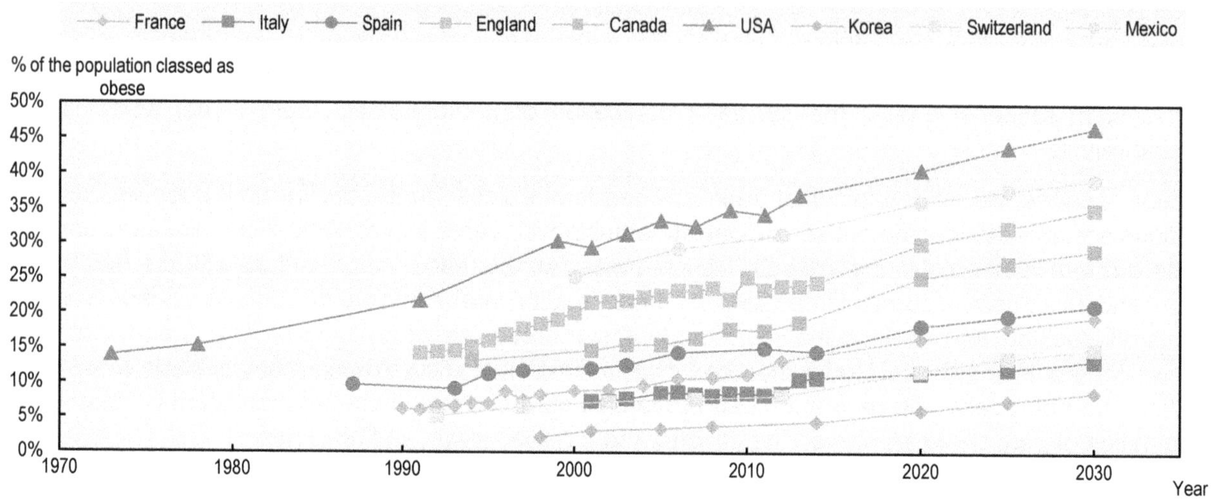

Note: Obesity defined as BMI≥30kg/m². OECD projections assume that BMI will continue to rise as a linear function of time.
Source: OECD (2017[22]), "Obesity Update", www.oecd.org/health/obesity-update.htm.

At the same time, some communicable diseases continue to pose a threat to populations globally. There are, for example, recurrent outbreaks of infectious diseases, such as recent measles outbreaks in unvaccinated populations in the United States and some European countries. In the United States, the annual number of reported measles cases went from 37 in 2004 to 667 in 2014 and 704 cases in the first half of 2019 (Patel et al., 2019[23]). In Europe, measles cases tripled between 2017 and 2018, rising from 25 863 in 2017 to more than 82 000 in 2018 (Thornton, 2019[24]). Over 90% of cases were in 10 countries, including France, Italy and Greece. Worldwide, the WHO reported that there has been a 300% increase in the number of measles cases in the first three months of 2019 (WHO, 2019[25]). A significant factor contributing to the outbreaks is misinformation within communities about the safety of vaccines. The primary health care sector has a greater role to play to increase vaccination rates by improving information to patients (Jacobson Vann et al., 2018[26]; EC, 2018[27]).

3.2.2. The involvement of primary health care practice in prevention activities is too low

As shown by the empirical literature, primary health care teams are in a unique position to meet the increasing health needs of an ageing population, a proportion of which suffer from chronic diseases, and to prevent the spread of infectious diseases. The primary health care team is expected to advise patients on healthy lifestyles and behaviour, to administer screening tests and other preventive care, and to manage and control the progress of chronic conditions.

However, recent data show that too many patients with chronic conditions do not receive the recommended preventive care. In 2014, across EU countries, 26% of patients suffering from certain chronic conditions did not receive any of the recommended preventive tests in the previous 12 months, this proportion was highest in Iceland reaching nearly 50% (Figure 3.2). Finland, Norway, Sweden, Romania, and Slovenia are also among countries where a high share (more than one-third) of people with chronic conditions did not receive the recommended tests in the previous 12 months, while Spain, Belgium, the Czech Republic, Luxembourg and Portugal are at the lower end of the scale (less than 20% of people with chronic conditions did not receive the recommended tests in the previous 12 months).

Figure 3.2. One-quarter of patients suffering from chronic conditions in EU countries did not receive any preventive tests in the past 12 months, 2014

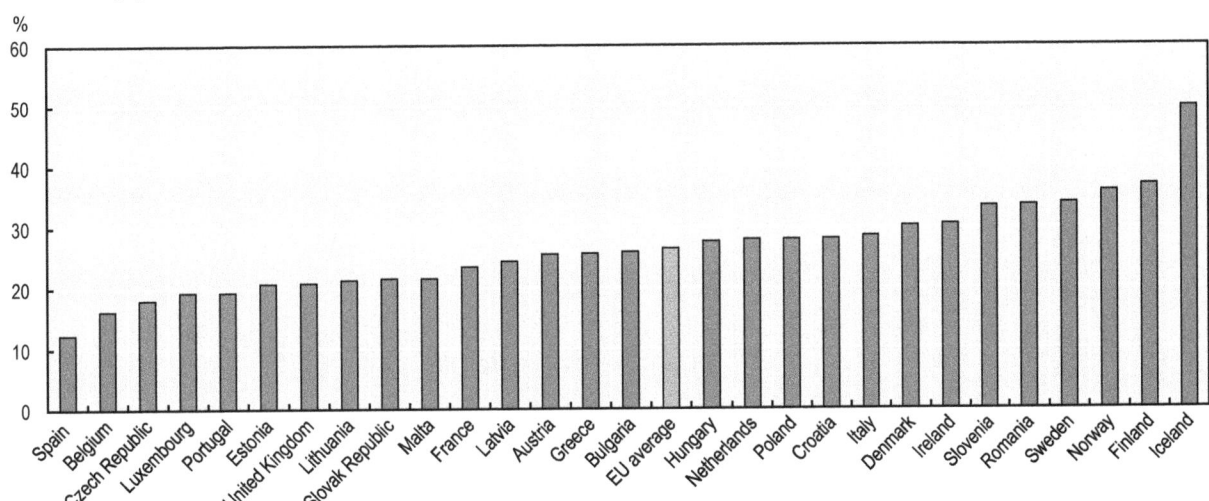

Note: The data refer to the proportion of people suffering from hypertension, myocardial infarction (or chronic consequences of myocardial infarction), stroke (or chronic consequences of stroke) or diabetes who did not receive any blood pressure measurement, blood sugar measurement or blood cholesterol measurement in the previous 12 months. Data corresponds to the year 2014, in which the United Kingdom was member of the European Union and therefore part of the EU average.
Source: OECD estimates based on EHIS-2.

In line with these findings, previous work suggests a decreased involvement in preventive care by primary health care teams (Figure 3.3) (Schäfer et al., 2016[28]). The involvement of general practice in preventive activities (including the measurement of blood pressure, the measurement of cholesterol, and providing health education) has decreased by 13% on average over the same period (Schäfer et al., 2016[28]). Italy, Poland, Finland, Portugal, Romania, Iceland, Denmark and Hungary saw the most significant decreases of more than 50% (Figure 3.3). The Netherlands[2], the Slovak Republic, Greece, Slovenia, the Czech Republic and Estonia are exceptions as they show relatively large increases in preventive activities.

Health services related to treatment of diseases have intensified in almost all European countries, except for the Czech Republic and the Slovak Republic. The increase in GP involvement in treatment of disease is particularly marked in Turkey (+32%), Romania (+26.7%) and Slovenia (+25.2). Under current conditions, additional participation in treatment may be one of the reasons why preventive care is not being delivered properly.

Physicians lack of time and obstacles in reimbursement arrangements are important factors hindering the implementation of preventive interventions in primary health care settings (Yarnall et al., 2003[29]; Geense et al., 2013[30]). Delivery of health education and disease prevention consume physician time. Evidence shows that while time spent in GP office visits has increased over the past decade, physicians continue to have difficulties in finding the time to perform preventive services. In the United States, Yarnall et al (2003) demonstrated that it is not feasible for physicians to deliver all the services recommended by the US Preventive Services Task Force to a representative panel of patients. More recently, Luquis and Paz (2015) showed that family physicians acknowledge that they could have an important role in providing health promotion, disease prevention and offering behaviour counselling. However, heavy workload related to paperwork and the use of EHR (as demonstrated in Chapter 2) and lack of time, are the most important factors hindering their ability to provide these services (Luquis and Paz, 2015[31]).

Figure 3.3. Involvement of primary health care practice in preventive activities has decreased by 13% on average over the past two decades

% relative change in disease treatment (▲) and in prevention (■) between 1993 and 2012

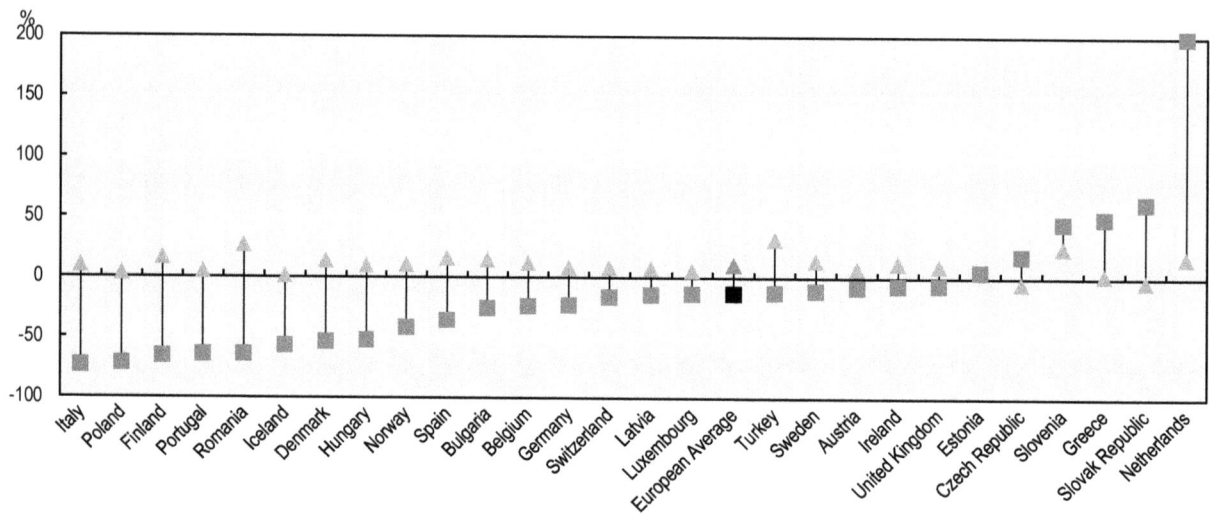

Note: Involvement in prevention includes the measurement of blood pressure, the measurement of cholesterol, and providing health education.
Source: Adapted from Schäfer et al (2016[28]), "Two decades of change in European general practice service profiles: Conditions associated with the developments in 28 countries between 1993 and 2012", https://doi.org/10.3109/02813432.2015.1132887.

3.2.3. Lack of care co-ordination between primary health care teams, specialists and hospitals is common across OECD countries

Co-ordination of care corresponds to an important dimension of patient-centred care (Santana et al., 2019[32]). Care co-ordination consists of organising patient care activities and sharing information among all providers to achieve safer and more effective care (WHO, 2018[33]). This requires a good flow of information and consistency of decisions across the different levels of care in the health system, including primary health care settings, specialist settings and hospitals.

For patients, uncoordinated care means duplication of information and diagnostic tests, which can also lead to adverse effects, particularly when there are poor transitions between hospital discharge and primary health care (Couturier, Carrat and Hejblum, 2016[34]). Fragmented, uncoordinated care is associated with lower care quality, leading to avoidable hospital admissions and higher health care costs (Frandsen et al., 2015[35]; Schneider et al., 2016[36]). Uncoordinated care is a particular problem for people with chronic conditions that require care and support, many of whom have multiple conditions associated with complex social needs (Frandsen et al., 2015[35]).

Evidence from patient-reported data indicates that there are high levels of care co-ordination problems between primary health care, specialists and hospitals. Figure 3.4 shows that between 29% and 51% of people surveyed in 11 OECD countries in 2016, reported having experienced problems of care co-ordination, which refers to: medical tests not being available at the time of appointment or that duplicate tests were made; specialist did not have basic information from GP or GP not informed about specialist care; and conflicting information from different providers. In addition, Figure 3.5 shows that problems in the flow of information between primary health care and specialist care explain a good part of these problems of co-ordination. Between 8% and 20% of people in these countries report that specialists did not have basic information or test results from their GP.

The recent synthesis of 21 papers published in peer-reviewed journals based on the international QUALICOPC dataset show that there is also room to improve the responsiveness of primary health care (Schäfer et al., 2019[37]). In two-thirds of EU countries, evidence shows a need to have more comprehensive consultations where multiple problems can be discussed during one consultation.

Figure 3.4. Problems with care co-ordination between different health care professionals are common across OECD countries, 2016

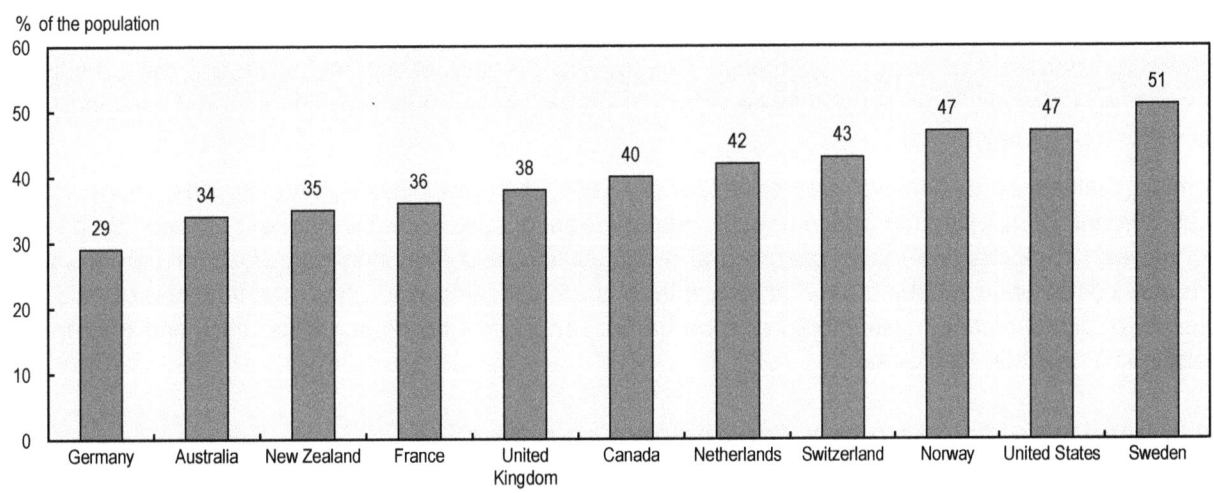

Note: Care co-ordination problems are defined as: test results/records not being available at appointment or duplicate tests ordered; specialist lacked medical history or regular doctor not informed about specialist care; and/or received conflicting information from different doctors or health care professionals in the past two years. The Swedish response rate in the Commonwealth Fund International Health Policy Survey is low, so cross-country comparability is low. The proportions are controlled for age, gender and health status.
Source: The Commonwealth Fund International Health Policy Survey 2016.

Figure 3.5. Basic information or test results from general practitioners not communicated to specialists, 2016

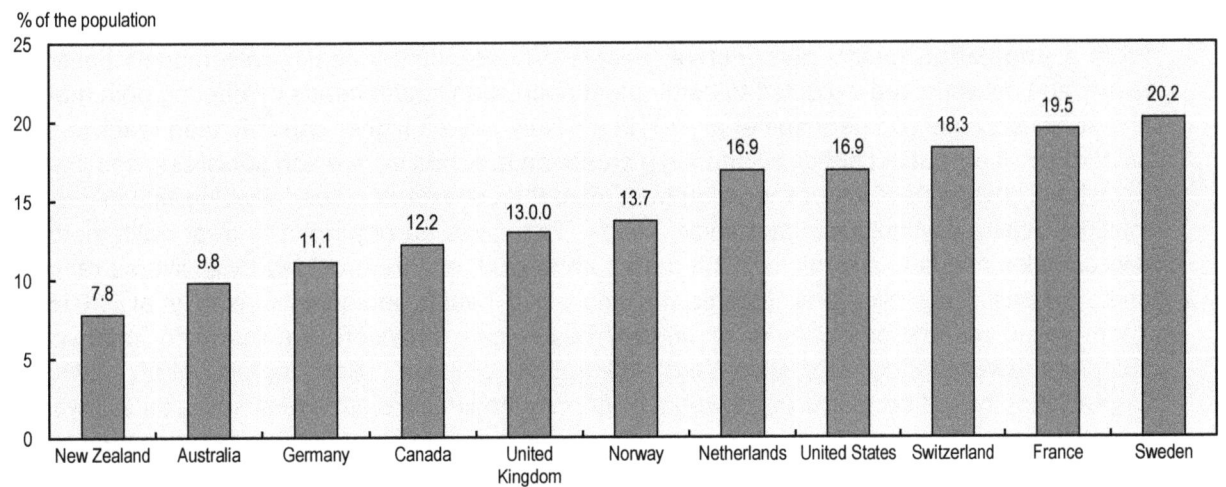

Note: The Swedish response rate in the Commonwealth Fund International Health Policy Survey is low, so cross-country comparability is low. The proportions are controlled for age, gender and health status.
Source: The Commonwealth Fund International Health Policy Survey 2016.

REALISING THE POTENTIAL OF PRIMARY HEALTH CARE © OECD 2020

3.3. Policy options to encourage greater effectiveness and responsiveness

This section looks at key policy levers to encourage effectiveness and responsiveness of primary health care systems. Policy options are divided into two categories: actions to improve prevention and care co-ordination, and those supporting greater self-management and responsiveness of primary health care[3].

A broad set of policy options have the potential to encourage more prevention and care co-ordination. Structural changes in organisation are foremost needed to shift from the traditional solo-practice primary health care model to a proactive, preventive and participatory approach. More teamwork between doctors and other primary health care professionals, backed by portable EHR, is required to improve comprehensiveness and care co-ordination. Changes to the incentives that determine the priorities of clinical practice would also support better care co-ordination, notably through bundled payments and population-based payments.

Promising initiatives to achieve greater responsiveness of primary health care include improving the measurement of quality and outcomes of primary health care (notably those reported by patients themselves), implementing health coaching and counselling, and exploring co-design for primary health care services to ensure people have an equal level of power relative to other health professionals. The potential of digital technologies should also be harnessed to provide personalised care and to empower users to live healthier lifestyles.

3.3.1. Improving disease prevention and care co-ordination

New models of people-centred primary health care delivery based on teams and networks deliver more co-ordinated and integrated care

Invest in better organisation to shift away from the reactive solo-practice primary health care models

In response to the growing complexity of health care needs, many OECD countries have intensified efforts to improve the comprehensiveness and the integration of the services provided within primary health care. Developing new models of primary health care delivery based on teams and networks is both a matter of striving for better health outcomes and an economic necessity:

- From a **population health perspective**, people-centred primary health care models based on teams and networks are expected to better meet population health needs by offering both medical and social services (Borgermans et al., 2018[38]). They have a higher capacity than reactive solo-practices to meet patient needs by offering a broad range of health care and social services. People often have several risk factors and suffer from more than one chronic condition, individuals present multiple health, psychological and social needs. This gives an argument to treat multi-morbidity and complex needs in a single and integrated framework of care provided by a diverse range of primary health care clinicians, technicians and allied health personnel (Jakab et al., 2018[39]). Team-based models or networks of primary health care providers are found to improve the comprehensiveness, co-ordination and integration of care (Schottenfeld et al., 2016[40]). Organisation based on teams or networks of primary health care providers, who can still work in solo-practice, is the best way to encourage communication and co-ordination between health care professionals.
- From an **economic perspective**, people-centred primary health care models based on teams and networks are found to offer economies of scale (Mousquès, 2011[41]). Integrating the primary health care workforce within a single organisation lowers transaction costs and reduces the health production cost because of shared use of inputs, such as equipment, human resources, and ICT, which also increases technical efficiency.

The 2018 OECD Policy Survey on the Future of Primary Care indicates that new models of primary health care delivery are being developed in 17 OECD countries (see Table 3.2). Models of care are expected to steer patients from immediate access to primary health care services for initial treatment to a continuous relationship with the primary health care team when needs become more complex. Most often, patients are split into groups allowing services to adapt to meet their particular social and medical needs. These new models of primary health care organisation often meet the following four characteristics:

- **Multi-disciplinary practices or interprofessional practices** with a different mix of primary health care professionals, different models of teamwork and different target populations (for example as seen in Australia, Canada, the United Kingdom and the United States). The policy survey indicates that there are a variety of existing models in the primary health care setting, with different combinations of GPs, family physicians, registered and advanced nurses, community pharmacists, psychologists, nutritionists, health counsellors, and non-clinical support staff, such as care co-ordinators or case managers.

- **Comprehensive health services in the community**, encompassing a range of services from disease prevention and health promotion, curative services, rehabilitation and management of chronic diseases, to support for self-management of chronic conditions (for example in Costa Rica). Care co-ordination between the care team is key to ensuring the appropriate care is provided at the appropriate place. This should favour the early detection of disease, reduce the exacerbation of disease, avoid duplication of services, and increase provider and patient satisfaction.

- **Population health management**, generally based on risk stratification using sophisticated IT systems (for example in Canada and Spain). Most patients will not require the capacities of a fully comprehensive primary health care team, it is therefore important to make sure that the composition of the primary health care team matches different levels of patient needs. The population health management approach helps teams understand the health and risk profiles of the community. It is increasingly used to implement proactive management of individuals and communities. Patients are stratified to identify opportunities for intervention before the occurrence of any adverse outcomes for individual health status. Patients are then grouped according to their health needs, and the support they receive ranges from those in good health, for whom the appropriate interventions are health promotion and screening, to those requiring ongoing interaction with the primary health care team because of complex needs. In Nova Scotia (Canada) for example, the planning for primary health care services is based on population need, where need is informed by data regarding material and psychosocial deprivation, provider-to-population ratios and population demographics and health status. It enables to consider variations across communities (e.g. employment and income, education, access to family physicians, material deprivation, health behaviours, emergency department visits) and supports strategic resource allocation for primary health care teams.

- **Engagement of patients in shared decision making,** (for example as seen in Israel). Consistent with a people-centred approach, team-based primary health care views patients as knowledgeable partners in their own care, and incorporates, as much as possible, their values, desires and preferences.

In most countries, integrated models of primary health care are community based to offer both medical and social services to patients having multiple chronic diseases and complex social needs, for example regarding food, housing, or substance abuse. Such integration between health and social care in the community goes beyond traditional health care services to address social determinants of health (see also Chapter 4). In addition, mobilising health and social care in the community enables the delivery of more efficient care, reducing hospital discharge delays and hospital readmissions (see also Chapter 2).

Table 3.2. New models of primary health care delivery have been established in 17 countries

Panel A. Name of primary health care organisations across OECD countries	
Countries	Name of the primary health care organisation recently established
Australia	Health Care Homes; Primary Health Networks
Austria	Primary care units
Canada	My Health Teams working with community health centres
Costa Rica	Basic Teams of Comprehensive Health Care (EBAIS)
Estonia	Primary care centres
France	Centres de Santé, Communautés Professionnelles Territoriales de Santé
Greece	Primary care facilities
Ireland	Primary care centres
Italy	Complex Primary Care Units (UCCPs)
Mexico	Health Centres with Extended Services
Norway	Intermediate care facilities
Slovak Republic	Integrated Primary care Centres
Slovenia	Primary care centres
Switzerland	Ambulatory Network
Sweden	Primary care centres
Turkey	Healthy Life Centres
United States	Patient-Centred Medical Home and Comprehensive Primary Care Plus
Panel B. Examples of services delivered and health professionals included	
Examples of services delivered	Examples of health professionals included
Prevention	General practitioners or family physicians
Health education	Registered or advanced nurses
Patient education	Community pharmacists
Self-management support	Psychologists
Curative services	Nutritionists
Disease management	Social workers
Specialist referral	Health counsellors
Care co-ordination	Other allied health professionals

Note: There is a lot of variation on the degree to which these health care services are delivered, and also a large heterogeneity in the combinations of health professionals included.
Source: OECD (2018[42]), Policy Survey on the Future of Primary Care.

Primary health care delivery based on teams or networks allows for a co-ordinated approach spanning primary health care, community services, hospital care and social care

Among the countries developing new models of primary health care delivery, the United States (with the Patient-Centered Medical Home, and the more recent Comprehensive Primary Care Plus), Australia (with Health Care Homes and Primary Health Networks), and Canada (with My Health Team) appear to be at the leading edge of this practice. These models of primary health care are highly integrated, team-based practices and promote patient-centred care through patient engagement and better access to treatment. Such models of organisation allow for a co-ordinated, whole system approach, spanning primary health care, community services, hospital care and social care. The foundation of such primary health care models is a high level of integration across the care team and care continuum resulting from an extensive use of EHR and new forms of communication (see also Section 3.1.2).

Australia is committed to delivering effective primary health care through the establishment of 31 Primary Health Networks (PHNs) as independent primary health care organisations, located throughout Australia. PHNs work to reorient and reform the primary health care system by taking a patient-centred approach to medical services in their regions. In addition, Health Care Homes are being developed as team-based models of primary health care. As at 30 June 2019, there were 132 Health Care Homes in Australia providing coordinated and flexible care to 10 255 patients. The Health Care Homes programme supports patients with chronic and complex health conditions to voluntarily enrol with a participating medical practice known as their 'Health Care Home'. The Health Care Home practice provides the patient a 'home base' for the ongoing co-ordination, management and support of their conditions (see Box 3.2).

> **Box 3.2. Health Care Homes in Australia**
>
> The overarching objectives of Health Care Homes are to:
> - more effectively identify patients with high co-ordination and multi-disciplinary needs and target services specifically for them;
> - improve the quality of care for people with multiple chronic diseases by providing patients with a clinical home base to improve continuity of care;
> - enhance care planning, team-based care and care co-ordination; and
> - enhance patient empowerment and health literacy. Patients are encouraged to play a greater role in their health care.
>
> The Health Care Home employs a risk stratification tool to identify potentially eligible patients and stratify them into one of three tiers based on the complexity of their needs. This tool is a software product that integrates with general practitioner's (GPs) clinical record systems. It comprises of two-steps: a predictive risk model to determine patients' risk of unplanned hospitalisation over the next 12 months, followed by an assessment with a clinician using a Hospital Admission Risk Program (HARP) questionnaire.
>
> Below are some of the key principles of Health Care Homes:
> - One care team – the patient has a committed care team, led by a nominated lead clinicians.
> - One shared care plan – with the support of the care team, the patient will develop a shared care plan. This plan helps the patient to have a greater say in their care and makes it easier for all the people involved, both inside and outside the Health Care Home, to co-ordinate that care.
> - Better access and flexibility – with a care team behind the patient, there is better access to care. Health Care Homes can also be more responsive and flexible. If the patient wants to talk to someone in the care team, it will not always be necessary to have an appointment with the GP, it may be possible to call or message the practice team.
> - Better co-ordinated – the care team will do more to co-ordinate all care from the usual doctor, specialists and other health professionals.
>
> Source: OECD (2018[42]), Policy Survey on the Future of Primary Care.

In Canada, several provinces have moved towards a team-based model for primary health care following the guidance of the Physician Integrated Framework (PIN) developed in 2006. The overarching objective was to encourage more care co-ordination and collaboration between primary health care physicians and clinics through greater use of EHR. The PIN initiative gave an impetus to the development of "My Health Team" (MyHTs) in several provinces of Canada, such as Manitoba or Ontario. Teams are typically made up of a physician, nurse practitioner and other allied health professionals, such as physiotherapists, dieticians, diabetes educators, pharmacists or social workers, depending on community need. It is considered as a one system approach for bridging the gap that currently exists between the Regional Health Authority and independent primary health care providers. It consists of a primary health care network for developing, planning, and operating all primary health care and related services. MyHTs encourage health organisations and providers to work collaboratively to form a network, aligning their goals, contributions, roles and responsibilities in order to achieve the best health outcomes for the population. With an appropriate management structure, MyHTs enable the formation of a strong primary health care network that shares a common vision and service standards. This entails the co-ordination of existing medical and social services and the care team, as well as the active involvement of all stakeholders. In Manitoba, the Center for Health Policy conducted a risk stratification study to understand the health and risk profiles of local communities. The study describes the patient populations that current and future MyHT could expect to serve, including where patients access primary health care in relation to where they live, in order to provide a more accurate description of patient populations. It also looks at whether patients are high users of services, are medically or socially complex, and the overlap between these three types of patients. Risk stratification data is used by MyHT service planning to update service plans, particularly relating to service co-ordination.

MyHT are working with Access Centres and Community Health Centres to offer services that are integrated, patient-centred, and often delivered close to home. These centres are publicly funded and include primary health care clinics, but may also include other core services, such as family and employment services. The overarching objective is to serve complex and vulnerable clients efficiently (see also Chapter 4).

Similar benefits are also seen in Shared Care, a model currently being implemented across several of the MyHTs. Shared Care is a mental health programme that involves family physicians working collaboratively with mental health counsellors and psychiatrists (see Box 3.3). The goal of this collaborative model is to assist individuals with mental health difficulties to access mental health services in a timely manner and to provide that care within the familiarity of their family physician's office and to be more efficient in how specialists' time is used. The Shared Care model improves care co-ordination and integration for people with mental disorders.

> **Box 3.3. Shared mental health care in Canada**
>
> Access to Shared Care services begins when a primary health care physician identifies that their patient is experiencing mental health difficulties. In these situations, the physician may refer the person to a mental health counsellor or a psychiatrist. The doctor, counsellor and/or psychiatrist will then work together with the person to identify the support and assistance they need to improve their mental health.
>
> Where possible, the family physician, mental health counsellor and psychiatrist work in the same office or clinic, so that care is co-ordinated. The mental health counsellor will provide individual, family or group counselling, depending on the needs of the individual. Services are short term and time limited. The psychiatrist will provide an assessment and consult the family physician to look for treatment options for those who need specialised mental health care.
>
> Source: OECD (2018[42]), Policy Survey on the Future of Primary Care.

The experience from the United States is also inspiring. The Primary Care Medical Home, also referred to as the Patient-Centered Medical Home, is a promising model for transforming the organisation and delivery of primary health care. As in Canada and Australia, the Patient-Centred Medical Home focuses on five functions and attributes:

- Comprehensive care – the care team is expected to meet the majority of each patient's physical and mental health care needs, including prevention, acute care and chronic care. The team most often includes physicians, advanced practice nurses, physician assistants, nurses, pharmacists, nutritionists, social workers, educators and care co-ordinators.
- Patient-centred care – the Primary Care Medical Home delivers care that is relationship-based with an orientation towards treating the whole person. It encourages partnership with patients and their families, supports patient's health literacy and patient's self-management.
- Co-ordinated care – the Primary Care Medical Home co-ordinates care across all elements of the broader health care system, including specialist care, hospitals, home health care and community services and support.
- Accessible services – health care services are accessible with shorter waiting times for urgent needs, enhanced surgery hours, around the clock telephone or electronic access to a member of the care team, and alternative methods of communication such as email and telephone care.
- Quality and Safety – the Primary Care Medical Home uses evidence-based medicine and clinical decision support tools to guide shared decision making with patients and families, whilst engaging in performance measurement and improvement.

In addition, the Centers for Medicare and Medicaid services (CMS) launched the Comprehensive Primary Care Initiative (CPC) in 2012. As part of the CPC, 502 practices across 7 regions had to implement new approaches to delivering primary health care. Primary health care practices had to implement the following 5 primary health care functions: enhanced access and continuity of care; planned and preventive care for chronic conditions; risk stratified care management; patient and caregiver engagement; and co-ordination of care with the patient's other providers. CPC supports the primary health care practices through enhanced payments, data feedback on patient outcomes, and learning support. Interestingly, as part of the initiative, there was no enforcement of any specific type of organisational structure. Practices had latitude in how they implemented changes to allow adaptation to their specific patient and practice characteristics. Recent evaluation shows that CPC practices reported improvements in primary health care delivery, including care management for high-risk patients and improved co-ordination of care transitions. Now the Comprehensive Primary Care Plus (CPC+) model is being implemented by 3 000 practices (Peikes et al., 2018[43]).

Very recently, France established the "*Communautés Professionnelles Territoriales de Santé*" (CPTS) as part of *MaSanté* 2022. CPTS consists of networks of health professionals working in the same geographical area who will work collaboratively to organise urgent primary health care, ensure more co-ordinated care between primary and secondary care, and encourage greater collaboration between physicians and other health professionals. As with MyHT in Canada, CPTS will link the primary health care team working in health care centres, called *Centres de Santé*, with individual primary health care physicians, home care providers and long-term care facilities (see Box 3.4). The overarching objective is to progressively eliminate solo primary health care practices that are often associated with isolation. Already in 2019, 200 CPTS have been established.

> **Box 3.4. Health Care Centers (Centres de santé) in France**
>
> Since the 19th century and still to a great extent today, primary health care in France has been performed by individual practitioners (physicians, nurses, auxiliaries, etc.) in private practices. But today, in order to ensure greater effectiveness and equity of interventions, there is a need for stronger cooperation and co-ordination between practitioners, inside an integrated system providing curative but also preventive and rehabilitative interventions (Ministère des Solidarités et de la Santé, n.d.[44]).
>
> Based on the initiatives of grouped practices known as "dispensaries" developed at a local level around World War II and also taking into account the latest actions, France has witnessed in recent years the development of multiprofessional grouped modalities for delivering outpatient primary health services, organised by private or public providers (Colin and Acker, 2009[45]). These new modes of primary health care delivery are called health care centres or "Centres de santé". They often group together several kinds of practitioners and serve local populations for which a comprehensive range of services is provided (IGAS, 2013[46]).
>
> In multiprofessional health centres, services are organised around general practitioners to help establish diagnosis (ex: medical imaging and biology), provide nursing and care (ex: nurses, physiotherapists, other community health workers, etc.) and specialised care or follow-up for patients (ex: rheumatology, cardiology, dermatology, etc.). Almost systematically, health care centres also provide preventive actions for the local population (ex: immunisation, screening, education for health, etc.). Dental care is also often provided as a specific part of primary health care. Moreover, centres are increasingly involved in research and innovation, as well as in medical education (resident physicians, student nurses, etc.).
>
> A considerable challenge is ensuring "internal" co-ordination among all the providers and units, but also "external" co-ordination with primary and secondary providers in a territory (ex: private practitioners, hospitals, maternal and child care, social services, etc.). Incentives and regulations were recently put in place in order to promote this co-ordination on a territorial basis (see for example the ENMR and the ROSP described in Chapter 2, and some recent experiments called *Paiement en Equipe des Profesionnels de Santé* and *Incitation à une Prise en Charge Partagée* described in this chapter) and to develop the exchange of health data between all the providers.
>
> In 2018, 1 831 health care centres were established in France (of which 407 multiprofessional and 97% in urban areas). The average staff number per centre is 33 persons of which 37% physicians, 10% dentist, 22% auxiliaries, 27% administrative staff (National Observatory of Health care Centers, 2018[47]).
>
> Source: The Fédération Nationale des Centres de Santé (FNCS).

Several studies in the United States show positive results. Primary Care Medical Homes have been found to improve care quality for a number of chronic conditions (Friedberg et al., 2015[48]; NCQA, 2017[49]; Schuchman, Fain and Cornwell, 2018[50]; Bates and Bitton, 2010[51]) and have improved patient experiences and increased staff satisfaction (NCQA, 2017[49]). They have also been linked with reduced costs, lower emergency department visits and fewer hospitalisations for patients with chronic conditions (Schuchman, Fain and Cornwell, 2018[50]; Bates and Bitton, 2010[51]; NCQA, 2017[49]).

In line with these findings, a recent literature review of 20 studies shows that inter-professional practice was associated with improved health outcomes and quality of life, notably for patients suffering from chronic diseases and cancer (NAP, 2019[52]). For example, inter-professional care improved diabetic patients' HgA1c by 10%, improved systolic blood pressure by 9% and decreased triglycerides levels by 62.6% (NAP, 2019[52]). Inter-professional primary health care also demonstrated cost-effectiveness and patient preferences.

There are also few evidence suggesting that advanced care teams in primary health care are more satisfying to clinicians and primary health care staff, when compared to more traditional single practice models (Sinsky and Bodenheimer, 2019[53]). Reviewing evidence from four interventions, Sinsky and Bodenheimer (2019) for example show that implementation of primary health care teams has led to a reduction in the number of after-hours work for family physicians and to a reduction in physician burnout (from 56% to 28% after one year of implementation). Advanced-care teams in primary health care have also been recognised as an effective way to improve provider and care team satisfaction. As perceived by the primary health care team, transforming primary health care using a team-based approach has resulted in higher levels of work-life balance (AHRQ, 2016[54]). New models of organisation based on teams or networks of providers is an improvement for primary health care staff, since it may save time, improve care quality and physician satisfaction notably by decreasing stress and improving work-life balance.

Strategies to support the implementation of team-based delivery of primary health care

Implementing team-based delivery of primary health care is not a simple undertaking given the traditional divisions of professional silos, and the fact that across many OECD countries, primary health care practices are owned by physicians themselves and operate as small enterprises. Primary health care physicians who want to create or migrate into group practices may need effective support from policy makers. Several publications highlight common barriers to the effective implementation of team-based delivery of primary health care (Schottenfeld et al., 2016[40]; Bodenheimer, 2007[55]; Socha-Dietrich, 2019[56]), including a culture of professional silos, lack of resources, inadequate payment systems and undefined relationships between team members. Recently, Socha-Dietrich (2019) has shown that there are two significant barriers to the effective deployment of teamwork in primary health care:

- Health workers are usually ill-prepared for teamwork, as both their training and work experience have been gained in very different (typically siloed and hierarchical) care models.
- Information on patients' expectations and experience of care is usually not included in the data used to identify who needs team-based care and what the team should offer. As a result, services risk being designed based on only a partial picture of patients' needs and the introduction of teams might be perceived by patients as disrupting the continuity of care with their primary health care physician.

To ensure effective team working, policy makers need to ensure that health professionals are well prepared for working in a team and to incorporate information on patients' expectations and care experiences into the team design. This requires support including: the preparation of business plans; access to loans to enable investment in practices; assistance in the selection, contract negotiation and training of support staff (see Box 3.5 for the Austrian example).

Team-based models of primary health care also require support through changes in payment systems, adjusting health system governance and implementing digital technologies. Integrating various services and utilising non-clinical workers is not traditionally reimbursed in a fee-for-service model, especially if payments are linked to the type of practitioner. Changes in payment methods are necessary, including a shift from fee-for-service to bundled services, for example, where payments are made for care over time (see below the section on bundled payments and shared saving models). Experiences from OECD countries also show that it is necessary to introduce flexibility into legal frameworks governing delivery of primary health care services, such as a national GP contract, in order to facilitate purchasing services from non-medical professionals by primary health care practices. In England for example, the general practice profession and NHS England developed a contractual framework which encourages and supports the development of multidisciplinary teams. Lastly, the availability and interoperability of information systems, in particular EHR, is a prerequisite to ensure the consistency and continuity in care within a team-based model of primary health care (Socha-Dietrich, 2019[56]).

Overall, the transition from solo-practice to team-based primary health care requires several changes including:

- changes in governance, reimbursement schemes and use of EHR
- changes in the culture and organisation of care, notably to allow for team meetings and more collaboration between professionals
- changes in the nature of interactions among colleagues and with patients to incorporate patients' expectations and experience of care into their care plan
- changes in education and training to ensure future and existing workers have the skills needed for interprofessional teamwork
- changes in the ways in which primary health care professionals and patients understand their roles and responsibilities.

> **Box 3.5. The strong focus on practical implementation is the guiding element in the current reform process in Austria aims at establishing primary health care units**
>
> Strengthening primary health care is a priority for Austria and constitutes one of the major objectives of the 2017 Austrian health reform. The reform aims to enhance primary health care capacity through the establishment of new multi-professional primary health care units, either in the form of primary health care centres at a single location or as a network of health professionals across several locations. The reform envisages the implementation of at least 75 such primary health care units by 2021. The multi-professional units should include at least a core team of GPs and qualified nurses but can also include pediatricians and other health and social professions such as physiotherapists or social workers. The reform further aims to increase access to primary health care by ensuring longer opening hours, particularly during evenings and weekends, in an attempt to reduce the burden on hospital outpatient departments. In June 2017 the National Council passed a bill on primary health care centres. The Health Reform Act regulates the necessary legal framework for the establishment of new multi-professional primary health care units and was one of the most important steps towards the strengthening of primary health care in Austria.
>
> The strong focus on practical implementation is the guiding element in the current reform process ("from the why and the what to the how"). This process is considered a best-practice for actual implementation and therefore is significantly supported by the European Commission's Structural Reform Support Service (SRSS). The European Commission supports activities and services to facilitate health professionals moving from single-handed practice to larger primary health care units. The overarching objective of the support is to establish multi-professional primary health care units and to increase awareness among stakeholders on the available technical and financial support.
>
> In particular, SRSS supports the following activities:
>
> - creating a start-up guide (in print and online) with information for health professionals
> - raising the attractiveness of primary health care for health profesionals
> - creating support materials and providing training sessions for the Social Health Insurance and Regional Governments
> - providing hands-on consultancy services to facilitate and support start up primary health care units
> - designing a website (www.pve.gv.at) and a comprehensive communication strategy.
>
> Currently 14 primary health care units are operational in 4 regions. Many more units are either in implementation or in a planning process for the upcoming years.
>
> Source: European Commission (2018[57]), "Structural Reform Support Service current activities and plans for a future Reform Support Service", https://ec.europa.eu/health/sites/health/files/non_communicable_diseases/docs/ev_20180928_co07_en.pdf and Information provided by the Austrian National Authority.

New ways of communicating with patients and portable EHR enable preventive work to be more proactive and support care team co-ordination

EHR for patients and computerised decision support systems can generate recommendations about individual patient's care based on their specific needs and clinical history characteristics. Systematic reviews indicate that computerised clinical decision support systems can potentially improve the efficiency of primary health care teams and clinical practice (OECD, 2017[58]) (see also Chapter 2).

In particular, keeping EHR enables primary health care teams to work on prevention in a more structured way. EHR generates clinical reminders to help physicians track preventive and ongoing care services for patients with chronic diseases. Such tools can have a major effect on patient safety and the overall quality of the care delivered by increasing compliance with guidelines and protocol-based care, reducing medication errors and adverse drug effects particularly in the management of chronic diseases such as asthma, diabetes or heart failure (Chaudhry et al., 2006[59]; Campanella et al., 2016[60]). In Finland, for example, the POTKU model provides GPs with the locally developed Evidence-Based Medicine electronic Decision Support (EBMeDS) system, which is matched with patient records to provide personalised care guidance (Hujala Anneli et al., 2016[61]). The system also generates automated reminders and warnings. As a medical support tool, EHR has been associated with the workflow, policy, communication and cultural practices recommended for safe preventive primary health care.

To identify and better manage high-risk patients, team-based models of primary health care need to rely on data analysis based on EHR. The use of such data is paramount to help assess risks, aid diagnosis of different symptoms, to direct patients to the most appropriate services for their needs and to improve co-ordination between health care professionals[4]. Spain, for example, uses risk stratification by unifying EHR with various data sources, including demographics, primary health care, hospital care and prescription data. Risk stratification and case finding allow alignment in the delivery of preventive services for groups at higher risk of worse health outcomes and to elaborate needs-based care plans[5] (see also Chapter 2).

To be effective, EHR needs also to be portable across the care continuum, and integrated with functionalities, such as: electronic scheduling of appointments, secure communication between patient and clinical teams, providing reference information on self-management of chronic conditions, electronic prescriptions and dispensing of drugs. Such well-structured EHRs facilitate the distribution of patient health information among all health providers. It allows providers to be notified when a patient has been in hospital, allowing them to proactively follow up with the patient. Each provider will have the same up-to-date information about patient care. Portable EHRs and new ways of communicating within care teams allows the process of care to be streamlined and increases the likelihood that patients are receiving appropriate, co-ordinated, and timely care.

In Israel, for example, all the health funds have comprehensive EHR in community care, which support the sharing of information among physicians, laboratories, diagnostic centres, hospitals and patients. EHRs are used across the community care setting and they capture detailed patient-level information, including demographics, diagnostic and testing information, and drug utilisation data. They also capture key clinical and public health quality monitoring data, including chronic disease management and some risk factor information. As Clalit (the largest health fund in Israel) has its own network of hospital services, its patient records are linked across community and hospital care. These electronic systems are used to support delivery of care processes, which is especially important for patients who see several health professionals and who make transitions between care settings.

In the United Sates, Kaiser Permanente implemented HealthConnect between 2004 and 2010. It is now the largest EHR in the United States. Health Connect enables all Kaiser Permanente clinicians to electronically access their patients' medical records. The EHR has many other functionalities: it integrates the clinical record with appointments, ancillary and specialty services, registration, and billing. It also enables performance benchmarks of all professionals in the network to be generated. Primary health care providers and medical offices can review entire medical records, check laboratory results, immunisation records, history of medical visits, ordering of prescriptions, and referrals. Best-practice research for health professionals is also accessible. Patients are empowered with easy and convenient access to their health information and health management tools, such as the ability to email their care teams or to refill prescriptions.

Many of these functionalities have been found to improve effectiveness of care among diabetes and hypertension patients. An impact evaluation of the introduction of secure messaging between physician and patients with diabetes showed that, when compared to a control group, there was 11.1 percentage points (pp) improvement in blood sugar control (HbA1c<9%), 10.5 percentage points improvement in cholesterol control (LDL-C<100mg/dl), and 6.6 percentage points improvement in blood pressure (BP<140/90) (Zhou et al., 2010[62]). The use of EHR has also been found to help clinicians to better target treatment changes, and follow-up testing for patients with diabetes mellitus (Reed et al., 2012[63]). Ultimately, the use of an EHR was associated with improved HbA1c and LDL-C levels among all patients.

Bundled payments and shared saving models have been shown to improve care co-ordination

Predominant forms of payment, such as fee-for-services and capitation, in their pure form, are not well suited to meet the challenges posed by ageing populations and the rising burden of chronic conditions (OECD, 2016[64]). Such models of payment are predominantly used for "siloed" financing of health providers, they struggle to support new models of care that are better equipped to achieve people-centred care stretching across several health providers and different levels of care, including primary health care centres, specialist clinics and hospitals. Several countries have, however, taken steps to adapt and blend these payment systems. Beyond implementing paying for prevention and paying for co-ordination schemes (see Chapter 2), some countries have introduced bundled payments and population-based payments with shared savings.

Bundled payments have been effective in improving care quality for chronic conditions

Bundled payments in primary health care settings have been introduced to improve quality of care for chronic conditions. These consist of one payment per patient with a chronic illness to cover the cost of all health care services provided by the full range of providers during a specific time period. As demonstrated by OECD (2016), bundled payments lead to better collaboration within and across care settings and can contribute to a greater standardisation of care and to the development of sophisticated IT systems. Evidence indicates that bundled payment programmes have been effective in containing rising costs, while leading to increased performance in terms of care quality, higher patient satisfaction and better adherence to medication and treatment protocol (OECD, 2016[64]; Hussey et al., 2012[65]). In the Netherlands, for example, the bundled payment for diabetes showed improvements in care quality for most process indicators (HbA1c, BMI checked, blood pressure checked, improvement in kidney function and cholesterol tests), it has led to more effective collaboration among health care providers and to better adherence to care protocols (Struijs and Baan, 2011[66]; de Bakker et al., 2012[67]).

Findings from the 2018 OECD Policy Survey on the Future of Primary Care indicate that paying for an episode of care through a bundled payment model is currently implemented in six OECD countries (Figure 3.6). Although the design and characteristics of bundled payments differ between OECD countries, the models developed in Australia and Canada could be of particular interest to other OECD countries and are worthy of consideration. In these countries, the bundled payment accounts for patient complexity, which is an important prerequisite to encourage the participation of primary health care providers (Stokes et al., 2018[68]).

Figure 3.6. Bundled payments and population-based financing are not widely adopted across OECD countries

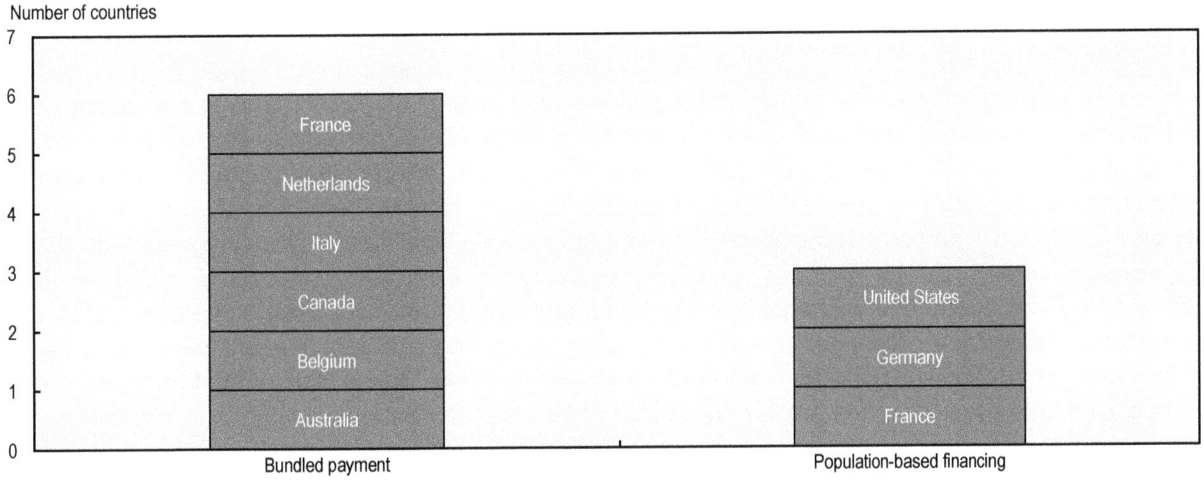

Bundled payment	Population-based financing
France	United States
Netherlands	Germany
Italy	France
Canada	
Belgium	
Australia	

Source: OECD (2018[42]), Policy Survey on the Future of Primary Care.

In Australia, funding for Health Care Homes is bundled into periodic payments. Three levels of payment are proposed. The amount paid is linked to each patient's level of complexity and need, with the highest amount paid for the most complex and high-need patients. The payment values represent an average payment for each level of complexity and recognise the individual variations in service delivery that patients will require at each level. Monthly payments are made to the practices on a retrospective basis. Each Health Care Home can determine how they use these payments, but are required to provide all general practice health care related to a patient's chronic and complex condition.

In Canada, the province of Manitoba, introduced Comprehensive Care Management (CCM) tariffs to physicians in 2017. This is a bundled payment that supports physicians to provide care to patients with complex needs in order to promote continuity, co-ordination and access to care, whilst also making care more comprehensive and patient-centred. The tariffs encourage the use of interprofessional teams and promote preventive care. The overarching objective is to encourage physicians to treat more patients suffering from diabetes, asthma, chronic obstructive pulmonary disease (COPD), congestive heart failure (CHF), hypertension, and coronary artery disease who typically require longer GP visits and more time to co-ordinate care. Five tariffs became available as of 1 April 2017 to pay eligible physicians for the annual management of primary health care for enrolled patients, and these payments are scaled according to complexity. CCM tariffs also include data requirements that help track the quality of care and registration of patients with complex needs.

In France, a new five-year pilot programme was launched in 2019 to experiment with bundled payments. The programme is called *Paiement en Equipe des Profesionnels de Santé* (PEPS). The objective is to ensure greater care integration, improved patient care pathways, and greater care co-ordination between primary health care and secondary care providers. The bundled payment will substitute the fee-for-service schemes, and will only apply for patients followed by a GP in a multi-professional health care centre (*Centres de Santé*). The pilot targets diabetes patients and elderly patients (aged 65 years and over), but also includes all patients having a named GP. Bundled payments will eventually be rolled out nationally from 2023 if evaluations show positive results.

Although bundled payments have not been introduced in Belgium, the interprofessional Integrated Needs-based Capitation is an innovative payment scheme which deserves attention. The Integrated Needs-Based Capitation model, which goes beyond flat capitation, was developed with 42 variables describing the needs of the patients (such as age, gender, socio-economic status, morbidity, functional status, etc) on the list of each community health centre. The model takes into account the demographical and epidemiological transition that affect primary health care system. As described by De Measeneer (2017), the Integrated Needs-Based Capitation System is well-fit to pay interprofessional primary health care team because it stimulates prevention and health promotion, task-shifting, collaboration between health care professionals and co-ordination of care (De Maeseneer, 2017[69]).

As shown by previous studies, the impact of the bundled payments on care co-ordination and quality of care might depend on the scope of the payment in relation to the range of providers involved and services covered (Stokes et al., 2018[68]). As bundled payments transfer the financial risk from insurers to providers, diverging interest between providers and fear of bearing financial risks can impede the participation of primary health care providers. This is particularly the case when patients have multiple needs, requiring a number of health care services, which can be provided by a diverse range of clinicians, technicians and allied health professionals. The successful implementation of bundled payments is more likely to happen within large-scale primary health care organisations with strong governance and sufficient financial reserves to assume the financial risk. In addition, and as seen in Canada and Australia, it is equally important to ensure that bundled payments account for the greater complexity of treatment for patients having multi-morbidity.

Population-based payments with shared savings provide a good incentive to improve care co-ordination and quality

Population-based payments are made to groups of health providers, such as, independent primary health care physicians, specialists, practice networks, hospitals, as well as management companies, and these payments cover most health care services for a defined group of the population. Similarly, as for bundled payments, the overarching objective is to overcome care fragmentation through greater care co-ordination. Rather than paying providers in "silos", the money follows the patients across providers, covers most health care services and has a more comprehensive view of population well-being.

The innovation with population-based payments is the possibility for providers to share the savings generated for the financers if they are able to reduce treatment costs while meeting pre-defined quality requirements. Providers participating in the network will be encouraged to collaborate if the scheme provides opportunities for joint savings. A prospective budget for a population is defined, and providers are financially rewarded if they can keep total costs below the benchmark value. This means that all costs for the patients participating in the integrated care programme are registered and retrospectively compared to historic figures or a benchmark, to determine if savings have been made.

Such innovative – and rather complicated models – of financing are still uncommon across OECD countries (see Figure 3.6). Several population-based payments with a shared saving approach are operating in the United States. The 2010 Affordable Care Act gave impulsion to the development of Accountable Care Organisations (ACOs), groups of health care providers that are collectively accountable for the organisation of health care and take financial responsibility for care provision. The Centers for Medicare and Medicaid Services (CMS) contract with ACOs for the care of a defined population of Medicare patients. Providers forming an ACO include primary health care providers and hospitals, but can also extend to specialists, long-term care facilities and home care. Although there are different programmes designed by CMS, for all models savings can only be earned when quality targets are being met.

In Germany, the Gesundes Kinzigtal GmbH is a joint venture contracted by two statutory health insurance funds to run a population-based integrated care model in rural southwest Germany. It serves middle- to lower-income populations with a high proportion of chronic diseases. The model includes strong stakeholder engagement, electronic integration across providers, patient involvement and empowerment, and data-driven management. The contracts are based on the virtual budget for each fund from the Central Health Fund total allocation. A network of doctors owns two-thirds of Gesundes Kinzigtal and a health management company (Optimedis AG) owns the remaining part. Potential savings are calculated between the virtual budget and actual cost of the whole population insured with the two health insurers in these regions. Around 86 providers have contracts with Gesundes Kinzigtal including GPs, outpatient specialists, hospitals, nursing homes, physiotherapists, pharmacies, providing coverage to 46% of the total population. Providers contracted by Gesundes Kinzigtal are paid by health insurers in the traditional way (fee for services). Doctors who are co-owners of Gesundes Kinzigtal will receive additional payments in case of financial success, and this is not dependent on explicit quality targets. The model puts strong emphasis on prevention, health promotion, and public health to generate value for the population in the long run.

Pimperl et al (2017), show that over 11 years, the integrated model of care resulted in sustained improvements in health outcomes, such as lower hospitalisation rates, higher life expectancy, and higher mean age at the time of death than the control group (Pimperl et al., 2017[70]). Patient satisfaction has increased, and financial results have proved reliable with cost reductions of 7% per insured person since 2014.

France launched a five-year pilot programme called *Incitation à une Prise en Charge Partagée* (IPEP), which is similar to shared savings population-based financing. It takes a population responsibility approach, similar to the Accountable Care Organisation in the United States. The collective payment is complementary to existing payment mechanisms. Shared savings are conditional on quality performance, and health professionals are free to use the savings as they wish. The objective is to improve the way health care professionals work in networks in order to meet the needs of patients in a given geographical area and to improve patient pathways through the health care system. Health care providers, such as primary health care physicians, community health agents, hospitals and social workers, need to collaborate to improve the care of patients based on quality and efficiency indicators.

3.3.2. Improving patient self-management and the responsiveness of primary health care

Efforts must be strengthened to monitor primary health care and ensure that the care it delivers is effective

Compared to the hospital sector, health care systems know little about the quality and outcomes achieved within primary health care. The data generated in most health care systems remains concentrated on inputs and activities. Although nearly all OECD countries report structure indicators, such as the number of primary health care physicians and the number of consultations, only a handful of OECD countries systematically report primary health care quality measures at the national level. Robust reporting information systems are needed to detect, measure and learn from inappropriate and poor primary health care quality. A rich information system is a prerequisite to achieving a good understanding of how, where or why inappropriate and poor primary health care quality exists. These measurements will be developed into actions for quality improvement.

The 2018 OECD Policy Survey on the Future of Primary Care indicates that 18 OECD countries reported having implemented policy measures to collect nationwide performance metrics to monitor the performance of primary health care (Figure 3.7). Such plans are still being discussed in Greece, Italy, the Netherlands, Slovenia and Switzerland. While in Ireland (and Luxembourg) there is no ongoing plan to collect performance metrics in primary health care, the country already collects performance metrics in respect of primary health care. As part of the performance assurance process, an overall analysis of key performance data is provided on a monthly basis to the Department of Health in Ireland. The activity data reported is based on Performance Activity and Key Planning Indicators, with performance monitored against planned activity as outlined in the National Service Plan. It is however generally accepted that there remains scope to improve data reporting from the primary health care sector, and work is ongoing in relation to developing system capacity in this regard.

Figure 3.7. 18 OECD countries have implemented policy measures to collect nationwide performance metrics to monitor the performance of primary health care

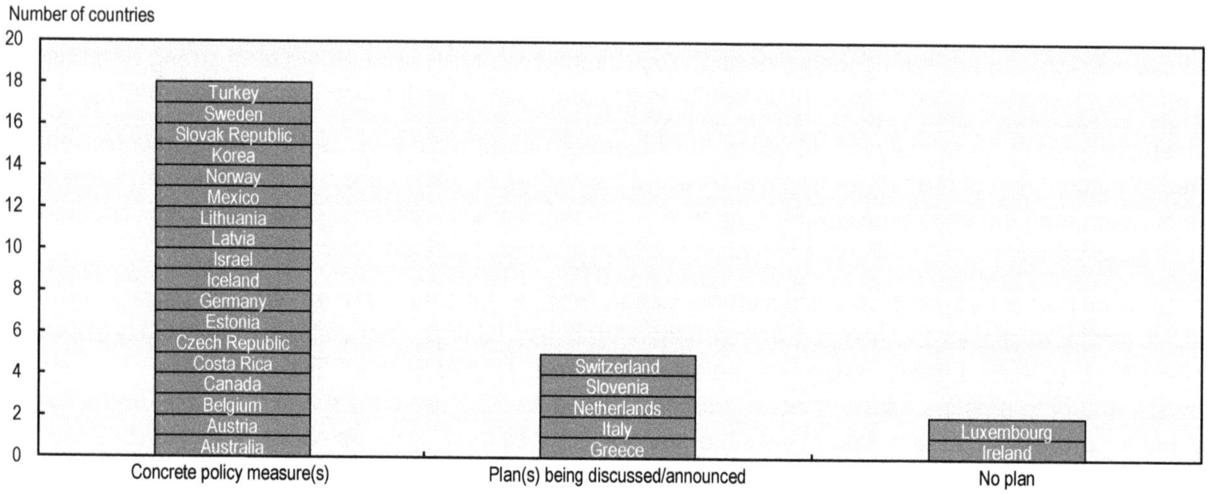

Concrete policy measure(s): Turkey, Sweden, Slovak Republic, Korea, Norway, Mexico, Lithuania, Latvia, Israel, Iceland, Germany, Estonia, Czech Republic, Costa Rica, Canada, Belgium, Austria, Australia

Plan(s) being discussed/announced: Switzerland, Slovenia, Netherlands, Italy, Greece

No plan: Luxembourg, Ireland

Source: OECD (2018[42]), Policy Survey on the Future of Primary Care.

Linking primary health care data to other data sources is necessary for assessing the patient care pathway

Essential to measuring health care quality and performance assessment is the ability to track patients as they progress back and forth through the health care system, the "care pathway". In these pathways, primary health care plays a pivotal role. However, the data landscape in many countries is fragmented: working with electronic records has become common for many primary health care providers, but to get a better view of what is happening in the health system, such data need to be linked across providers and levels of service, such as data from hospital care and social care.

To date, few countries link primary health care data systematically to other sources to assess performance of the health system. Across the OECD, primary health care data remains one of the least regularly linked data sources in health systems. In 2015, 10 out of 22 OECD countries reported that they can link primary health care data with other sources and only 2 countries (Korea and the United Kingdom) reported that primary health care data is regularly linked with other data sources to monitor health care quality and health system performance (OECD, 2015[71]).

In the United Kingdom, the Clinical Practice Research Datalink (CPRD) provides routine record linkages between primary health care data and a range of health-related patient datasets within England (see Box 3.6). CPRD also produces confidential reports designed to help GPs improve the quality of their prescribing, patient safety and to review care pathways.

In the future, all OECD health care systems should be capable of linking public health data with primary health care data. Linking primary health care data with public health data could be used to capture relationships between multiple behavioural factors and a particular set of conditions. Such information could be used to conduct specific targeted prevention actions towards disadvantaged or high-risk populations.

> **Box 3.6. The Clinical Practice Research Datalink in the United Kingdom**
>
> CPRD is a UK Government research service jointly supported by the Medicines and Healthcare products Regulatory Agency (MHRA), and the National Institute for Health Research (NIHR) to promote health care research and drive innovation through the use of patient electronic health records (EHR) (Wolf et al., 2019[72]; Herrett et al., 2015[73]).
>
> CPRD was the first to provide routine record linkages between primary health care data and a range of health-related patient datasets. Data linkage is undertaken by NHS Digital, the trusted third party of CPRD.
>
> Anonymised primary health care patient data can be individually linked to secondary care and other health and area-based datasets (including Hospital Episode Statistics, death registration, national cancer registration, mental health datasets, measures of relative deprivation and rural/urban classification). These linkages enable CPRD to provide a fuller picture of the patient care record to support vital public health research, informing advances in patient safety and delivery of care. CPRD is expanding its health care data and research services to increase both the cover of primary health care data and the number of datasets that are linked and made available on a routine basis to the research community.
>
> CPRD also produces confidential reports designed to help GPs improve the quality of their prescribing and patient safety. Reports show the practice performance, benchmarked against other participating GP practices.
>
> Source: Wolf et al. (2019[72]), "Data Resource Profile: Clinical Practice Research Datalink (CPRD) Aurum", https://doi.org/10.1093/ije/dyz034 and Herrett et al. (2015[73]), "Data Resource Profile: Clinical Practice Research Datalink (CPRD)", https://doi.org/10.1093/ije/dyv098.

Better primary health care data on clinical performance is a prerequisite to better monitoring and improvements in care

The availability and quality of primary health care data for performance assessment needs to advance in most countries. To ensure primary health care is effective, it is necessary to collect data on clinical performance and efficiency at individual provider level. This can then be used to provide feedback to providers, who may be able to compare themselves to their peers and access tools for performance improvement (OECD, 2017[74]).

Indicators could, for example, focus on:

- defined daily doses of antibiotic use in ambulatory care per 1 000 inhabitants
- prescription or referrals in accordance with guidelines
- percentage of individuals with COPD or asthma who have had a lung function measurement during the last 12 months
- percentage of diabetic population with blood pressure above 140/90 mmHg observed in the last 12 months.

Recent evidence shows that such clinical performance and efficiency indicators are available in only a limited number of OECD countries. Canada, Denmark, Estonia, Finland, France, Israel, Italy, Latvia, Lithuania, the Netherlands, Portugal, Slovenia, Spain, Sweden, the United Kingdom and the United States, are among these countries (Reynders et al., 2018[75]; OECD, 2017[74]; Chipman, 2019[76]). In Sweden, for example, the project called Primary Care Quality Sweden is a quality improvement system comprising around 150 quality measures and technical methods for collecting data automatically (Chipman, 2019[76]).

The overarching objective is to support quality improvement without causing any extra administrative work for the primary health care team (doctors, nurses, physiotherapists, occupational therapists, psycholgists and other primary health care professionals). The system covers indicators such as comorbidities, lifestyle habits and pharmaceutical treatment, diagnosis-specific indicators for 12 categories of conditions commonly seen in primary health care, as well as patient-reported data. In 2018, Primary Care Quality Sweden covered half of Sweden's 1 200 health centres (Chipman, 2019[76]). In Israel, the Quality Indicators in Community Healthcare programme captures more than 35 measures of quality of care on preventive measures, use of recommended care, and the effectiveness of care, including for asthma, cancer and diabetes management as well as cardiovascular health (OECD, 2017[74]).

Ideally, the information collected should be used systematically to identify inappropriate or poor primary health care and undertake actions for quality improvement. According to Reynders et al (2018)[36], performance measurement is embedded within the policy process to target areas of improvement in some regions of Italy and Spain. In the region of Lazio, for example, primary health care quality indicators are systematically used by the Health Plan Directorate to evaluate clinical performance for chronic conditions. The information is then used to set clinical and organisational objectives for health care providers and to link the level of achievement of these objectives to annual budget or contract extensions of health care professionals. Similarly, in Spain, performance indicators help to target strategic areas of improvement in health centres. Performance assessment is used to define national strategies for chronicity, health promotion, ischemic heart disease, COPD, diabetes and stroke (among others). These strategies resulted in slight improvements in some of the health problems which were prioritised (Reynders et al., 2018[75])

Collecting patient-reported measures enables monitoring of the effectiveness of primary health care from patients' perspectives

Health care systems know very little about whether the primary health care delivered succeeds in improving people's well-being and their ability to play an active role in society. It is only when we measure outcomes reported by patients themselves – such as quality of life – that important differences in the outcomes of care emerge.

Patient-reported indicators measuring both health status and the experience of receiving health care from the patients' perspective are essential to ensuring services are responsive to people's needs and preferences, and to improving the quality and outcomes of primary health care. Patient-reported indicators are also particularly useful for promoting and evaluating people-centred care. They are defined as:

- Patient-reported experience measures (PREMs), which capture the patient's view on health service delivery (e.g. communication with nurses and doctors, staff responsiveness, discharge and care co-ordination); whereas
- Patient-reported outcome measures (PROMs), provide the patient's perspective on their health status (e.g. symptom burden, side effects, mental health and social functioning).

It is essential that patients are consulted on the primary health care aspects that matter most to them. As primary health care is often the first point of contact with the health care system, taking into account patients' perspectives on their experiences with primary health care services, their values and perceptions, are all crucial elements for performance assessment. Collecting patient reported measures can help define quality, curb less successful practices and influence the direction of change, for example, by guiding decisions on the allocation of resources.

Yet, there is little effort nationally and internationally to survey patients' self-reported outcomes and experiences in order to improve them. In the area of primary health care, PREMs and PROMs are rarely collected at practice level. Among OECD countries, England and the United States are at the leading edge of this practice (Box 3.7). At national level however, PREMs are increasingly being collected through national population-based surveys or by participating in the Commonwealth Fund Survey. This is the case in Australia, Canada, Denmark, France, Germany, Ireland, Israel, Luxembourg, the Netherlands, New Zealand, Norway, Sweden, Switzerland, the United Kingdom and the United States (Fujisawa and Klazinga, 2017). In Australia for example, patients' experience with GP care is collected at national level through the Survey of Health Care. The Survey of Health Care is used to conduct national estimations on whether patients have a usual GP and/or place of care and how this continuity of care affects their experiences.

In 2017, the OECD launched the Patient-Reported Indicators Surveys (PaRIS) to address the need to understand the outcomes and experiences of people with chronic diseases (Box 3.8). PaRIS offers an opportunity to gather the evidence necessary to develop health systems centred on the needs of the people they serve. Comparing the performance of health systems will inform policy makers and help them understand to what extent their policies can deliver more people-centred health systems. This will also enlighten people with chronic conditions, helping them to understand how the outcomes and experiences of care in their own country compare with those in other countries. Ultimately, it will help open a dialogue with service providers about how to further improve the performance of health services and health systems to become more people-centred.

Box 3.7. Collecting PREMs at the practice level: Examples from the United States and England

In the **United States**, the Consumer Assessment of Health Care Providers and Systems programme (CAHPs), managed by the Agency for Health Care Research and Quality (AHRQ), helps policy makers and providers gain a better understanding of patient experience with health care. It consists of:

- assessing patient experience at practice level
- reporting survey results
- helping organisations use the results to improve the quality of care.

The CAHPS programme applies to different health care settings, including primary health care. CAHPS surveys ask patients to report on their experiences with a range of health care services at multiple levels of the delivery system. Patient survey measures can relate to patient's experiences with providers (e.g. accountable care organisations, home health care and nursing homes), with care for specific health conditions (e.g. mental health care), or with care delivered in facilities (e.g. home and community-based services).

In **England**, the GP Patient Survey assesses patient's experience of health care services provided by GP practices within the National Health Service (NHS) England. It assesses experience of access, making appointments, the quality of care received from health care professionals, patient's health and experience of their GP practice. The survey also includes a number of questions assessing patient's experience of NHS dental services. Around 2 million patients registered with a GP practice are surveyed twice a year. The Care Quality Commission uses the results from this survey in their regulation, monitoring, and inspection of GP practices in England. The GP Patient Survey website is remarkable. It offers a description of each GP practice and its performance based on the latest survey. The analysis tool also provides comparison of performance between GP practices.

Source: Based on 2019 GP Patient Survey, http://www.gp-patient.co.uk, and The Agency for Healthcare Research and Quality, https://www.ahrq.gov/cahps/index.html.

> **Box 3.8. The PaRIS survey**
>
> In 2017, the OECD launched the Patient-Reported Indicators Surveys (PaRIS) to address the need to understand the outcomes and experiences of people with chronic diseases. PaRIS offers an opportunity for gathering the evidence necessary to transform health care systems into patient-centred systems based on the needs of the people they serve.
>
> The initiative includes:
>
> - The OECD supporting countries in accelerating the adoption and reporting of validated, standardised, internationally comparable patient-reported indicators in three areas: hip and knee replacements, breast cancer care and mental health care.
> - Developing a new set of internationally comparable measures to help policy-makers assess to what extent their policies are on track to make health systems more people-centred. This new international survey focuses on patients with one or more chronic conditions, who are living in the community, and who are largely treated in primary health care or other ambulatory care settings.

Individual and group-based services in primary health care settings support better self-management

Supporting individuals to gain access to necessary information and to develop technical skills, will ensure a high level of self-efficacy and self-management which has been associated with better health outcomes and care experiences (Hibbard and Greene, 2013[77]). Clinical and non-clinical services to support self-management are varied, ranging from personalised care planning, one-on-one coaching and counselling in primary health care (Edwards, Dorr and Landon, 2017[78]; Olsen and Nesbitt, 2010[79]; de longh et al., 2015[80]; Housden, Wong and Dawes, 2013[81]; Liddy et al., 2014[82]). These services support the maintenance of an individual's skills and confidence to self-manage aspects of their care and to manage the wider social and lifestyle aspects of their health in the long term.

Personalised care planning

Personalised care planning is a formal process whereby practitioners and patients collaborate to create a longitudinal treatment plan (Edwards, Dorr and Landon, 2017[78]). Structured discussions to develop care plans in primary health care work to identify an individual's goals, provide relevant information, agree on any treatments or medications, and look at whether there are any appropriate structured education programmes. Care plans have been widely used, in some cases already for more than two decades, across Australia, Canada, Germany, the United Kingdom and United States (Young, Boyle and Mutch, 2016[83]). A systematic review of personalised care planning demonstrated improvements in: quality of care for people with diabetes, hypertension and asthma; improvements in self-efficacy and self-care; and some improvements in psychological and general health indictors. Moreover, interventions were most effective when they were integrated into routine care (Coulter A, Entwistle VA, Eccles A, Ryan S, Shepperd S et al., 2015[84]). A number of resources need to be available to support care planning, with templates, capacity building tools and support monitoring. The Well-being Star approach is an interesting example in this regard, it is a trademarked approach developed in the United Kingdom, designed to support the development of personal health plans for self-management. The tools available facilitate preparing plans jointly by a patient and health professional, as well as providing training for staff and tools for monitoring implementation (Outcomes Star, 2019[85]).

Health coaching and counselling

Beyond personalised care planning, there are health coaching and counselling services that can be provided in primary health care settings. Health coaching or counselling are interventions offering one-on-one focused self-management support for a patient to learn to be an active participant in the self-management of a chronic condition. Health coaching has been shown to achieve sustained behavioural change, including improved nutrition, physical activity, weight management and medication adherence (Liddy et al., 2014[82]; Olsen and Nesbitt, 2010[79]). When integrated with combined lifestyle intervention (CLI), health coaching and counselling are promising initiatives supporting self-management (DeJesus et al., 2018[86]). CLIs support people in initiating and maintaining healthier lifestyle behaviours, including physical activity, dietary and behavioural components. GPs, practice nurses, physiotherapists, psychologists or dieticians most often carry out CLIs. Previous studies have shown that CLIs have been effective in terms of weight reduction and health improvements, compared with standard care or drug treatment alone (van Rinsum et al., 2018[87]). Previous work also shows that when offered systematically in primary health care settings, counselling interventions also have the potential to generate large health and life expectancy gains (OECD, 2010[88]; Sassi, 2015[89]).

According to the 2018 OECD Policy Survey on the Future of Primary Care, 14 OECD countries reported counselling on lifestyle changes or disease prevention for non-treatment seeking patients in primary health care settings (Australia, Canada, the Czech Republic, Estonia, Germany, Greece, Italy, Korea, Latvia, Mexico, the Netherlands, Slovenia, Sweden and Turkey).

In the Netherlands, the Coaching on Lifestyles (Cool) intervention and the SLIMMER diabetes prevention lifestyle intervention in Dutch primary health care are remarkable. The Cool intervention has been implemented for people who are overweight or obese to help them achieve a sustained healthier lifestyle. The programme consists of 8 group sessions and between 4 and 10 individual sessions, targeting physical activity, dietary behaviours, sleep and stress. The longitudinal pre- and post-study reviews identify lifestyle change at 8 and 18 months after initiation. Positive and sustained changes among adults were found regarding behaviour and quality of life (van Rinsum et al., 2018[87]). In a similar vein, the SLIMMER diabetes prevention lifestyle intervention, implemented in Dutch public and primary health care, involved general practices, dieticians, physiotherapists and sports clubs. It consisted of both dietary and physical interventions in individual or group session consultations (also called shared medical appointments), and individual case management. A recent randomised control trial has shown that the SLIMMER programme improved body weight, clinical and metabolic risk factors, dietary intake, physical activity, and quality of life in the intervention group (Duijzer et al., 2017[90]). The intervention group, for example, showed significantly greater improvement in anthropometry and glucose metabolism. After 12 and 18 months, differences between the intervention and control group were -2.7 kg and -2.5 kg for weight and -12.1 pmole and -8.0 pmole for fasting insulin (Duijzer et al., 2017[90]).

Canada, the Czech Republic and Germany have introduced brief alcohol intervention in primary health care. Germany is currently working to target alcohol-related disabilities through brief interventions offered in primary health care settings and in the work place. In Italy, health education and support from primary health care physicians have been introduced to improve diets and physical activity. Japan also has a comprehensive programme aimed at improving healthy lifestyles – including dietary habits and physical activity – based on counselling in community centres. In Estonia, family physicians are expected to educate and advise patients on screening programmes, alcohol intake, HIV prevention and immunisation. In the Czech Republic, GPs provide health promotion, particularly within regular preventive checks. Since 2000, colorectal cancer screening using faecal occult blood testing has been established in GPs offices and they are also involved in vaccination programmes.

Peer support groups, most often included in community-based programmes, can also provide an important source of education, emotional support and practical problem-solving assistance among people facing similar challenges. This may take the form of peer listening, education, tutoring or mentoring, built on shared personal experience and empathy. Peer support groups have been used widely for the treatment and management of chronic diseases (Jakab et al., 2018[91]), with well-studied experiences for mental health and anxiety in Australia, Canada, New Zealand, the United Kingdom and the United States. In Nova Scotia (Canada), Your Way to Wellness programme is a self-management programme for those living with chronic disease (cancer, cardiovascular diseases or diabetes for example). It helps people with chronic conditions and their caregivers overcome daily challenges, take action and live a healthy life. Groups meet weekly for two and half hours for six weeks and are led by trained volunteers, most of whom have chronic conditions themselves. Participants learn how to set goals and problem solve, improve communication with health care providers, family and friends, eat healthier, manage symptoms, fear and frustration and improve self-confidence. Peer support is associated with better self-management for cardiovascular disease, diabetes, mental health, and other chronic conditions (de Iongh et al., 2015[92]; Patil et al., 2018[93]; Ferrer, 2015[94]) and has also contributed to higher quality of life among breast cancer patients (Taleghani et al., 2012[95]).

Technology-based platforms linking patients to primary health care teams show promise in improving self-efficacy and health behaviour

In less than a decade, the percentage of people from European countries seeking health information online has increased rapidly, nearly doubling from 28% in 2008 to 51% in 2017 (Figure 3.8) (OECD/EU, 2018[96]). Similarly, recent OECD data show that seeking health information ranks second, just after online purchases, among most frequent activities by Internet users (see Chapter 2). Importantly, this proliferation in use of the Internet has lessened early pitfalls of Internet-based solutions and their potential to contribute to a socio-economic "digital divide" among those less likely to have access to or feel comfortable using computers.

Figure 3.8. The percentage of people seeking health-related information online is increasing in all European countries, 2008-17

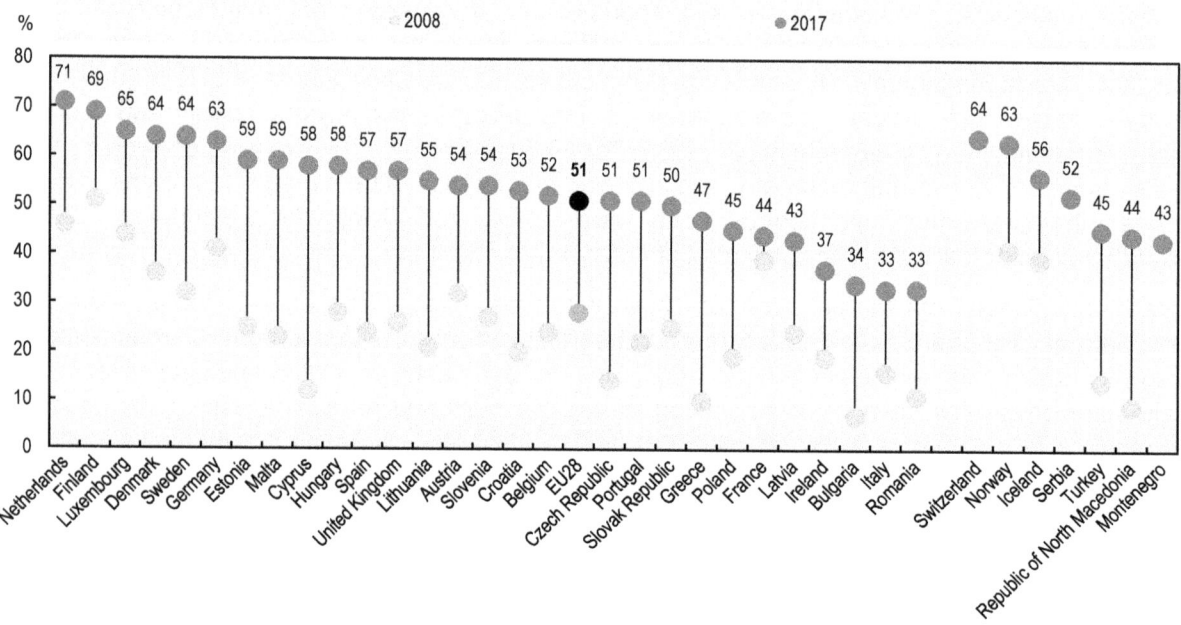

Note: Data corresponds to the years 2008-17, in which the United Kingdom was member of the European Union and therefore part of the EU average.
Source: OECD/EU (2018[96]), *Health at a Glance: Europe 2018: State of Health in the EU Cycle*, https://doi.org/10.1787/health_glance_eur-2018-en.

The increased use of the Internet and technology-based platforms for health-related information (also called mobile health or mHealth) presents a vital medium for self-management support (see also Chapter 2). Online self-management resources and programmes hold several inherent advantages: patients can control when and where they participate; technology can overcome isolation due to distance; and data storing and processing is streamlined, among other advantages. More recently, mobile technology has shown increasing potential to integrate self-management support seamlessly into daily life. Smartphone software and mobile phone and tablet apps that not only remind patients about self-monitoring tasks but also send the results directly to their medical team show promise for improving self-efficacy, health behaviours and clinical outcomes (Whitehead and Seaton, 2016[97]; Bender et al., 2011[98]). To date, many online self-management support services in primary health care are those linking patients and providers, including patient-provider portals, smartphone applications and telephone or Internet-based consultations and monitoring.

Patient-provider portals

Health portals are websites that also provide secure online access to personal health records, linking patients and health providers so they can make appointments, share test results and communicate electronically (Health Council of Canada, 2012[99]). Review data suggests the success of web-based patient portals depends on user-friendly designs, attention to data security when messaging, available guidance on how to use the portal and easy-to-use and understand health information. In Finland, the Oulu Self Care Service is an electronic platform providing self-care services, including secure communication, chatting with nurses or booking appointments (see Box 3.9). In Canada, a number of regional online portals have increased patient-provider communication through secure messaging such as the miHealth application; a Canadian-made app initially designed and piloted for northern Ontario and now expanded for wider use (see Box 3.8). In Estonia, patients have access to their personal health information from home, giving them the possibility to reference a wide range of relevant health information based on their health status and treatment plans. The patient portal also provides general information on their condition, relevant lifestyle changes and frequently asked questions by patients. In Turkey, the E-pulse patient portal has been established by the Turkish Ministry of Health. It is a personal health record system that integrates the information systems of all health institutions. Thanks to E-pulse, people can access their lab results, medical images, prescription, medication and diagnosis details, and health records. They can share their medical records with their doctor(s), make medical appointments, and can also enter data manually to aid condition monitoring.

> **Box 3.9. Patient-provider portals in Finland and Canada**
>
> **The Oulu Self Care Service in Finland**
>
> In Finland, in 2010 the Oulu Self Care Service was launched in the City of Oulu, northern Finland. It is a web-based communication platform for patients and professionals. It makes information available to encourage healthier life styles and disease prevention (Lupiañez-Villanueva, Sachinopoulou and Theben, 2015[100]). The e-service platform also provides self-care services including secure communication, live-chat with nurses, booking appointments, checking laboratory results, accessing personal information, a self-care library with content for diabetes, asthma and blood pressure, electronic health checks and digital coaching (e.g. for sleep, stress, weight and exercise). The Oulu Self Care Service has been recognised as a key enabler of the chronic care model to improve health outcomes, and make care more efficient through a shared use of data among health and social care providers. By 2018, the platform had registered approximately 110 000 users, with approximately 14 200 locals using the service each month. The City of Oulu continues to look for opportunities to expand the range of services, and to scale up the services to the entire region over the long term.

> **miHealth application in Canada**
>
> In Canada, the miHealth application is a secure platform for patients and physicians to chat. It allows primary health care practitioners to check in on patients and stay up-to-date with their medical history and patients the ability to access their personal health information, direct message with physicians and view test results. The application works on a subscription basis and allows a patient to hold their health data electronically and link between providers.
>
> Source: OECD (2018[42]), Policy Survey on the Future of Primary Care.

Self-monitoring using smartphones

Smartphone software can be used to remind patients about self-monitoring tasks, but also to send the results of these tasks directly to their medical team. Smartphone applications demonstrate promising results when applied to self-monitoring of physical activity (Ormel et al., 2018[101]), increasing adherence to dietary programmes (Payne et al., 2018[102]), and increasing access to mental health services (Chandrashekar, 2018[103]). Review data on key success factors for smartphone-based apps highlight the importance of individual tailoring and adaptive learning, feedback systems, clinician, peer and technical support and self-monitoring features (Chandrashekar, 2018[103]; Hind and Sibbald, 2015[104]).

The Symptom Checker established in Australia, is an online tool that helps guide consumers to the most appropriate health care and provides evidence-based information and advice for their health issues. It helps patients understand symptoms and possible signs of illness, causes and complications. Patients can find out more about their symptoms and possible causes and get advice on the next steps for their health care, whether it is self-care or talking to a health professional. In the United Kingdom, Babylon Health can deliver personalised health assessments, treatment advice and face-to-face appointments with a doctor 24 hours a day, 7 days a week. The service also allows users to receive drug prescriptions, referrals to health specialists, and to book health examinations. Through the app, patients can get answers about lifestyle and family history to create a health report and get practical insights to make positive lifestyle changes.

Telephone or Internet-based monitoring

Telehealth interventions to support self-management are a widely used and studied modality of services (see also Chapter 2). These include Internet-based and telephone-based monitoring and education, telemedicine or telehealth kiosks (de longh et al., 2015[92]). Review data reports the effectiveness of telehealth technologies in improving self-care skills and self-monitoring behaviours, and increasing clinical outcomes among older adults with chronic conditions (Guo and Albright, 2018[105]; Hanlon et al., 2017[106]).

A number of countries have experience with the use of telehealth services. Denmark is one of the most active countries in telemonitoring, with a range of services delivered through two programmes: TeleCare North and the Virtual Hospital (Cravo Oliveira Hashiguchi, 2020[107]). TeleCare North is a telemonitoring programme involving the North Denmark regional authority, its hospitals, GPs and 11 municipalities. The programme combines home resources, including tablets and step counters, videos and e-logs to store and send measurements taken from home, with monthly video conferencing to assess progress. Since 2013, 1 400 patients have been monitored in the context of COPD. The success of this initiative has contributed to its expansion across the country and widened its use to other conditions (Dinesen, Huniche and Toft, 2013[108]; World Health Organization Regional Office for Europe, 2016[109]). The Virtual Hospital programme monitors women with pregnancy complications in their own homes. The project will be scaled nationally in 2020. It allows families with preterm babies to be followed at home using a tablet, a customised scale for weighing the infant and a measuring tape to monitor the growth of the baby's head, plus families can also request video consultations (Cravo Oliveira Hashiguchi, 2020[107]).

Other OECD countries providing telemonitoring programmes include Austria (as part of the Health Dialogue Diabetes Mellitus campaign which is only offered for a selected group of insured people), the Czech Republic (with telemonitoring programmes on chronic heart failure and diabetes), Ireland (with a telemonitoring programme on epilepsy) and Lithuania (with a telemonitoring programme for palliative care) (Cravo Oliveira Hashiguchi, 2020[107]).

Exploring co-design can make primary health care more responsive to the needs of service users

Co-design (also called "Experienced-based co-design") is an approach that enables staff and patients to co-design services and care pathways, together in partnership. Co-designing services ensures people with experience of a condition to have an equal level of power and influence relative to other health professionals involved.

This involves gathering experience from patients and staff through in-depth interviewing, focus groups or group discussions and identifying priorities for improvement in the delivery of health care services. The material is then presented to staff and patients to explore the findings and work together to identify an improvement strategy.

The method has been applied to a range of clinical services including cancer care, diabetes care, drug and alcohol treatment and mental health care. In Australia, Canada and England, experienced-based co-design already shows promise to improve care quality and change some key aspects of health care delivery. Australia, for instance, used experience-based co-design to improve patient's experiences of mental health services as they transition through tertiary services to primary health care and self-management support. The overarching objective was to understand the experiences of patients, to identify opportunities for service redesign and integration and to develop initiatives aimed at improving consumer experiences of transitions. Three main outputs resulted from the project: i) design and develop consumer information; ii) design, implement and evaluate a consistent post discharge follow-up process; and iii) increase awareness and understanding of the role of community mental health integration projects. Overall analysis of referral patterns between secondary and primary health care appeared to indicate improvements in appropriateness and timeliness of mental health care (AHHA, 2018[110]).

Incentives on the demand side can be used to change patient's behaviour

Incentives may facilitate sought after changes for the delivery of self-management services in primary health care. Different demand-side financing and incentive schemes have been applied in some OECD countries, with the common aim of increasing an individual's choice over preventive care and control over their health and health care. Examples of these different approaches include the following:

- **Health care vouchers or coupons** provide free access or reduce the cost of health care services. This scheme has been used in Florida in the United States for health-related products such as over-the-counter medications where beneficiaries receive vouchers when seeking preventive health services, such as obtaining a flu shot. California's Medicaid programme introduced non-health-related incentives, such as movie tickets or gift certificates, to reward patients who keep up with scheduled well-child visits for their infants and adolescents (The Commonwealth Fund, 2019[111]). In Texas, the Medicaid programme is working to pilot "individual health rewards" to volunteer beneficiaries if they participate to smoking cessation or weight loss programmes. These credits could then be used to purchase additional health services (The Commonwealth Fund, 2019[111]). This model of incentives has proven especially effective for reaching vulnerable population groups. For example, in Germany, to increase the uptake of services for newly arrived refugees, a model of health care vouchers for accessing primary health care services was introduced (Rolke, Wenner and Razmun, 2018[112]). The vouchers are collected or received via email on a quarterly basis and aim to ensure individuals that would otherwise not have free access to primary health care are able to visit local primary health care providers; decreasing the burden on free inpatient and emergency care (Rolke, Wenner and Razmun, 2018[112]).

- **Personal health budgets** are characterised as a sum of money, typically determined based on a personalised care plan, to support an individual's health and well-being needs (e.g. funding a personal assistant to help with personal care at home or for equipment such as a wheelchair). The modality works by enabling an individual to have the choice and control over decisions about their care and services. The model has been applied in England to support people with long-term conditions (NHS England, 2018[113]; NHS England, 2017[114]). The model is expected to continue to be rolled out with a new target of 200 000 people by 2023-24. Evidence from pilots between 2009 and 2012 found the use of personal health budgets for people using mental health services and for a range of long-term conditions contributed to improved quality of life and well-being, greater choice and control, and reduced total spending for people with high levels of need (Jones et al., 2018[115]).

- **Conditional cash transfers** which were first implemented in low- and middle-income countries, consist of providing cash benefits to families on the condition they engage in activities that generate long-term benefits, such as using preventive care services (Lagarde, Powell-Jackson and Blaauw, n.d.[116]). They work to minimise direct and indirect costs for seeking health services while also addressing more entrenched demand-side obstacles, such as failure to perceive the benefits of preventive health interventions. In the United States, recent evaluation showed that conditional cash transfers led to positive improvements in the health of poor families, notably through greater use of preventive health services (Courtin et al., 2018[117]). In Germany, supporting self-management is backed by financial resources; statutory health insurance companies pay EUR 1.05 per insured person to promote self-help (Trojan, Kofahl and Nickel, 2017[118]). Review data finds the use of conditional cash transfers can increase the uptake of preventive services. There is also data that suggests participation increases with the amount of the incentive (Agency for Healthcare Research and Quality, 2014[119]).

3.4. Conclusions

A large body of evidence shows that strong primary health care is associated with improved health outcomes and more people-centred care. As the first point of contact with the health care system, and as a trusted source of information, primary health care teams are in a unique position to advise patients on lifestyles and health behaviour, to administer preventive care, and to manage and control the progress of chronic conditions (notably through self-management, health coaching and counselling). This is ever more needed, particularly in OECD countries, where citizens' expectations about services are high, societies are ageing; and complex cases are costly.

Yet, despite this strong evidence-base, recent international data show that too many patients with chronic conditions do not receive the recommended preventive care and that there are significant problems with care co-ordination between primary health care, specialists and hospitals. To make sure primary health care realises health gains, more needs to be done to encourage both the effectiveness and responsiveness of primary health care.

A broad set of policy options should be adopted by policy makers. Structural changes in the organisation of care are foremost needed to shift from the traditional solo-practice primary health care model to a proactive, preventive and participatory approach, based on a teams or networks of providers. More teamwork between doctors and other primary health care professionals, backed by portable EHRs, is required to improve prevention and care co-ordination. Changes to the incentives that determine clinical practice would also support better care co-ordination, notably through the use of bundled payments and population-based payments.

Better measurements of quality and outcomes of primary health care, notably those reported by patients themselves, health coaching and counselling, and implementing co-design for primary health care services are crucial components in supporting greater responsiveness in primary health care. The potential of self-management services offered by technology-based platforms should also be harnessed to provide personalised care to empowers users to live healthier lifestyles.

References

Agency for Healthcare Research and Quality (2014), "Wellness and health promotion programs use financial incentives to motivate employees AHRQ.", *Agency for Healthcare Research and Quality*.. [119]

AHHA (2018), *Experience Based Co-Design: a toolkit for Australia*, AHHA, https://ahha.asn.au/experience-based-co-design-toolkit. [110]

AHRQ (2016), "Team-Based Primary Care: Convergence of Improving Engagement, Safety, and Enhanced Joy in Practice", *AHRQ Pub. No. 16-0035*, https://micmrc.org/system/files/BEllin%20teambased-1_0.pdf. [54]

Bates, D. and A. Bitton (2010), *The future of health information technology in the patient-centered medical home*, http://dx.doi.org/10.1377/hlthaff.2010.0007. [51]

Bender, J. et al. (2011), "Can pain be managed through the Internet? A systematic review of randomized controlled trials", *Pain*, http://dx.doi.org/10.1016/j.pain.2011.02.012. [98]

Bodenheimer, T. (2007), "Building Teams in Primary Care : Lessons Learned", *California HealthCare Foundation*. [55]

Borgermans, L. et al. (2018), "How Leapfrogging in primary care can contribute to upscaling NCD core services", *Eurohealth*, Vol. 24/1. [38]

Campanella, P. et al. (2016), *The impact of electronic health records on healthcare quality: A systematic review and meta-analysis*, http://dx.doi.org/10.1093/eurpub/ckv122. [60]

Campbell, R. et al. (2003), "Cervical cancer rates and the supply of primary care physicians in Florida", *Family Medicine*. [15]

Chandrashekar, P. (2018), "Do mental health mobile apps work: evidence and recommendations for designing high-efficacy mental health mobile apps", *mHealth*, http://dx.doi.org/10.21037/mhealth.2018.03.02. [103]

Chaudhry, B. et al. (2006), "Systematic review: impact of health information technology on quality, efficiency, and costs of medical care", *Annals of internal medicine*, http://dx.doi.org/10.7326/0003-4819-144-10-200605160-00125. [59]

Chipman, A. (2019), *Value-Based Healthcare In Sweden: Reaching the next level*, Economist Intelligence Unit Limited, https://eiuperspectives.economist.com/sites/default/files/value-basedhealthcareinswedenreachingthenextlevel.pdf. [76]

Colin, M. and D. Acker (2009), "Les centres de santé : une histoire, un avenir", *Santé Publique*, Vol. 21, pp. 57-61, http://dx.doi.org/DOI : 10.3917/spub.090.0057. [45]

Conejo-Cerón, S. et al. (2017), *Effectiveness of psychological and educational interventions to prevent depression in primary care: A systematic review and meta-analysis*, Annals of Family Medicine, Inc, http://dx.doi.org/10.1370/afm.2031. [6]

Coulter A, Entwistle VA, Eccles A, Ryan S, Shepperd S, P. et al. (2015), "Personalised care planning for adults with chronic or long- term health conditions (Review)", *Cochrane Database Syst Rev*, http://dx.doi.org/10.1002/14651858.CD010523.pub2.Copyright. [84]

Courtin, E. et al. (2018), "Conditional cash transfers and health of low-income families in the US: Evaluating the family rewards experiment", *Health Affairs*, http://dx.doi.org/10.1377/hlthaff.2017.1271. [117]

Couturier, B., F. Carrat and G. Hejblum (2016), "A systematic review on the effect of the organisation of hospital discharge on patient health outcomes", http://dx.doi.org/10.1136/bmjopen-2016. [34]

Cravo Oliveira Hashiguchi, T. (2020), "Bringing health care to the patient: An overview of the use of telemedicine in OECD countries", No. 116, OECD, Paris, https://dx.doi.org/10.1787/8e56ede7-en. [107]

de Bakker, D. et al. (2012), "Early results from Adoption of bundled payment for diabetes care in the Netherlands show improvement in care coordination", *Health Affairs*, http://dx.doi.org/10.1377/hlthaff.2011.0912. [67]

de Iongh, A. et al. (2015), *A practical guide to self-management support. Key components for successful implementation*, The Health Foundation, London, https://www.health.org.uk/publications/a-practical-guide-to-self-management-support. [92]

de Iongh, A. et al. (2015), *A practical guide to self-management support : Key components for successful implementation*, The Health Foundation, London, https://www.health.org.uk/publications/a-practical-guide-to-self-management-support. [80]

De Maeseneer, J. (2017), *Family Medicine and Primary Care : At the Crossroads of Societal Change*, LannooCampus, Leuven. [69]

DeJesus, R. et al. (2018), "Impact of a 12-week wellness coaching on self-care behaviors among primary care adult patients with prediabetes", *Preventive Medicine Reports*, http://dx.doi.org/10.1016/j.pmedr.2018.02.012. [86]

Dinesen, B., L. Huniche and E. Toft (2013), "Attitudes of COPD patients towards tele-rehabilitation: A cross-sector case study", *International Journal of Environmental Research and Public Health*, http://dx.doi.org/10.3390/ijerph10116184. [108]

Duijzer, G. et al. (2017), "Effect and maintenance of the SLIMMER diabetes prevention lifestyle intervention in Dutch primary healthcare: A randomised controlled trial", *Nutrition and Diabetes*, http://dx.doi.org/10.1038/nutd.2017.21. [90]

EC (2018), *Vaccination programmes and health systems in the European Union. Expert Panel on effective ways of investing in Health (EXPH)*. [27]

Edwards, S., D. Dorr and B. Landon (2017), *Can personalized care planning improve primary care?*, http://dx.doi.org/10.1001/jama.2017.6953. [78]

European Commission (2018), *Structural Reform Support Service current activities and plans for a future Reform Support Service*, https://ec.europa.eu/health/sites/health/files/non_communicable_diseases/docs/ev_20180928_co07_en.pdf (accessed on 4 July 2019). [57]

Ferrante, J., E. Gonzalez and R. Roetzheim (2000), "Effects of Physician Supply on Early Detection of Breast Cancer", *Journal of the American Board of Family Practice*, Vol. 13, pp. 408-14. [16]

Ferrer, L. (2015), "Engaging patients, carers and communities for the provision of coordinated/integrated health services: strategies and tools.", *Copenhagen: WHO Regional Office for Europe.*. [94]

Frandsen, B. et al. (2015), "Care fragmentation, quality, and costs among chronically Ill patients", *American Journal of Managed Care*, Vol. 21/5. [35]

Friedberg, M. et al. (2015), "Effects of a medical home and shared savings intervention on quality and utilization of care", *JAMA Internal Medicine*, http://dx.doi.org/10.1001/jamainternmed.2015.2047. [48]

Geense, W. et al. (2013), "Barriers, facilitators and attitudes influencing health promotion activities in general practice: An explorative pilot study", *BMC Family Practice*, http://dx.doi.org/10.1186/1471-2296-14-20. [30]

Guanais, F. et al. (2019), "Primary Health Care and Determinants of the Perception of the Health System and Quality of Care in 17 Countries in LAC and the OECD", in Guanais, F. et al. (eds.), *From the Patient's Perspective: Experiences with primary health care in Latin America and the Caribbean*, Inter-American Development Bank, Washington, DC. [8]

Guo, Y. and D. Albright (2018), "The effectiveness of telehealth on self-management for older adults with a chronic condition: A comprehensive narrative review of the literature", *Journal of Telemedicine and Telecare*, http://dx.doi.org/10.1177/1357633X17706285. [105]

Hanlon, P. et al. (2017), *Telehealth interventions to support self-management of long-term conditions: A systematic metareview of diabetes, heart failure, asthma, chronic obstructive pulmonary disease, and cancer*, http://dx.doi.org/10.2196/jmir.6688. [106]

Hansen, J. et al. (2015), "Living in a country with a strong primary care system is beneficial to people with chronic conditions", *Health Affairs*, http://dx.doi.org/10.1377/hlthaff.2015.0582. [4]

Hartley, L. (2002), "Examination of primary care characteristics in a community-based clinic", *Journal of Nursing Scholarship*, Vol. 34/4, pp. 377-382, http://dx.doi.org/10.1111/j.1547-5069.2002.00377.x. [12]

Health Council of Canada (2012), *Self-management support for Canadians with chronic health conditions: a focus for primary health care*, Health Council of Canada, Toronto. [99]

Herrett, E. et al. (2015), "Data Resource Profile: Clinical Practice Research Datalink (CPRD)", *International Journal of Epidemiology*, http://dx.doi.org/10.1093/ije/dyv098. [73]

Hibbard, J. and J. Greene (2013), "What the evidence shows about patient activation: Better health outcomes and care experiences; fewer data on costs", *Health Affairs*, http://dx.doi.org/10.1377/hlthaff.2012.1061. [77]

Hind, J. and S. Sibbald (2015), "Mini-Review Article : Smartphone Applications for Mental Health – A Rapid Review WURJ", *Western Undergraduate Research Journal: Health and Natural Sciences*, http://dx.doi.org/10.5206/wurjhns.2014-15.16. [104]

Housden, L., S. Wong and M. Dawes (2013), "Effectiveness of group medical visits for improving diabetes care: A systematic review and meta-analysis", *CMAJ*, http://dx.doi.org/10.1503/cmaj.130053. [81]

Hujala Anneli et al. (2016), *The POTKU project (Potilas kuljettajan paikalle, Putting the Patient in the Driver's Seat), Finland*, http://www.icare4eu.org/pdf/POTKU_Case_report.pdf (accessed on 20 May 2019). [61]

Hussey, P. et al. (2012), "Closing the quality gap: revisiting the state of the science (vol. 1: bundled payment: effects on health care spending and quality).", *Evidence report/technology assessment*. [65]

IGAS (2013), *Les centres de santé : Situation économique et place dans l'offre de soins de demain*, IGAS, Rapport RM2013-119P, http://www.igas.gouv.fr/IMG/pdf/RM2013-119P-Centres_de_sante.pdf. [46]

Jacobson Vann, J. et al. (2018), *Patient reminder and recall interventions to improve immunization rates*, http://dx.doi.org/10.1002/14651858.CD003941.pub3. [26]

Jakab, M. et al. (2018), *Health systems respond to noncommunicable diseases: time for ambition*, WHO Regional Office for Europe, Copenhagen. [91]

Jakab, M. et al. (2018), "Health systems respond to NCDs: the opportunities and challenges of Leap-frogging", *Eurohealth*. [39]

Jones, K. et al. (2018), *Personal health budgets: Targeting of support and the service provider landscape*, http://www.pssru.ac.uk. [115]

Kringos, D. et al. (2013), "Europe's strong primary care systems are linked to better population health but alsoto higher health spending", *Health Affairs*, Vol. 32/4, pp. 686-694, http://dx.doi.org/10.1377/hlthaff.2012.1242. [3]

Lagarde, M., T. Powell-Jackson and D. Blaauw (n.d.), *Managing incentives for health providers and patients in the move towards universal coverage*, http://www.hsr-symposium.org. [116]

Levine, D., B. Landon and J. Linder (2019), "Quality and Experience of Outpatient Care in the UNited States for Adults with and Without Primary Care", *JAMA Internal Medicine*, Vol. 179/3, pp. 363-372. [9]

Liddy, C. et al. (2014), "Health coaching in primary care: A feasibility model for diabetes care", *BMC Family Practice*, http://dx.doi.org/10.1186/1471-2296-15-60. [82]

Lupiañez-Villanueva, F., A. Sachinopoulou and A. Theben (2015), *Oulu Self-Care (Finland) Case Study Report*, European Commission Joint Research Centre, Luxembourg, http://dx.doi.org/10.2791/692203. [100]

Luquis, R. and H. Paz (2015), "Attitudes About and Practices of Health Promotion and Prevention Among Primary Care Providers", *Health Promotion Practice*, http://dx.doi.org/10.1177/1524839914561516. [31]

MacInko, J., B. Starfield and T. Erinosho (2009), *The impact of primary healthcare on population health in low- and middle-income countries*, http://dx.doi.org/10.1097/JAC.0b013e3181994221. [2]

Macinko, J., B. Starfield and L. Shi (2003), "The contribution of primary care systems to health outcomes within Organization for Economic Cooperation and Development (OECD) countries, 1970-1998", *Health Services Research*, http://dx.doi.org/10.1111/1475-6773.00149. [1]

Ministère des Solidarités et de la Santé (n.d.), *National program « Ma santé 2022 »*, https://solidarites-sante.gouv.fr/systeme-de-sante-et-medico-social/ma-sante-2022-un-engagement-collectif/ (accessed on 2 September 2019). [44]

Mousquès, J. (2011), "Le regroupement des professionnels de santé de premiers recours : quelles perspectives économiques en termes de performance ?", *Revue française des affaires sociales*, Vol. 2-3, p. pages 253 à 275. [41]

NAP (2019), *State of the science: a synthesis of interprofessional collaborative practice research*, National Academies of Practice, Lexingtion, https://napractice.org/Portals/0/NAP%20State%20of%20the%20Science%20-%20Final%20for%20publication.pdf. [52]

National Observatory of Health care Centers (2018), *Les chiffres nationaux 2018 de l'observatoire des CDS*, https://www.fncs.org/les-chiffres-nationaux-2018-de-l-observatoire-des-cds (accessed on 2 September 2019). [47]

NCQA (2017), *Patient-Centered Medical Home Recognition*. [49]

NHS England (2018), *Personal health budgets (PHBs) NHS England.*. [113]

NHS England (2017), *Personal health budgets and Integrated Personal Commissioning National expansion plan*, NHS Policy Document 06627. [114]

Oderkirk, J. (2017), "Readiness of electronic health record systems to contribute to national health information and research", *OECD Health Working Papers*, No. 99, OECD Publishing, Paris, https://dx.doi.org/10.1787/9e296bf3-en. [120]

OECD (2018), *Policy Survey on the Future of Primary Care*. [42]

OECD (2017), *Caring for Quality in Health: Lessons Learnt from 15 Reviews of Health Care Quality*, OECD Reviews of Health Care Quality, OECD Publishing, Paris, https://dx.doi.org/10.1787/9789264267787-en. [74]

OECD (2017), *New Health Technologies: Managing Access, Value and Sustainability*, OECD Publishing, Paris, https://dx.doi.org/10.1787/9789264266438-en. [58]

OECD (2017), *Obesity Update 2017*, OECD, Paris, http://www.oecd.org/health/obesity-update.htm. [22]

OECD (2016), *Better Ways to Pay for Health Care*, OECD Health Policy Studies, OECD Publishing, Paris, https://dx.doi.org/10.1787/9789264258211-en. [64]

OECD (2015), *Cardiovascular Disease and Diabetes: Policies for Better Health and Quality of Care*, OECD Health Policy Studies, OECD Publishing, Paris, https://dx.doi.org/10.1787/9789264233010-en. [21]

OECD (2015), *Health Data Governance: Privacy, Monitoring and Research*, OECD Health Policy Studies, OECD Publishing, Paris, https://dx.doi.org/10.1787/9789264244566-en. [71]

OECD (2010), *Obesity and the Economics of Prevention: Fit not Fat*, OECD Publishing, Paris, https://dx.doi.org/10.1787/9789264084865-en. [88]

OECD/EU (2018), *Health at a Glance: Europe 2018: State of Health in the EU Cycle*, OECD Publishing, Paris/EU, Brussels, https://doi.org/10.1787/health_glance_eur-2018-en. [96]

Olsen, J. and B. Nesbitt (2010), "Health Coaching to Improve Healthy Lifestyle Behaviors: An Integrative Review", *American Journal of Health Promotion*, http://dx.doi.org/10.4278/ajhp.090313-lit-101. [79]

Ormel, H. et al. (2018), "Self-monitoring physical activity with a smartphone application in cancer patients: a randomized feasibility study (SMART-trial)", *Supportive Care in Cancer*, http://dx.doi.org/10.1007/s00520-018-4263-5. [101]

Or, Z., J. Wang and D. Jamison (2005), "International differences in the impact of doctors on health: A multilevel analysis of OECD countries", *Journal of Health Economics*, http://dx.doi.org/10.1016/j.jhealeco.2004.09.003. [20]

Outcomes Star (2019), "well-being Star: The outcomes star for adults self-managing health conditions", *Triangle Consulting Social Enterprise Limited*. [85]

Patel, M. et al. (2019), "Increase in Measles Cases — United States, January 1–April 26, 2019", *MMWR. Morbidity and Mortality Weekly Report*, http://dx.doi.org/10.15585/mmwr.mm6817e1. [23]

Patil, S. et al. (2018), *Effect of peer support interventions on cardiovascular disease risk factors in adults with diabetes: A systematic review and meta-analysis*, http://dx.doi.org/10.1186/s12889-018-5326-8. [93]

Payne, J. et al. (2018), "Defining Adherence to Dietary Self-Monitoring Using a Mobile App: A Narrative Review", *Journal of the Academy of Nutrition and Dietetics*, http://dx.doi.org/10.1016/j.jand.2018.05.011. [102]

Peikes, D. et al. (2018), "The Comprehensive Primary Care Initiative: Effects on spending, quality, patients, and physicians", *Health Affairs*, http://dx.doi.org/10.1377/hlthaff.2017.1678. [43]

Pimperl, A. et al. (2017), "Case Study: Gesundes Kinzigtal, Germany - Accountable care in Practice: Global perspectives", *Research Gate - Technical Report*. [70]

Reed, M. et al. (2012), "Outpatient electronic health records and the clinical care and outcomes of patients with diabetes mellitus", *Annals of Internal Medicine*, http://dx.doi.org/10.7326/0003-4819-157-7-201210020-00004. [63]

Reynders, D. et al. (2018), *A new drive for primary care in Europe rethinking the assessment tools and methodologies : report of the Expert Group on Health Systems Performance Assessment*, Publications Office of the European Union. [75]

Roetzhiem, RG; Pal, N; Gonzalez, EC; Ferrante, JM; Van Durme, D. (1999), "The Effects of Physican Supply on the Early Detection of Colorectal Cancer", *The Journal of Family Practice*. [17]

Rolke, K., J. Wenner and O. Razmun (2018), "Organization of access to primary health care for newly arrived refugees in Germany: a case study in the federal state of North Rhine-Westphalia.", *Public Health Panorama*, Vol. 4/4, pp. 491-735. [112]

Sans-Corrales, M. et al. (2006), *Family medicine attributes related to satisfaction, health and costs.*, http://dx.doi.org/10.1093/fampra/cmi112. [5]

Santana, M. et al. (2019), *Measuring patient-centred system performance: A scoping review of patient-centred care quality indicators*, BMJ Publishing Group, http://dx.doi.org/10.1136/bmjopen-2018-023596. [32]

Sassi, F. (ed.) (2015), *Tackling Harmful Alcohol Use: Economics and Public Health Policy*, OECD Publishing, Paris, https://dx.doi.org/10.1787/9789264181069-en. [89]

Saver, B. (2002), "Financing and Organization Findings Brief", *Academy for Research and Health Care Policy*, Vol. 5/1-2. [11]

Schäfer, W. et al. (2016), "Two decades of change in European general practice service profiles: Conditions associated with the developments in 28 countries between 1993 and 2012", *Scandinavian Journal of Primary Health Care*, Vol. 34/1, pp. 97-110, http://dx.doi.org/10.3109/02813432.2015.1132887. [28]

Schäfer, W. et al. (2019), "Are people's health care needs better met when primary care is strong? A synthesis of the results of the QUALICOPC study in 34 countries", *Primary Health Care Research & Development*, Vol. 20, p. e104, http://dx.doi.org/10.1017/S1463423619000434. [37]

Schneider, A. et al. (2016), "Costs of coordinated versus uncoordinated care in Germany: Results of a routine data analysis in Bavaria", *BMJ Open*, http://dx.doi.org/10.1136/bmjopen-2016-011621. [36]

Schottenfeld, L. et al. (2016), *Creating Patient-Centered Team-Based Primary Care*, Agency for Healthcare Research and Quality, https://pcmh.ahrq.gov/page/creating-patient-centered-team-based-primary-care. [40]

Schuchman, M., M. Fain and T. Cornwell (2018), "The Resurgence of Home-Based Primary Care Models in the United States", *Geriatrics*, http://dx.doi.org/10.3390/geriatrics3030041. [50]

Shi, L. (2005), "Primary Care, Specialty Care, and Life Chances", *International Journal of Health Services*, http://dx.doi.org/10.2190/bduu-j0jd-bvex-n90b. [13]

Shi, L. and B. Starfield (2005), "Primary Care, Income Inequality, and Self-Rated Health in the United States: A Mixed-Level Analysis", *International Journal of Health Services*, http://dx.doi.org/10.2190/n4m8-303m-72ua-p1k1. [10]

Sinsky, C. and T. Bodenheimer (2019), "Powering-Up Primary Care Teams: Advanced Team Care With In-Room Support", *Ann Fam Med*, Vol. 17/4, pp. 367-371, http://dx.doi.org/10.1370/afm.2422. [53]

Socha-Dietrich, K. (2019), *Interprofessional Teams for Complex Patients in Primary Health Care: Patients' and health professionals' experience. Fast Track Paper presented at the 25th Session of the Health Committee*, OECD, Paris. [56]

Starfield, B., L. Shi and J. Macinko (2005), "Contribution of Primary Care to Health Systems and Health", *The Milbank Quaterly*. [14]

Stokes, J. et al. (2018), *Towards incentivising integration: A typology of payments for integrated care*, http://dx.doi.org/10.1016/j.healthpol.2018.07.003. [68]

Struijs, J. and C. Baan (2011), "Integrating Care through Bundled Payments — Lessons from the Netherlands", *New England Journal of Medicine*, http://dx.doi.org/10.1056/nejmp1011849. [66]

Taleghani, F. et al. (2012), "The effects of peer support group on promoting quality of life in patients with breast cancer", *Iranian Journal of Nursing and Midwifery Research*. [95]

The Commonwealth Fund (2019), *Public Programs Are Using Incentives to Promote Healthy Behavior*, https://www.commonwealthfund.org/publications/newsletter-article/public-programs-are-using-incentives-promote-healthy-behavior. [111]

Thornton, J. (2019), "Measles cases in Europe tripled from 2017 to 2018", *BMJ (Clinical research ed.)*, http://dx.doi.org/10.1136/bmj.l634. [24]

Triantafillidis, J. et al. (2017), *Screening for colorectal cancer: The role of the primary care physician*, http://dx.doi.org/10.1097/MEG.0000000000000759. [19]

Trivedi, D. (2017), *Cochrane Review Summary: Interventions for improving outcomes in patients with multimorbidity in primary care and community settings*, Cambridge University Press, http://dx.doi.org/10.1017/S1463423616000426. [7]

Trojan, A., C. Kofahl and S. Nickel (2017), "Patient-Centered Medicine and Self-Help Groups in Germany: Self-Help Friendliness as an Approach for Patient Involvement in Healthcare Institutions", in *Patient Centered Medicine*, InTech, http://dx.doi.org/10.5772/66163. [118]

van Rinsum, C. et al. (2018), "The coaching on lifestyle (CooL) intervention for overweight and obesity: A longitudinal study into participants' lifestyle changes", *International Journal of Environmental Research and Public Health*, http://dx.doi.org/10.3390/ijerph15040680. [87]

Whitehead, L. and P. Seaton (2016), *The effectiveness of self-management mobile phone and tablet apps in long-term condition management: A systematic review*, http://dx.doi.org/10.2196/jmir.4883. [97]

WHO (2019), *New measles surveillance data for 2019*, Surveillance data, https://www.who.int/immunization/newsroom/measles-data-2019/en/. [25]

WHO (2018), *Continuity and coordination of care A practice brief to support implementation of the WHO Framework on integrated people-centred health services*, http://dx.doi.org/Licence: CC BY-NC-SA 3.0 IGO. [33]

Wolf, A. et al. (2019), "Data Resource Profile: Clinical Practice Research Datalink (CPRD) Aurum", *International Journal of Epidemiology*, http://dx.doi.org/10.1093/ije/dyz034. [72]

World Health Organization Regional Office for Europe (2016), *Lessons from transforming health services delivery: compendium of initiatives in the WHO European Region*, http://www.euro.who.int/pubrequest. [109]

Yano, E. et al. (2007), "Primary care practice organization influences colorectal cancer screening performance", *Health Services Research*, http://dx.doi.org/10.1111/j.1475-6773.2006.00643.x. [18]

Yarnall, K. et al. (2003), "Primary care: Is there enough time for Prevention?", *Am J Public Health*, Vol. 93/4, pp. 635–641. [29]

Young, C., F. Boyle and A. Mutch (2016), "Are Care Plans Suitable for the Management of Multiple Conditions?", *Journal of Comorbidity*, http://dx.doi.org/10.15256/joc.2016.6.79. [83]

Zhou, Y. et al. (2010), "Improved quality at Kaiser permanente through e-mail between physicians and patients", *Health Affairs*, http://dx.doi.org/10.1377/hlthaff.2010.0048. [62]

Notes

[1] The analysis is controlled for health needs and overall health system characteristics.

[2] The Netherlands' large increase is in part due to the low score for 1993 (0.05). The figure almost tripled by 2012 (0.14) but is still below the average (0.19).

[3] Improving health literacy is also a key strategy to support individuals in their health behaviour and improve health outcomes for all. This topic is further explored in Chapter 4 of this report.

[4] As already mentioned in Chapter 2, OECD countries vary greatly in the degree to which GPs are using EHR. In 2017, 15 countries reported that at least 90% of primary health care physician's offices were capturing patient diagnosis and treatment information in EHR (Oderkirk, 2017[120]). By contrast, Mexico and Poland reported that less than one-third of primary health care physician's offices were using EHR.

[5] Spain uses risk stratification as part of its integrated care programme implemented in the Basque Country. Care delivery is managed by Integrated Care Organisations (ICO) which oversee primary and hospital care for a defined population and provide preventive interventions and personalised medical care. There are three important health care providers as part of the ICO: hospital-based professionals, primary health care teams and a 24 hours, 7 days a week nurse-led call centre.

4 Less inequalities and more inclusive societies

This chapter builds on available evidence to present a comprehensive set of policy actions to reduce social health inequalities and promote more inclusive societies by leveraging primary health care. The first section of the chapter presents the evidence base associating strong primary health care and lower social health inequalities. This is followed by an assessment of the many financial, structural, and personal barriers impeding access to primary health care across OECD countries, which can result in or exacerbate social health inequalities. Section 4.3 presents several policy actions on both demand and supply sides to tackle social health inequalities. Special emphasis is devoted to organisation changes in primary health care necessary to bring care closer to people and communities that are typically underserved, and to enable patients to make the best of their health by addressing social and economic barriers to care.

Key Findings

- There is a robust evidence base associating strong primary health care and lower health inequalities. The published literature shows how strong primary health care is associated with better access to primary health care, reaching a broad population base when it effectively serves as the first point of contact with the health care system. Strong primary health care is better oriented than other levels of care to provide effective health promotion and prevention interventions based on the medical and social needs of patients. This helps tackle risk factors for health and other social determinants of health.
- International experience across OECD countries shows that, under current service models, primary health care is not succeeding in delivering equal access to care across different levels of socio-economic status or geographical location. For example, international figures show that in ten out of 33 OECD and EU countries, primary health care services are not affordable for more than 15% of the population, and people with lower incomes consistently have lower-utilisation rates of preventive services in virtually all EU and OECD countries.
- There are many financial, structural, and personal barriers impeding access to primary health care. Tackling health disparity and inequalities in access to care thereby requires interventions on both demand and supply sides.
  - On the supply side, reorganising primary health care and making it accessible around the clock is one way to reduce inequalities in health and access to care. Such interventions bring care closer to people and communities which are typically underserved.
    - Revisiting how health professionals are utilised (e.g. nurse practitioners, community pharmacists, and community health workers) can improve access to high quality primary health care services in remote or underserved areas where there is a shortage of primary health care physicians (as seen in Australia, France, Switzerland and the United States).
    - Digital consultation can save a lot in time and convenience for patients and primary health care physicians (as seen in Canada, Costa Rica, Korea, Norway and the United Kingdom). With appropriate governance and quality monitoring, digital consultation can effectively bring primary health care closer to where people live or work and reduce geographical barriers to care.
    - Mobile clinics have a critical role to play in providing high quality primary health care to disadvantaged populations. Not only do mobile primary health care clinics gain the trust of vulnerable populations, they also contribute to better health outcomes through improved access to screening (as seen in Germany, Latvia and Portugal), better management of chronic diseases such as mental health (as seen in France), and by addressing social determinants of health (as seen in Mexico and the United States).
  - On the demand side, addressing social and economic barriers to primary health care is critical to enabling patients to make the best of the available care.
    - User charges or other types of cost sharing for using primary health care exist in one third of OECD countries. This is not appropriate given the persisting inequalities in health and access to care. The provision of free primary health care at the point of utilisation, and reducing patient contributions, is a prerequisite for improving financial access to primary health care (as seen recently in Belgium, Greece and Iceland).
    - Integrating medical and social care is critical to addressing social determinants of health. Community health centres can specifically be designed and structured to eliminate

system wide barriers to accessing health care, such as poverty or social exclusion (as seen in Canada and the United States). It is important to provide incentives for primary health care providers to invest in social interventions or to carry out specific activities to improve disease prevention. Add-on payments for providers associated with these specific policy goals are possible options for consideration.

- Providing both culturally and linguistically adapted information about rules for access to care and available services helps patients from different social and economic backgrounds access and use primary health care services in a more timely and appropriate way. Online tools and information sessions or education courses are key policy options to improve health literacy skills for disadvantaged populations (as seen in Greece, Ireland and the Netherlands).

- Improved connections between primary health care and occupational health are critical to reducing the detrimental labour market impact of ill-health, and contributing to tackling social health inequalities for better lives and more inclusive economies. As seen in Sweden, increasing the role of primary health care providers to protect and improve the health of workers goes hand in hand with adequate education and workplace adaptations offering workers the best opportunity to fulfil their role.

4.1. Strong primary health care can improve the equity of health systems

This section shows that, according to many studies, primary health care physicians and primary health care teams are a suitable setting from which to tackle health inequalities. Overall, the literature shows that strong primary health care is associated with better access to and quality of care because it is the first point of contact with the health care system, which in turn improves the equity of outcomes. Evidence also suggests that continuous and comprehensive primary health care can provide effective health promotion and prevention interventions based on the medical and social needs of patients. This helps tackle risk factors for health and other social determinants of health, in particular for the most deprived populations.

4.1.1. As the first point of contact primary health care is able to access a larger number of people than any other specialty

A gatekeeping system, whereby primary health care physicians are controlling and orienting the patient's entry into secondary care, is becoming a key feature in several OECD countries. Gatekeeping systems are strong when there is a referral system and a patient-registration system. In the latter case, the primary health care physician acts as a care practitioner, a guide and a case manager. Strong gatekeeping systems are seen as a way to ensure that patients receive the best possible care for their conditions and for achieving greater appropriateness and co-ordination of care. In such systems, primary health care has a broader population coverage than any specialty and has a better platform for accessing a large number of people. It has direct contact with patients, and most patients will see their primary health care physician as the first point of contact within the health service. By this definition, primary health care has been found to support health equity (Chetty et al., 2016[1]).

In 18 OECD countries, primary health care physicians are the first point of contact and have the ability to refer patients to secondary care when necessary. Registering with a primary health care physician, who serves as the focal point for co-ordinating care, is mandatory in 14 OECD countries. In nine OECD countries, there is both a referral system and a patient-registration system (Table 4.1). As shown by previous studies (Starfield, Shi and Macinko, 2005[2]; Reibling and Wendt, 2013[3]; Kringos et al., 2010[4]), social inequalities in the use of health care services are lower in countries where primary health care practitioners play a more dominant role, for example, by being the first level of contact.

Table 4.1. Gatekeeping systems across OECD countries

		Are patients required or encouraged to register with a primary health care physician or practice?			
		Yes, patients are required to register	Patients are not required to register, but there are financial incentives to do so	No incentive and no obligation to register	Total number of countries
Do primary health care physicians control access to secondary care?	Yes, a referral is required	Chile, Estonia, Finland, Israel, Italy, Norway, Portugal, Slovenia, Spain,	New Zealand	Australia, Canada, Hungary, Ireland, the Netherlands, Poland, Sweden, the United Kingdom[1]	18
	Patients are not required to obtain a referral, but there are financial incentives to do so	Latvia, Lithuania, the Slovak Republic, Iceland	Belgium, Denmark, France, Switzerland	Mexico, the United States	10
	No incentive and no obligation to obtain a referral	Turkey	Germany	Austria, the Czech Republic, Greece[2], Japan[3], Korea, Luxembourg	8
	Total number of countries	14	6	16	36

1. In England, primary health care is the usual way of accessing secondary care, but in certain circumstances, patients can refer themselves for some secondary care services without consulting a GP. 2 In Greece, primary health care is in a transitional phase where people can register in primary health care facilities and thus need a referral to access specialist care. Those not yet registered can still access specialist services directly. Direct access to specialists will gradually be faded out, with the expectation that primary health care physicians will become the first point of contact for all residents.3. In Japan, patients who visit medical doctors in large hospitals without any referral will have to pay an additional fee.

Source: OECD (2016[5]), Health System Characteristics Survey, http://www.oecd.org/els/health-systems/characteristics.htm.

Empirical evidence indicates that inequalities of access to primary health care are lower than those of access to specialised care across OECD countries. Standardising for health needs, 67% of people in the lowest income quintile have seen a GP in the past 12 months, compared to 72% in the highest income quintile, which is a rather small difference (see Figure 4.1) (OECD, 2019[6]). Inequalities are significantly more pronounced when it comes to the probability of seeing a specialist: a person with low income is 12 percentage points less likely than a person with high income to see a specialist (OECD, 2019[6]).

Figure 4.1. The probability of a GP visit in the past 12 months differs by only 5 percentage points between the lowest and highest income quintiles, 2014 (or more recent data)

32 European and OECD countries

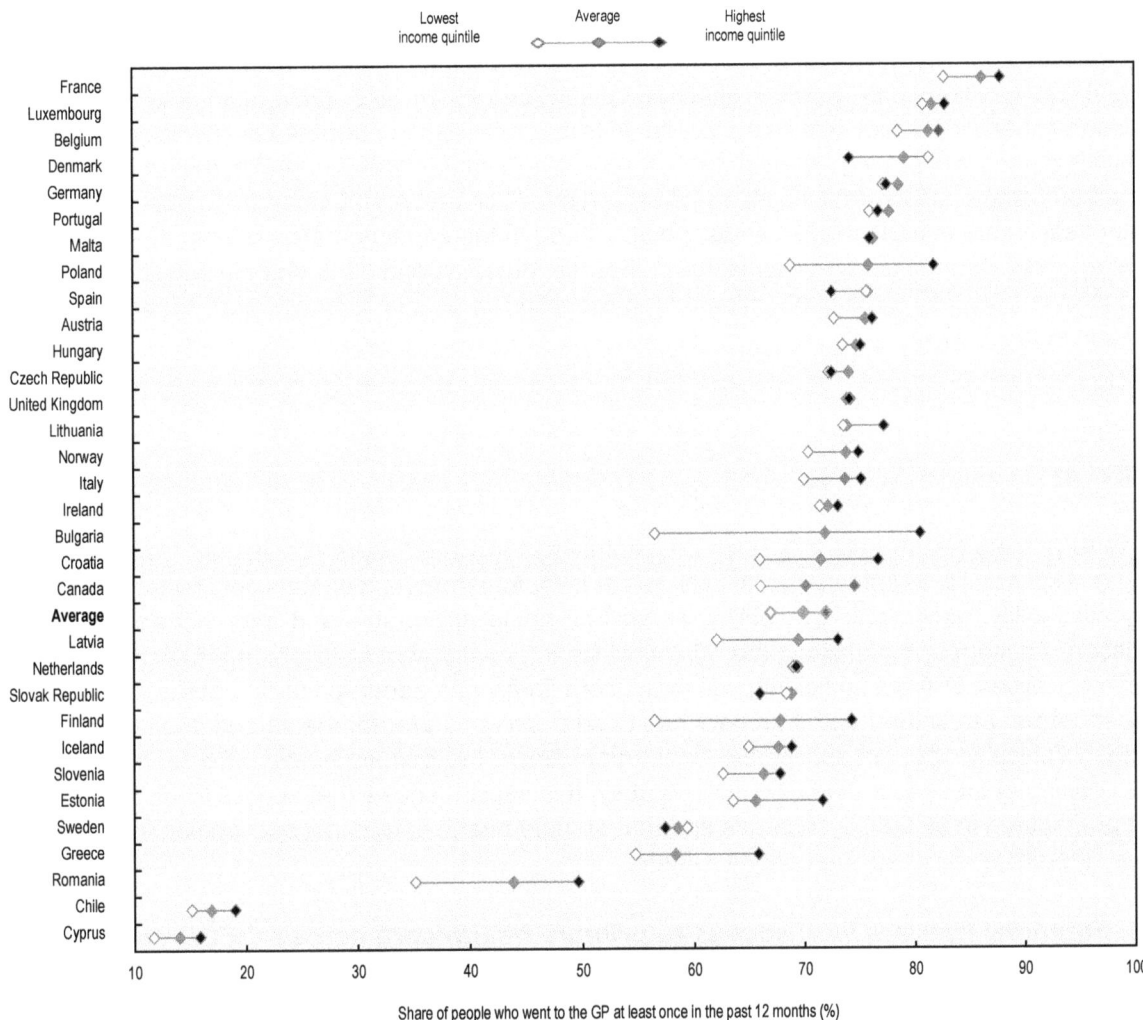

Note: Chile: visits refer to the past three months; excluded from the average. Probabilities are indirectly standardised for health care needs.
Source: OECD (2019[6]), *Health for Everyone?: Social Inequalities in Health and Health Systems*, https://dx.doi.org/10.1787/3c8385d0-en.

4.1.2. Risk factors for health and other social health determinants can be more effectively tackled with a comprehensive primary health care system and good continuity of care

By providing comprehensive and continuous care, primary health care systems can improve health equity (Chetty et al., 2016[1]; Ruano, Furler and Shi, 2015[7]). A strong primary health care sector implies a primary health care team who knows the medical history and social situation of patients. The primary health care team provides not only curative, but also preventive care to patients in their own communities. There must be a good understanding of the social context in which their patients live, which can help tackle risk factors for health and other social determinants of health. Primary health care is more able than any other specialty to provide health promotion and modify care provision based on the needs of the people they serve (Chetty et al., 2016[1]; Salmi et al., 2017[8]).

This is particularly important for vulnerable and disadvantaged people, who have an increased likelihood of poor health status than those who are better off, which is, among other things, explained by a higher exposure to risk factors detrimental to their health and lower access to preventive and health care services. Indeed, in most OECD countries, the distribution of obesity is unequally distributed among the least educated. Smoking rates are also twice as high for people in the lowest education group, compared to those in the highest group, on average across 33 countries (OECD, 2019[6]). Strong, continuous and comprehensive primary health care, that does not discern between gender, socio-economic conditions or geographical location, can provide effective health promotion and prevention interventions to the population generally (for example using mobile units in rural areas), or targeted at specific conditions (such as district nurses performing cervical cancer screening), or for specific health determinants (such as targeted smoking cessation for deprived communities) (Salmi et al., 2017[8]). In England, strengthening primary health care in underserved areas, notably through the implementation of effective intervention for secondary prevention of cardio-vascular heart disease, diabetes and other chronic conditions, has helped to reduce the absolute socio-economic gaps in mortality amenable to health care from 2007 and 2011 (Cookson et al., 2017[9]).

4.2. Accessibility of primary health care services is a challenge in many OECD countries

Access to primary health care has been conceptualised in varied ways (Levesque, Harris and Russell, 2013[10]). Accessibility to primary health care has at least four important dimensions: financial accessibility, timely availability, geographic availability, as well as being acceptable and approachable for the target population. These four dimensions are all critical for improving access to primary health care to reduce health inequalities. Without sufficient availability, both timely and geographically, access to primary health care cannot be guaranteed and if primary health care services are affordable and available (both timely and geographically), but not acceptable for the population, the primary health care service might not be used. Looking at these four dimensions separately, this section shows that access to primary health care is not guaranteed in all OECD countries and that primary health care is not succeeding in delivering care across different levels of socio-economic status.

4.2.1. Financial barriers limit access to primary health care across OECD countries

Affordability of primary health care services is critical to ensuring equitable access to primary health care. This relates to the economic capacity of people and their willingness to pay to use primary health care services. Financial accessibility to primary health care is generally measured by the proportion of the population covered by primary health care services, and by the type and scope of coverage within primary health care services. Indeed, co-payments, deductibles or cost sharing arrangements can constitute financial barriers to receiving primary health care, which limit access, further deteriorating a person's health status (OECD, 2019[6]). In addition, the 2008 global financial crisis which resulted in growing unemployment rates and increased cost of living, has worsened financial burdens for many sectors of the population. This has created an opportunity cost of seeking care in health care systems where access to primary health care is not granted for free at the point of care. In such health care systems, individuals decrease their demand for health care, and sometimes postpone seeking health care (Eurofound, 2014[11]).

In ten out of 33 countries, primary health care services are not affordable for more than 15% of the population

The Quality and Costs of Primary Care (QUALICOPC) survey shows that on average, across 35 countries, around 15% of adults postponed or abstained from a visit to the general practitioner (GP) when they needed one. Among them, 12% did so because they did not have insurance or because of other financial reasons (Figure 4.2). This proportion varies from more than 25% in Romania, Greece, New Zealand, Cyprus, Ireland and Bulgaria, to less than 5% in Austria, England, Denmark, the Netherlands, Canada, Switzerland and Finland. Overall, it appears that in 30% of European and OECD countries (ten countries out of 33), primary health care services are not affordable for more than 15% of the population. This is excessively high and not acceptable given that health inequalities persist across all OECD countries.

Figure 4.2. In ten out of 33 countries, primary health care services are not affordable for more than 15% of the population, 2013

33 European and OECD countries

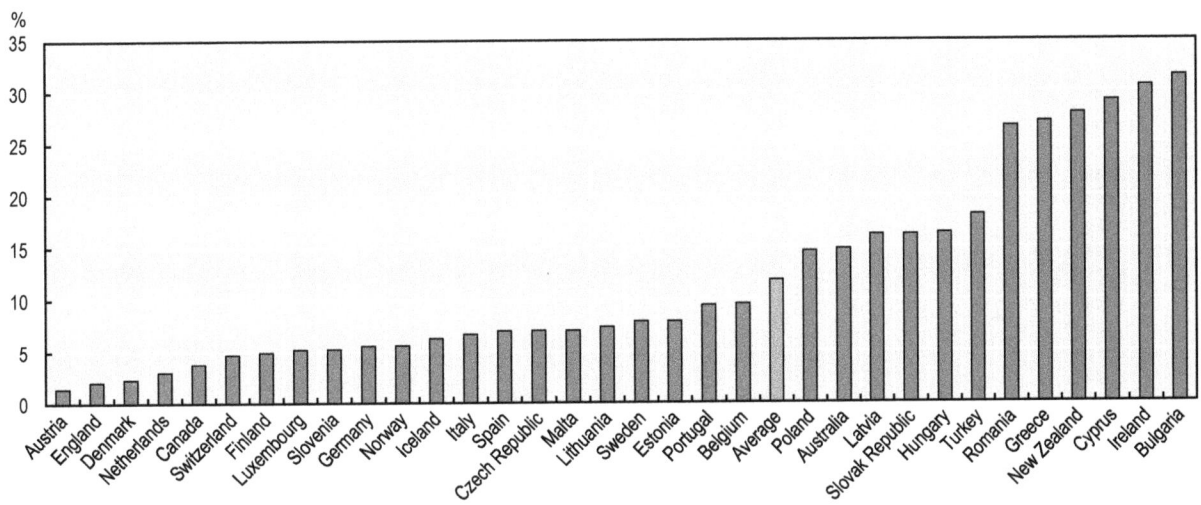

Note: There are no available data for France and Israel. The proportion refers to the adult population who have postponed or abstained from a visit to the GP when they needed one because they did not have insurance or because of other financial reasons.
Source: OECD estimates based on QUALICOPCs.

People with lower incomes have lower probability of undergoing screening

While previous work generally found no difference by income level in the probability of a GP visit (for the same level of needs) (OECD, 2019[6]), recent estimations across EU and OECD countries suggest that people with the lowest income consistently have lower utilisation rates of preventive services. Recommended preventive care is thereby not delivered equally across different socio-economic groups.

In particular, for cervical, breast and colorectal cancers, the likelihood that people in the target population and in the lowest income quintile will have undergone screening in the recommended period is significantly lower than that of people in the highest-income quintile. For instance, only 61% of women with the lowest income had cervical cancer screening, compared to 78% of women with the highest. Figure 4.3 presents the rate of cervical cancer screening, showing large income-related inequalities in screening uptake in many EU and OECD countries.

Figure 4.3. Prevalence of cervical cancer screening, by income quintile, 2014 (or more recent data)

Share of women aged 20-69 years who had a pap smear test in the past three years in 32 European and OECD countries

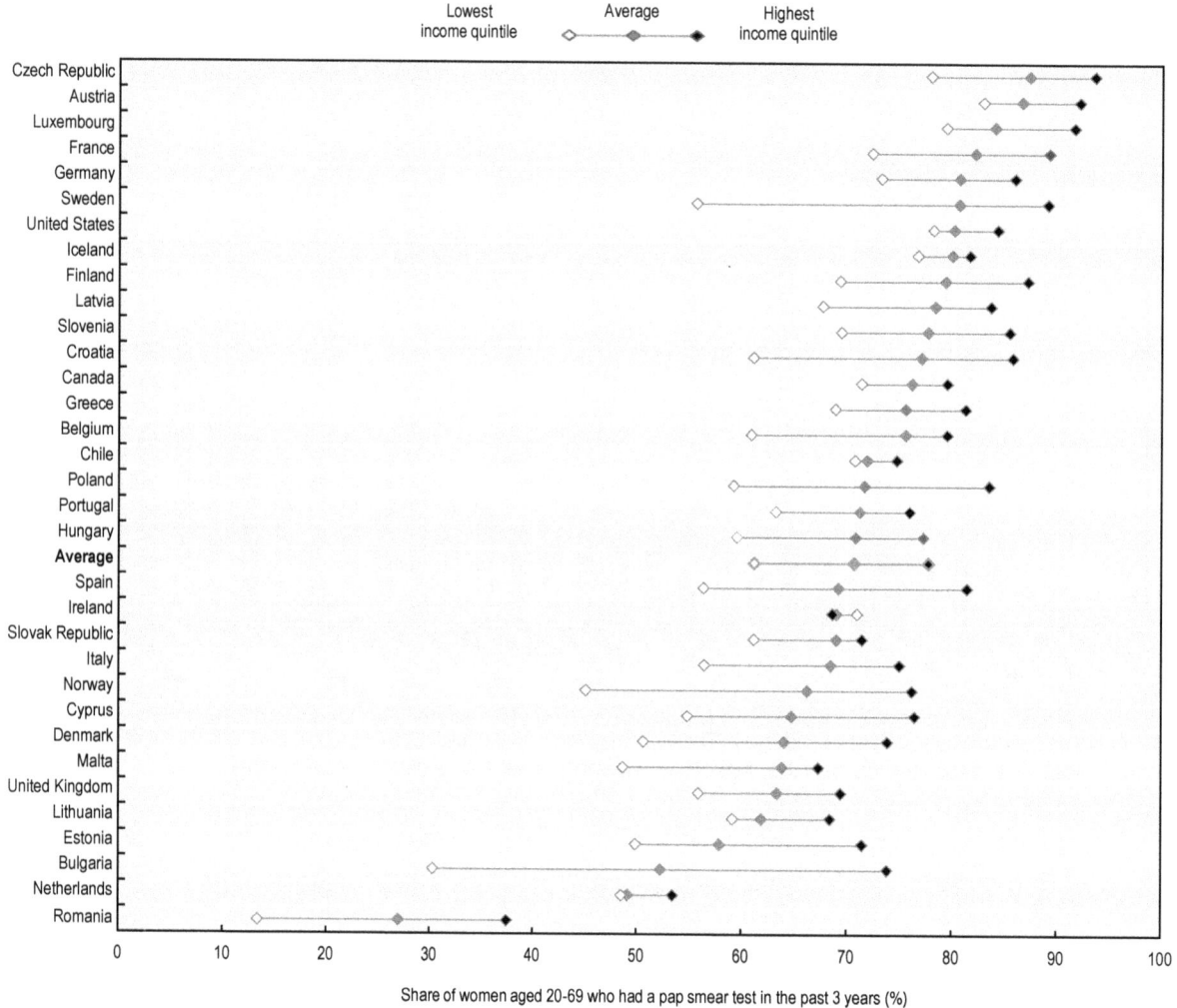

Note: Small sample size in Bulgaria (about 300 individuals per income group for this analysis). Screening rates in the Netherlands are higher based on national surveys.
Source: OECD (2019[6]), *Health for Everyone?: Social Inequalities in Health and Health Systems*, https://dx.doi.org/10.1787/3c8385d0-en.

4.2.2. Primary health care is not always available when it is needed

It is not enough to experience affordable primary health care services to actually make use of primary health care services. Access to primary health care also depends on timeliness. Primary health care services need to be available, around the clock, either in person or virtually, for all individuals when they need it. As shown by previous studies, most OECD health systems report key challenges in providing primary health care services outside working hours in an accessible and safe way (Berchet and Nader, 2016[12]). This has been also confirmed empirically using data from the QALICOPC survey. Between 2011 and 2013, 30% of people, on average, across European and OECD countries reported that it is too difficult to see a GP during evenings, nights and weekends (Figure 4.4) and in the Slovak Republic, Cyprus, and Lithuania, this number rose to more than 50%. Challenges to provide primary health care services outside normal working hours partly relate to primary health care providers' reluctance to practise due to high workload and insufficient remuneration (Berchet and Nader, 2016[12]).

Seeing a GP is also becoming more of a challenge, as patients often suffer from long waiting times to get a consultation. The QUALICOPC survey showed that more than 15% of people in 12 countries waited more than a week to get a consultation with their GP or the primary health care team (Figure 4.4). This proportion ranges from less than 3% in Belgium, the Czech Republic, Ireland, Luxembourg, the Netherlands, New Zealand, the Slovak Republic and Malta, to more than 25% of the population in Canada, Finland, Iceland, Portugal, and Sweden. Without corrective action, this problem is likely to grow in the future with increasing health care needs and expected shortage of workforce (Scheffler and Arnold, 2019[13]).

Figure 4.4. In many European and OECD countries, general practitioners are not available when patients need them, 2013

% of the adult population who reported that it was too difficult to see a GP out-of-hours (OOH), and who waited more than a week for a GP consultation in 33 European and OECD countries

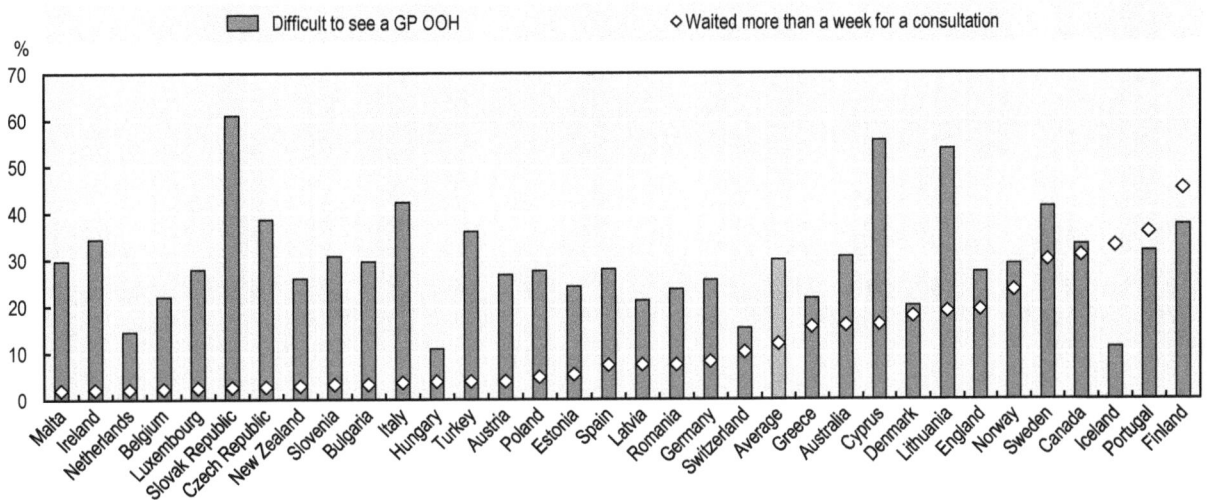

Note: There are no available data for France and Israel. The proportion refers to the adult population who reported that it was too difficult to see a GP out-of-hours (OOH), and the proportion of the adult population who waited more than a week for a GP consultation.
Source: OECD estimates based on QUALICOPC.

As a result of unavailable primary health care services, there is a high proportion of people who go to the emergency department instead of going to the GP (see Chapter 2) (OECD, 2017[14]). These emergency department visits can be costly and potentially harmful to patients. They consume emergency department inputs and jeopardise the prompt treatment of more seriously ill patients. They also lead to overcrowding and disrupt patient flow within hospitals, which might adversely affect the quality of care.

4.2.3. Geographical constraints are a barrier for access to primary health care

Access to primary health care also requires an adequate number and proper distribution of doctors in all parts of the country. Concentration of doctors in one region and shortages in others can lead to inequities in access, such as longer travel or waiting times. When the availability of health care resources in rural and remote areas is poor, geography constitutes a barrier of cost, time and inconvenience for patients. This is a source of concern since it can lead to delays in care, compromise patient safety and result in health complications. Patients living in rural and underserved areas will have to travel long distances to reach the primary health care team or will experience long waiting times, which can impede people from seeking primary health care assistance.

As shown by international figures, the density of physicians is consistently greater in urban regions. There are particularly large differences in the distribution of doctors between predominantly urban and rural regions in Canada, Hungary and the Slovak Republic, although the definition of urban and rural regions varies across countries (OECD, 2019[15]). The distribution of physicians between urban and rural regions is more equal in Japan and Korea, but there are generally fewer doctors in these two countries (Figure 4.5).

Figure 4.5. The density of physicians is consistently greater in urban regions across OECD countries, 2016 (or nearest year)

Physicians per 1 000 population in urban and rural areas across 16 OECD countries

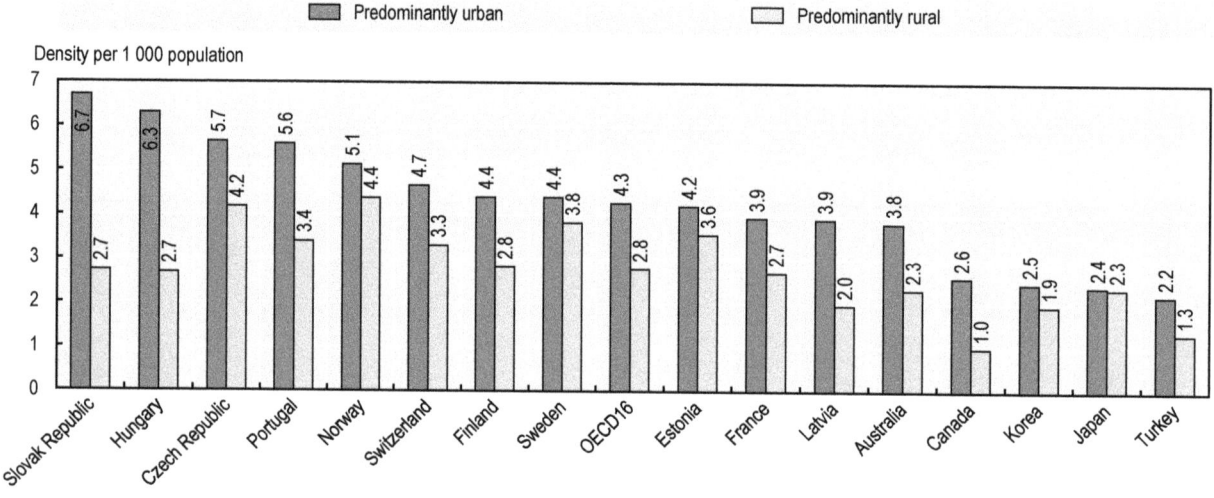

Source: OECD (2019[15]), *Health at a Glance 2019: OECD Indicators*, https://doi.org/10.1787/4dd50c09-en.

Many people across OECD and European countries postponed or abstained from a visit to their GP because they could not physically get there. In Australia, Canada, Greece, Poland, the Slovak Republic and Slovenia, at least 20% of people did not visit a primary health care practice when they needed to because they could not physically get there (Figure 4.6). In a similar vein, around 10% of people think that their GP practice is too far away from where they live or work. This proportion ranges from less than 4% in England to more than 25% in the Slovak Republic (Figure 4.6).

As shown by previous studies, people living in rural and remote areas are often the most economically deprived populations, they experience inequitable access to primary health care contributing to poorer health status than urban residents. In Australia, for example, people living in rural and remote areas have lower access to primary health care, which can be associated with higher morbidity and mortality rates. Residents from remote areas of the Northern Territory are, for example, 50% more likely to be hospitalised than those from non-remote areas (Wakerman et al., 2017[16]). Similar health disparities linked to poor access to primary health care are found in Canada and United States where there are important scattered rural and remote communities (Bosco and Oandasan, 2016[17]; Cossman, James and Wolf, 2017[18]).

Figure 4.6. In many European and OECD countries, general practitioners are not easily reached by their patients, 2013

% of the adult population who have postponed or abstained from a visit to the GP because they could not get there and % who say their local GP is too far from where they live in 33 European and OECD countries

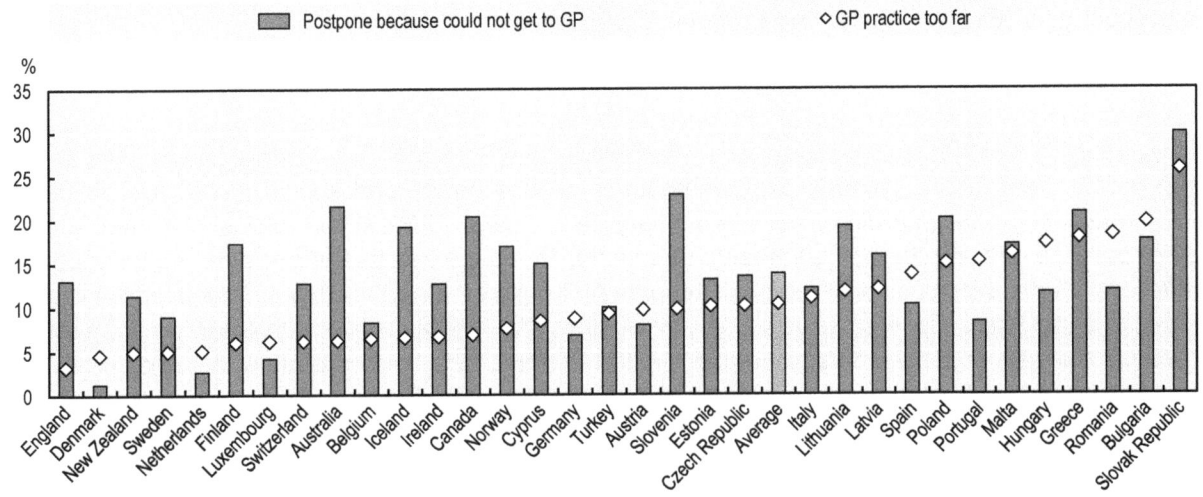

Note: There are no available data for France and Israel. The proportions refer to the adult population who have postponed or abstained from a visit to the GP when they needed one because they could not get there and to the adult population who reported that their GP practice was too far from where they lived.
Source: OECD estimates based on QUALICOPC.

4.2.4. Low health literacy may limit the acceptability and approachability of primary health care services for patients

Acceptability is an important quality component of a people-centred primary health care system. It refers to the conformity to the wishes, desires and expectations of patients and their families (Dyer, Owens and Robinson, 2016[19]). It relates to cultural and social factors and attributes of providers and patients (for example, age, gender, ethnicity and religion). Complementary to the notion of acceptability is the notion of approachability. Patients, regardless of social and ethnic origin, should be able to identify some form of services and reach them (Levesque, Harris and Russell, 2013[10]). However, primary health care services are not automatically known by the population due to a low level of health literacy, which refers to an "individual's knowledge, motivation and skills to access, understand, evaluate and apply health information" (Moreira, 2018[20]).

Individuals with low health literacy levels have particular difficulty in accessing, interpreting and navigating health information provided in or outside of health care settings. Recent estimations show that in two-thirds of European countries more than half of the people have poor levels of health literacy (Moreira, 2018[20]). Across OECD countries, at least one-third of populations have low health literacy. Low levels of health literacy are exacerbated among the most marginalised and vulnerable groups of the population (the less educated, elderly people or migrant populations, among others) (Moreira, 2018[20]). Low health literacy is associated with lower participation rates in vaccination programmes (Biasio, 2017[21]), difficulties in communicating with health providers (Schillinger et al., 2004[22]), poor adherence to medication guidelines, and more often suffer from patient safety incidents (e.g. related to medication) (Schillinger et al., 2005[23]). As a result, individuals with low health literacy have worse health outcomes (Bostock and Steptoe, 2012[24]) and experience a lower quality of care, compared to individuals with higher health literacy levels. Therefore, low health literacy strongly exacerbates health inequalities.

In addition, low health literacy has major cost implications for the health system, particularly due to increased hospital admissions and primary health care visits, suboptimal health choices and inadequate medication use by individuals with low health literacy (Moreira, 2018[20]; PriceWaterhouseCoopers, 2017[25]). A Dutch study showed that low health literacy costs the health system EUR 264 million annually, while overall societal costs reach nearly EUR 1 billion (PriceWaterhouseCoopers, 2017[25]). In the United States, additional costs related to low health literacy range between 3% to 5% of the total health care cost per year (Eichler, Wieser and Brügger, 2009[26]).

4.3. Leveraging primary health care to reduce health inequalities

Health policies and health systems can contribute to reduce health and social related inequalities by improving access to the four dimensions of primary health care. This section shows that there are two types of policy leveraging the primary health care sector to reduce health and social related inequalities. On the supply side, this consists of reorganising primary health care and making it more accessible. Such interventions bring care closer to people and communities that are typically underserved due to distance, or because they are otherwise disadvantaged. On the demand side, this consists of enabling patients to make the best of their health by addressing social and economic barriers to care.

4.3.1. Changing the organisational model of primary health care is central to improving the availability of services

This section reviews interventions that bring care closer to people and communities that are typically underserved due to distance, or because they are otherwise disadvantaged.

Readjusting the role of health care professionals to better serve the needs of remote communities

Revisiting how health care professionals are utilised, and in some cases changing their scope of practice, can improve access to primary health care services in remote or underserved areas where there is a shortage of primary health care physicians. This strategy is widely recommended to help manage the increasing demands for health care, while reducing geographical inequalities in access to care. A positive trend that is apparent in some OECD countries is the growing role of nurse practitioners and community pharmacists in carrying out patient education, disease prevention, chronic disease management and immunisations traditionally carried out only by doctors (also in Chapter 2). The development of Community Health Agents in primary health care settings is also a good policy option to improve access for people living in remote areas. Such strategies fill gaps and alleviate workforce shortages.

In Australia, the Allied Health Rural Generalist Programme is rather unique across OECD countries. It is a practical, work-integrated development programme, for early career professionals designed to meet the needs of rural and remote health services. The programme has been developed in Queensland and implementation started in 2014. The programme addresses requirements for training, development, and ongoing support (see Box 4.1). It targets health professionals in their early careers as occupational therapists, pharmacists, radiographers, nutritionists, podiatrists or physiotherapists working in rural or remote health settings. There is also a Rural Generalist medical programme for GPs in their early careers (two years clinical experience). In the latter case, this enables GPs to be upskilled so they can perform some specialist roles including, for example, anaesthetics and obstetrics. Another approach adopted in Australia is that of nurse practitioners, called remote area nurses (RAN). RAN are recognised as forming the backbone of rural and remote primary health care. They can work as part of a small team or work independently. They are available 24 hours a day, seven days a week, and have a broad scope of practice across the course of their careers. They have to work across acute, emergency, aged, palliative, mental health, family and community health care areas.

> **Box 4.1. The Allied Health Rural Generalist Program in Australia**
>
> Allied Health Rural Generalist Training Program consists of two year temporary positions to assist early career professionals to kick-start their careers in rural and remote practice in supportive and development-focused roles. Positions are supported in a team with an experienced practitioner of the same profession. This may include on-site support and development opportunities.
>
> All Allied Health Rural Generalist Training Positions benefit from:
>
> - a structured development plan.
> - up to 20% of work time allocated to training and participation in service development activities.
> - funding to undertake professional development activities such as clinical placements and workshops. Allied Health Rural Generalist Training Position sites implement innovative service development initiatives designed to improve access to high quality health care for their rural and remote communities. Initiatives can include supported telehealth service delivery, expanded scope of practice and delegation to support workers.
>
> Source: OECD (2018[27]), Policy Survey on the Future of Primary Care, completed with information taken from the Services for Australian Rural and Remote Allied Health.

In the United States, nurse practitioner roles have emerged as a solution to the existing shortage of primary health care physicians. Buerhaus (2018[28]) shows that nurse practitioners are significantly more likely than primary health care physicians to care for vulnerable populations (including ethnic minorities, women, indigenous people, the uninsured or those with low incomes). Indeed, nurse practitioners show a higher likelihood of accepting Medicaid recipients, providing care for the uninsured and accepting lower payments than physicians. Interestingly, the cost of care provided by nurse practitioners to rural populations was significantly lower than equivalent care provided by physicians. However, in many states nurse practitioners are held back by laws and regulations that restrict their scope of practice, impeding access to primary health care for many vulnerable populations (Buerhaus Peter, 2018[28]). Indeed, people in states with more restrictive legislation for nurse practitioners had significantly less geographic access to primary health care. This is also confirmed by Maier and Aiken (2016[29]) who show that restrictive regulations had unintended consequences on access and cost of health care in the United States (Maier and Aiken, 2016[29]). Allowing nurse practitioners to practice to the fullest extent of their training and ability, and removing restrictions that limit their scope of practice, is a key policy option for consideration.

Community health workers have also been developed in the United States, notably to address social determinants of health, and to promote health care access for vulnerable and hard to reach populations (Hartzler et al., 2018[30]). Community health aides, for example, provide primary health care services in remote Alaskan villages, whose population would otherwise have no access to appropriate health care delivery (Golnick et al., 2012[31]). They are the first point of contact with the health care system for the population living in these very remote villages. They work under the supervision of community health practitioners, and there is an integrated referral system that includes physicians, regional hospitals and a tertiary hospital (Golnick et al., 2012[31]). The range of primary health care services delivered by community health aides mostly includes care for chronic and preventive treatment, and emergency visits (often for respiratory distress and chest pain) (see also Chapter 2 for additional examples).

As in other OECD countries, France is currently extending the role of nurses and pharmacists, which is seen as a key policy lever to improve access in underserved areas where the number of primary health care physicians is decreasing. Compared to Australia and the United States, France is in the early stages of implementation. The new decree establishing the profession of Advanced Nurse Practitioner (*Infirmière en Pratique Avancée*) was issued in June 2018. The Advanced Nurse Practitioner will work within a primary health care team to manage patients having chronic conditions and take the lead in prevention and co-ordination. In parallel, the role of community pharmacists is gradually increasing. Community pharmacists are allowed to perform three rapid diagnostic orientation tests: the capillary blood glucose test for diabetes screening; the oropharyngeal tests for influenza; and the group A streptococcal tonsillitis test. The objective is to determine if antibiotic treatment is necessary and if a visit to the doctor is required for a prescription. The community pharmacist can also participate in punctual screening programmes for chronic obstructive pulmonary disease (COPD). The pilot vaccination programme in community pharmacies in the regions of Auvergne-Rhone-Alpes and Nouvelle-Aquitaine was also a success. Recent evaluation showed that the scheme increased convenience for people with no adverse consequences for patient safety. The programme is now extended in the regions of Haut de France and Occitanie. While these initiatives are welcomed in recognising that pharmacists should play a fundamental role in providing urgent primary health care for patients with minor self-limiting illnesses and preventive care, it will be important to build patient awareness around these initiatives. Policy makers need to communicate to ensure that patients are well aware of the services offered by community pharmacists.

To face a relative shortage of GPs in Switzerland, the Swiss Pharmacist's Association (pharm-suisse) has developed Netcare. The objective is to offer opportunities to pharmacists to provide primary triage using a structured decision tree for 24 common conditions. If needed, community pharmacists can request a real-time video-consultation with a physician (see Box 4.2). All pharmacists offering NetCare have to complete two training courses: one course covering the most common medical conditions observed in primary health care, and one course on all the decision trees.

Recent evaluations show that NetCare pharmacists could resolve around 75% of the cases presented to them, and nearly 20% of conditions were managed by the pharmacist with physician backup via the telemedicine centre (Erni et al., 2016[32]). Among the latter, 88% of cases were solved after teleconsultation. Overall, findings show that if pharmacists and physicians are equally successful in treating common conditions, the NetCare service is substantially less costly than comparators. The NetCare programme, which was initially in a pilot phase in 2013 and 2014, is now rolled-out nationally. By 2017, 309 pharmacies were enrolled in the NetCare project. The position of community pharmacists as gatekeepers to the health care system has been recognised through the integration of NetCare pharmacies into some health insurance schemes.

As shown in Chapter 2, community pharmacists in Finland, Italy and the United Kingdom also carry out patient education, preventive treatments, chronic disease management or immunisations traditionally carried out only by doctors.

While there is compelling evidence on the effectiveness and safety of care provided by nurse practitioners and pharmacists, experience from OECD countries shows that embracing workforce flexibility and expansion of clinical roles is difficult to implement. Policy makers need to ensure that primary health care staff uses their competencies, and are not held back by laws and rigidities that restrict their scope of practice (see also Chapter 2). Not doing so would exacerbate barriers of access to care and lead to a dramatic waste in human capital.

> **Box 4.2. Collaboration between physicians and pharmacists in primary health care in Switzerland: The NetCare programme**
>
> Assessment of a patient's medical condition consists of a two-step process. The first step consists of checking for the exclusion criteria, which relates to patients with severe co-morbidities, unclear clinical situations, or alarming symptoms. The second step consists of assessing the patient's medical condition with the specific decision tree, which can result in:
>
> - Management by the pharmacist (counselling and dispensing of over the counter drugs), the pharmacist will also make a follow-up call to check the patient's condition three days after the assessment.
> - Management by the pharmacist with physician backup via the telemedicine centre with a secure video consultation. If appropriate, a prescription is sent to the pharmacy.
> - Referral to either an emergency room or GP for a face-to-face consultation.
>
> Source: OECD (2018[27]), Policy Survey on the Future of Primary Care and Erni et al (2016[32]), "netCare, a new collaborative primary health care service based in Swiss community pharmacies", https://doi.org/10.1016/j.sapharm.2015.08.010.

Improved use of alternatives to face-to-face consultations can save time and be more convenient for patients and providers

As long-distance travel, together with a lack of primary health care providers, can create barriers of access to primary health care, several OECD countries introduced alternatives to face-to-face consultation through the use of telemedicine. Telemedicine involves the use of information and communication technologies to deliver health care at distance. Telemedicine, through video consultation for example, makes primary health care services available to patients closer to their home or work. It allows communication between patients and medical staff, as well as the transmission of medical records and other data between different locations. Teleconsultation is a very promising way to improve access – both timely and geographically – and to relieve pressure on primary health care physicians.

The policy survey indicates that 16 countries out of 26 have implemented policy measures to promote the use of telemedicine for primary health care delivery (Australia, Belgium, Canada, Costa Rica, the Czech Republic Estonia, France, Germany, Iceland, Israel, Ireland, Italy, Mexico, the Netherlands, Switzerland and Turkey). Most often, this takes the form of real-time or asynchronous telemedicine services, in either the public or private sector.

In Norway, the University of Tromsø piloted the first applications from the end of the 1980s in the north and west of the country, where populations are isolated. Health insurance providers in Norway finance the practice. In primary health care, video consultations are performed, for example, for COPD patients at risk of exacerbation or for adults with mental health problems (Zanaboni, Knarvik and Wootton, 2014[33]). In Sweden, since 2018, access to primary health care over the internet is free via DoKtor.se. Patients will first consult a nurse who will assess their medical needs. Patients not suitable for digital consultations will be advised to seek face-to-face consultation with a primary health care physician. In Finland, patients in remote areas where the supply of primary health care providers is limited, can use "health uts" to access remote primary health care services (Cravo Oliveira Hashiguchi, 2020[34]). In Costa Rica, telemedicine has also been utilised for more than five years for patients living in remote areas where access is difficult. In the Czech Republic, the private International Center for Telemedicine offers services in cardiology and diabetes.

In Canada, the province of Saskatchewan has been using telehealth technology for over a decade to reach rural and remote locations[1]. Telehealth connects patients to health care professionals using live, two-way videoconferencing technology and equipment. This secure service is available in many health care facilities across the province and allows patients and doctors to communicate, both verbally and visually, from two completely separate areas of the province. Patients can receive primary health care by visiting the nearest telehealth site and meeting with a professional in a virtual exam room. Telehealth can connect to available diagnostic peripherals, such as stethoscopes, vital signs monitors and ultrasound equipment, making real-time diagnosis and patient monitoring possible. In rural and remote areas, telehealth services are particularly used for mental health and addiction appointments, for prescription refills and chronic disease management.

In addition, as of 2017, Saskatchewan began piloting remote presence technology for a number of northern communities. Remote presence technology (RPT) is an advanced telemedicine technology that allows an expert (physician, nurse, pharmacist, etc.) to be "present" in the community. Essentially, it allows the team in the community to have access to expertise on demand. This provides increased patient access to health services, regardless of location, and gives the patient the ability to access these services without leaving their own community, even from within their own home.

Similar services exist in Lithuania, with the Dermtest application which allows physicians to send dermatological images to specialists. In Portugal, since 2018, primary health care physicians are required by law to attach pictures of any skin lesion when referring a patient to a first dermatology consultation at the hospital.

In Korea, medical doctors may give digital consultations in a remote area by using ICT, such as computers or visual communication systems. A pilot medical outreach programme has been in operation since September 2014. It targets medically underserved areas and utilises the Digital Health Innovation System (DHIS). In Japan, teleradiology and telepathology are also widely used.

Ireland has recently established pilot mental telehealth sites. In addition, the Sláintecare Action Plan (a ten-year programme to implement a Citizen Care Plan) has targeted the development of telehealth solutions and work with stakeholders is ongoing.

In France, the 2018-22 National Health Strategy gives new impetus to telemedicine, with sufficient funding to promote its development. Developing telemedicine is part of the national strategy to improve access to health care and reduce health inequalities related to workforce shortages in remote and rural areas. The *2018 Loi de Financement de la Sécurité Sociales* (Art.36) allows the funding of teleconsultations and tele-expertise in France. Starting in autumn 2018, video consultations (between medical doctors and patients) and tele-expertise (between medical doctors) became nationally available after several years of ad-hoc trials (see Box 4.3 for an example of video-consultation in France). The national health insurance fund and medical professions' representatives have agreed on a set of tariffs for telehealth. Key policy levers helped accelerate the deployment of telemedicine in France including the provision of financial support; organisational support; and reductions in administrative procedures.

Other similar services exist in the United Kingdom (PushDoctor and Babylon GP at Hand[2], see also Chapter 2 for further details), in Germany (Medlanes), in Switzerland (Medgate) or in Belgium (ViVIDoctor). While digital GP services have great potential to improve access to primary health care services, policy makers need to ensure these new services offer safe and high-quality care, and usage levels are appropriate. The Care Quality Commission in England for example conducts annual inspection of digital services. The 2019 inspection has shown that PushDoctor delivers safe, effective, and responsive services (Care Quality Commission, 2019[35]). Areas of outstanding practice include investment in staff training and development, encouraging team work, listening to patient feedback and implementing a continuous quality improvement audit programme. From the patient perspective, digital consultations also appear very convenient and of easy access. A recent independent evaluation has found high patient satisfaction rates with Babylon GP at Hand, and feedback on aspects of the quality of care was good (Quigley, Hex and

Aznar, 2019[36]). However, Babylon GP at Hand has found an increase in demand for teleconsultations, notably for younger and healthier patients, which questions the suitability of the service for some patients (Iacobucci, 2019[37]). Indeed, patient's experiences were less positive for patients with complex needs (Quigley, Hex and Aznar, 2019[36]).

> **Box 4.3. LIVI is one of the new digital GP services to deliver an alternative to face-to-face consultations in France**
>
> The overarching objective of LIVI is to meet the growing demand for unplanned care. The LIVI digital service aims at reducing pressure on general practitioners (GPs) and emergency departments, as well as improving access to care for those living in areas characterised by provider shortages and geographical mal-distribution. The Digital GP service targets patients with minor self-limiting illness, who could not get a consultation with their GP within 48 hours.
>
> LIVI provides non-face-to-face consultation with a graduate GP practicing in France, registered with the National Council of Physicians.
>
> Invoiced at the same price as a face-to-face consultation, a LIVI teleconsultation costs EUR 25 and is reimbursed by the French Social Security.
>
> LIVI is also present in other OECD countries including Norway, Spain, Sweden and the United Kingdom. In France, there are many other platforms providing non-face-to-face consultation including, among others, Doctolib, Qare, or MedecinDirect.

Together, such evidence demonstrates the need for policy makers to ensure that video-consultation and other digital health services are well-regulated to provide an equally safe and high quality service as face-to-face consultations, and sub-optimal use should not be encouraged (Cravo Oliveira Hashiguchi, 2020[34]). Health care quality inspections of digital GP services that monitor and assess the care delivered is a step in the right direction. Monitoring care quality delivered as part of GP digital services is critical to ensure that such innovations offer value for OECD health care systems.

Yet, there are too few evaluations demonstrating the impact of non-face-to-face consultation on health care quality, patient satisfaction and physician workload. Caffery et al (2017[38]) show that telemedicine improves health outcomes among indigenous communities by increasing access for rural and remote patients suffering from multiple chronic conditions and limited resources (Caffery et al., 2017[38]). A recent evaluation based on interviews with GPs, other staff members and patients in the United Kingdom showed that patients appreciated the efficiency and convenience offered by alternatives to face-to-face consultations (Atherton et al., 2018[39]). In the United States, current studies show that the availability of online tools has allowed providers to offer high quality care for their patients, and that it provided convenient medical care, notably after-hours care. Video consultation provided immediate and convenient solutions for people who otherwise would have to travel or wait for a face-to-face clinical evaluation (Pearl, 2014[40]). A recent umbrella review of systematic reviews and meta-analysis of telemedicine in OECD countries shows that telemedicine can lead to gains in effectiveness, efficiency and equity in the health system (see also Chapter 2) (Cravo Oliveira Hashiguchi, 2020[34]). It shows the evidence base associating telemedicine with improvements in access to care, reduced travelling costs and better equity for rural and indigenous populations (Cravo Oliveira Hashiguchi, 2020[34]). As noted, the challenge is that patients who would most likely benefit from digital technology are also those most likely to face difficulties in accessing and using it. This is the case of rural populations (whose broadband access is not always appropriate), but also the elderly, and people in the lowest income quintiles or lowest education groups.

Mobile facilities can be particularly relevant to reach the most deprived and marginalised populations

Primary health care services may not be appropriately designed and organised to reach the most vulnerable populations in the best way. People with low income, rural populations, homeless or other minority groups, often have poorer health, have multiple risk factors for diseases and face a higher number of barriers in accessing health care services (OECD, 2019[6]). The health care system needs to redesign the service delivery model to better reach out to these population groups. Mobile health clinics are an innovative model of health care delivery that can help alleviate health disparities in the most vulnerable populations (Peritogiannis et al., 2017[41]; Yu et al., 2017[42]).

Mobile health clinics provide a wide range of primary health care services (including preventive care, mental health or dental care services) from a bus or a van equipped with all of the necessary technology to provide clinical services in underserved or disadvantaged areas. Such facilities provide community-tailored care to vulnerable populations, both in urban and rural areas, to overcome barriers of time, money, or distance. They are particularly effective in providing urgent care or preventive health care, and for initiating chronic disease management. Although continuity of care can be difficult to maintain under such models of care, specific arrangements may be implemented to overcome this limitation. For example, mobile health care facilities may be equipped with the information and resources to help patients navigate through the health care system, and to connect them with the medical and social services in their community. Mobile health care facilities provide accessible and sustainable high-quality care, such as that performed in more traditional health care settings.

Empirical findings show that mobile clinics in the United States have a critical role to play in providing high quality primary health care at a low cost to vulnerable populations (Yu et al., 2017[42]). Mobile primary health care clinics have been shown not only to be able to engage with and gain the trust of vulnerable populations, but also to improve individual health outcomes through improved access to screening, preventive care, and management of chronic diseases, such as mental health issues. Interestingly, mobile primary health care facilities have also been shown to address social determinants of health through the delivery of social services.

In Mexico, there are 50 Health Windows, one in each of the consulates, plus two Mobile Windows in Kansas City and New Jersey, which provide timely information and access to community centres with cultural sensitivity for Mexican families in the United States. Mobile health care facilities have the objective of extending primary health care to localities that do not have access to health services due to their geographic dispersion or characteristics of the population. In Germany and Portugal, mobile health clinics are being implemented in some rural areas to guarantee adequate primary health care and to help alleviate workforce shortages.

In some other OECD countries, mobile health care units provide specific services. In Latvia, mobile primary health care facilities are specifically designed to perform mammogram screening, and physical health and dental checks in rural areas. In France, mobile health care units target mental health care needs. The service called *équipes mobiles psychiatrie précarité* (EMPP) aims at reaching the most vulnerable populations, including the homeless, migrants, marginalised people or minority groups, who are particularly at risk of mental disorders. EMPP provide prevention services, and are responsible for the identification of needs to orient patients and ease access to care if medically required. The service is recognised as an interface between the primary health care sector and psychiatric sectors, enabling co-ordination of care teams between, and across, the health and social sector. In a similar vein, Greece provides community mental health services in rural areas through the development of Mobile Mental Health Units (MMHUs). MMHUs were introduced in rural and remote areas of the mainland and in several of the numerous Greek islands. MMHUs use the resources and infrastructure of the primary health care system to provide a range of services, including: diagnosis and evidence-based treatment, enhancing patient skills, education and support for families, and educational programmes for the community. All services are free of charge. The team consists of nine members: one psychiatrist, two psychologists, two nurses, two health visitors and two social workers. The MMHU provides visits to the eight primary health care centres in the catchment area once a week, and also provides home visits. As shown by previous evaluations, MMHU has contributed to the reduction of hospitalisations and to ease access to care for patients with psychotic disorders (Peritogiannis et al., 2017[41]).

4.3.2. Addressing social and economic barriers to care

On the demand side, there are interventions aimed at enabling patients to make the best of the available care by addressing social and economic barriers to care. These consist of guaranteeing affordable primary health care services, building community efforts to provide both social and medical services, engaging health activities in the workplace and increasing patient health literacy. These policies targeting patients matter when it comes to make primary health care services affordable, approachable and acceptable.

Expanding coverage of primary health care services

As shown in Section 2.1, financial barriers to primary health care are still too significant across OECD countries. Co-payments, deductibles or cost sharing arrangements constitute financial barriers to receiving primary health care especially for low- and middle-income groups.

Responses from the 2016 OECD Health System Characteristics Survey show that user charges or other types of cost sharing for using primary health care exist in 12 countries out of 32 countries (see Figure 4.7). In Belgium, France, Luxembourg and Switzerland, for example, patients have to pay the full cost of health services and get reimbursed for covered services afterwards. In Finland, Iceland, Japan, Latvia, Norway, Portugal, Slovenia and Sweden patients pay user fees or co-payments. In only 20 out of 32 countries, patients receive free services at the point of care (Australia, Austria, Canada, Chile, Costa Rica, the Czech Republic, Denmark, Estonia, Germany, Greece, Ireland, Israel, Italy, Lithuania, Mexico, the Netherlands, Poland, Spain, Turkey and the United Kingdom).

The 2018 OECD Policy Survey on the Future of Primary Care also shows that in at least one-third of responding countries (Belgium, the Czech Republic, Germany, Iceland, Italy, Latvia, Mexico, Sweden and Switzerland), there are plans to increase, or introduce, user charges or other types of cost sharing for using primary health care. This is not appropriate given the persisting inequalities in health and access to care. The population in some OECD countries already face high levels of co-payment per visit to the primary health care physician. As of 2016, co-payment per visit ranges from EUR 1 in France, EUR 1.42 in Latvia, to around EUR 14 in Norway (NOK 136) and Finland (FIM 82). In Ireland, out-of-pocket payments for primary health care services are dramatically higher and patients are required to pay up to EUR 60 to see the GP, unless they have a medical card. Applications for the medical card are means-tested and application forms need to be signed by a GP. In Australia, Medicare data show that, while most GP visits are free for the patient at the point of care (for 86% of attendances in 2017-18), out-of-pocket contributions have increased by 20% since 2013-14, and from AUD 35.83 to AUD 37.39 on average between 2016-17 and 2017-18 (The Royal Australian College of General Practitioners, 2018[43]; Australian Government Department of Health, 2019[44]).

Although exemptions to pay co-payments exist in many OECD countries for the poorest patients and/or to patients with chronic conditions, cost-sharing policies, even where minimal, remain an obstacle to accessing primary health care services, including for middle-class households.

Figure 4.7. In 20 OECD countries out of 32, patients receive free primary health care services at the point of care

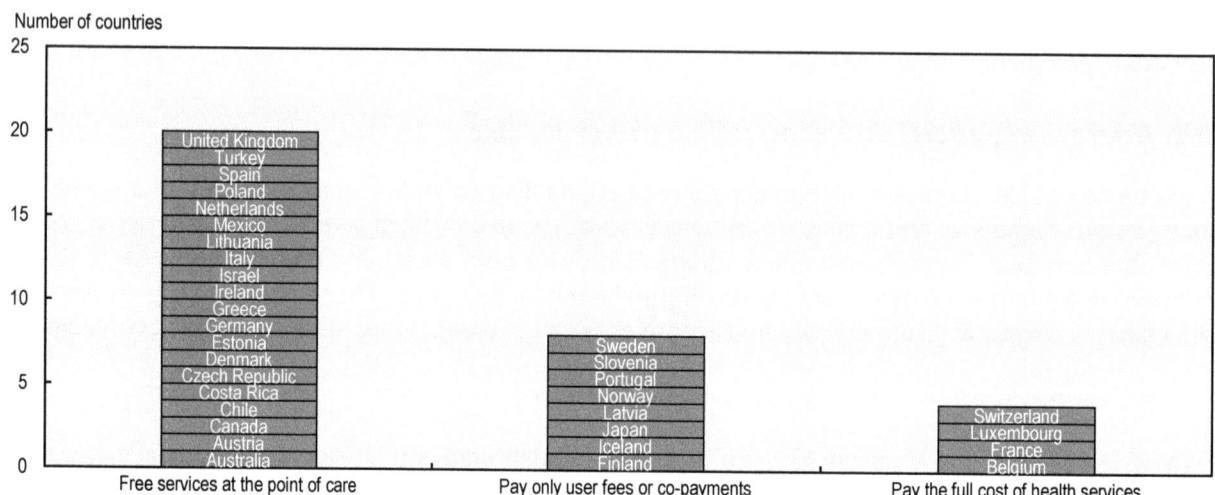

Note: In Australia, Medicare provides all Australians with subsidised or no-cost access to a wide range of primary health care services (through provision of fee-for-service patient benefits) and prescription medicines. In Belgium, France, Luxembourg and Switzerland, patients pay the full cost of primary health care services and get reimbursed for covered services afterwards.
Source: OECD (2016[5]), Health System Characteristics Survey, http://www.oecd.org/els/health-systems/characteristics.htm.

Previous work shows that covering health care costs for populations not previously covered increases their use of health care services, which also improves health outcomes, particularly among the poorest populations and children (Bourgueil, Jusot and Leleu Henri, 2012[45]). For that reason, several OECD countries are taking steps to remove financial barriers that impede access to primary health care. These strategies range from making primary health care free at the point of care (as seen in Greece in 2016) to reducing the amount of out-of-pocket payments or setting a ceiling (as seen in Belgium and Iceland in 2017).

In Greece, coverage used to be mainly linked to employment status through social health insurance for employees and their families. With the 2008 financial crisis, a lot of Greek citizens had fallen out of insurance coverage through unemployment or because they were unable to keep up contributions. Over 2 million people were still not able to access publicly financed services by 2015. The problem was solved in 2016 as the coverage has become universal thanks to legislation to ensure that all Greek citizens can again access the health benefits package. All Greek citizens were given the right to primary health care. Achieving universal coverage with primary health care services is the best option for improving access to care for the entire population.

Belgium implemented another strategy by introducing a bill to prevent patients from paying out-of-pocket payments above a certain threshold. In 2017, the government in Iceland introduced a new system of setting user charges in order to reduce the cost of health care for frequent users. The new system defines a maximum amount to be paid every three months. When the upper limit is reached, patients will only pay a low fixed sum every month using the primary health care service.

Expanding coverage of primary health care services by making primary health care free at the point of care, or by reducing co-payments or cost sharing exemptions, should be a priority in all OECD countries.

Integrating primary health care and social care can address important social health determinants

Beyond ensuring affordable access to primary health care, integrating primary health care and social care is necessary to address social determinants of health. Community health centres are specifically designed and structured to eliminate system wide barriers to accessing health care such as poverty, social exclusion and housing, which are generally associated with mental health issues.

In the Scotland, the Links Worker Programme makes links between people and their communities through their GP practice. The programme, funded by the Scottish Government, aims at mitigating the impact of the social determinants of health in people that live in areas of high socio-economic deprivation. The programme uses social prescribing approaches to support general medical practices to link people with local community resources (such as group learning, healthy eating advice, sports associations, cookery or art activities) that could help them to live well in their communities. From April 2014, the programme was tested in seven general medical practices serving very deprived populations in Glasgow with a further eight similar practices acting as a comparison group. An evaluation of the programme, commissioned by NHS Health Scotland, showed some improvement in health outcomes regarding anxiety symptoms, depressive symptoms, and self-reported exercise levels (Mercer et al., 2017[46]).

In Canada, the Access Centres and Community Health Centres are non-profit organisations that provide primary health care and health promotion programmes for individuals, families and communities. The overarching objective is to strengthen people's capacity to take more responsibility for their health and well-being, by providing education and advice. Community health centres work together with others on health promotion initiatives within schools, in housing developments and in the workplace. An interesting characteristic is the fact that they are bridging together families and individuals with support or self-help groups that offer peer education, support in coping or are working to address social conditions that affect health. Health promotion programmes that contribute to the development of healthy communities, include stress management, parenting education, counselling and education related to weight. For the youth aged between 14 and 24, specific programmes offered by the Community Health Centres include addressing risks associated with poverty, teen pregnancy, sponsorship of community kitchens, self-help groups related to family violence, support to find employment, and family counselling.

Similarly, in the United States, community efforts have been deployed to effectively manage patients with complex clinical and social needs by integrating primary health care and social services. Social needs include housing, food insecurity, and assistance with utilities or transportation. The development of such innovative service delivery models has been initiated by bottom-up innovations driven by community-led efforts. As of 2018, 301 community partnerships across the United States have been identified. To facilitate peer learning, the Center for Medicare and Medicaid Innovation has recently launched the Accountable Health Communities Program (Amarasingham et al., 2018[47]). This is a five-year programme which aims at supporting service delivery approaches that will link beneficiaries with community services that may address their health-related social needs, for example, housing instability, food insecurity, utility needs, domestic violence, and transportation needs (Amarasingham et al., 2018[47]).

Efforts at community level to address both medical and social needs have great potential to tackle social determinants of health and reduce health inequalities. As part of this process, it is equally important to issue incentives for providers to encourage investment. As documented in Chapter 2, add-on payments could encourage primary health care providers to invest in social interventions or to carry out specific activities to improve preventive care.

Primary health care actions conducted in the workplace help to promote more inclusive economies

Engaging primary health care action in the workplace is a key policy lever to tackle social health determinants and encourage fulfilment of employees. Physical and mental risk factors at work are important determinants of health, with direct consequences on current and future health status, as well as on future employment prospects. Currently, exposure at work to injuries, noise, carcinogenic agents, airborne particles and ergonomic risks accounts for a substantial part of the burden of chronic diseases (for example 37% of all cases of back pain and 11% of asthma) (WHO, 2017[48]).

Connecting primary health care and occupational health is thereby critical for better prevention of chronic conditions (such as musculoskeletal or mental health disorders) that lead to absenteeism or early departure from the labour force (James, Devaux and Sassi, 2017[49]). Through closer integration between primary health care and work, health policies can play an important role in reducing the detrimental labour market impact of ill-health, contributing to reducing social health inequalities and promoting better lives and more inclusive economies.

Primary health care could take a more proactive role in this direction. Yet in 2018, only ten out of 24 countries that participated in the OECD Policy Survey on the Future of Primary care had implemented concrete measures aimed at strengthening the role of primary health care in protecting and improving workers health (Figure 4.8). This is despite evidence suggesting the effectiveness of primary health care interventions to protect workers' health (Nicholson and Gration, 2017[50]). It will be vital to increase focus on prevention activities in the workplace across OECD health care systems.

Figure 4.8. Less than half of OECD countries implemented concrete policy measures aimed at strengthening the role of primary health care in protecting and improving workers' health

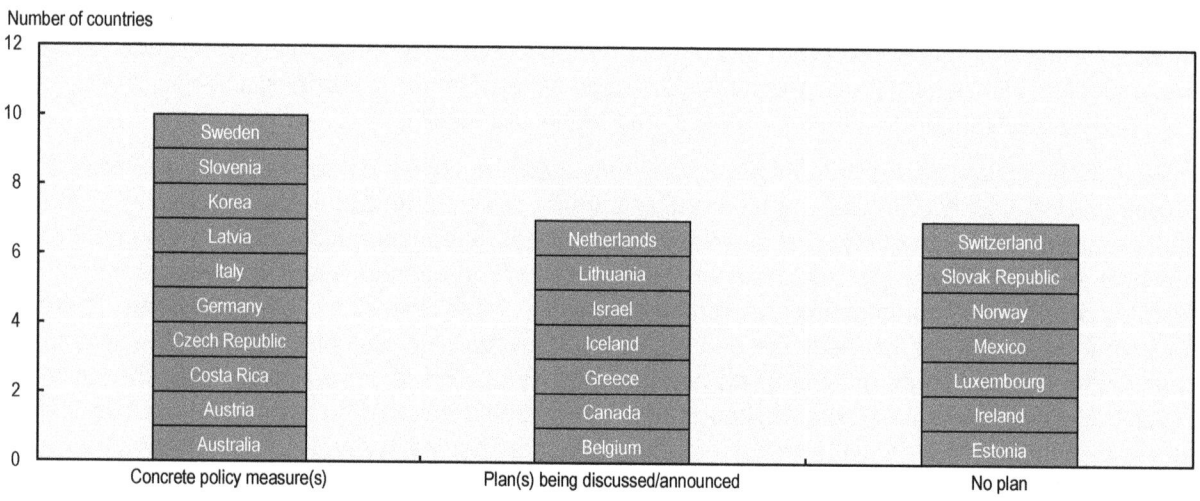

Note: Countries were asked whether policy measures aimed at strengthening the role of primary health care in protecting and improving workers' health were introduced in recent years.
Source: OECD (2018[27]), Policy Survey on the Future of Primary Care.

Primary health care needs to do more to protect workers' physical and mental health. This could include strategies promoting mental and physical health awareness amongst managers, changes to the physical working environment, improving social relations at work, and offering programmes dedicated to encouraging disabled people to return to work. Equally important is the health surveillance of workers, through assessing and responding to mental stress and physical strain at work.

Among OECD countries, the few good examples include Belgium, Germany and Sweden, which all focus on prevention of mental distress at work and on return to work programmes for people who suffer from a disabling experience. Sweden has recently developed a new function for primary health care called "the rehabilitation coordinator" whose job is to enhance return to work opportunities for patients with common mental disorders. The overarching objective is to develop a model for return to work for patients with stress related disorders, which includes both the workplace and the Swedish primary health care setting. This initiative could guide other OECD countries in the process of increasing the role of primary health care in protecting workers' health. In Belgium, prevention advisors, who specialise in psychosocial problems, give guidance to workplaces on psychological well-being, and support the preparation of risk assessment plans to minimise stress and violence at work (Samele, Frew Stuart and Urquia Norman, 2013[51]). In Germany, the 2015 Preventive Health Care Act strengthens the role of the occupational medical doctor. Accordingly, occupational medical doctors are expected to work in collaboration with the primary health care team in order to promote people's health and employability. The objective is to improve the focus of health promotion and disease prevention at work.

In Australia, Safe Work Australia and its state and territory affiliates have responsibility for supporting employers to protect workers' physical and mental health through providing them with tools to implement effective occupational health and safety practices and through strengthening worker access to primary health care services.

Increasing the role of primary health care providers to protect and improve the health of workers should go hand in hand with adequate education and tool development to offering primary health care providers the opportunity to fulfil their role. OECD health care systems should supply primary health care providers with information, guidance and training on the management of health and work (see Chapter 2).

Improving the availability of health information and improving health literacy skills for deprived populations

Providing clear information about rules for access to care and about primary health care services helps patients from different social and economic backgrounds access and use primary health care services in a more timely and appropriate way (OECD, 2018[52]). The provision of sufficient information about health care entitlements and available primary health care services is a key element to making primary health care services more approachable and improving health literacy skills. It is important that these initiatives reach their target audience, such as certain population groups, the migrant population for example, or specific diseases, such as those suffering with mental health problems or other chronic conditions.

Australia, France, Greece, Spain, Sweden and the United States provide examples of how to improve transparency on health information and primary health care services through telephone-based interpreter services, online tools, information sessions or education courses.

In Australia, Healthdirect provides every Australian with 24 hours a day, seven days a week, access to the trusted information and advice they need to manage their own health and health related issues. The nurse-led telephone helpline and website is a core national service. Although the majority of services managed by Healthdirect Australia are designed to assist people living in rural and remote locations who have difficulty in accessing health services, the national website provides important information on the availability of general practice services, with contact details, opening hours, billing services and other information. Similar official government-led websites exist in other OECD countries (for example, Austria, France, Germany and the United States) to provide either general public health information, or information targeting certain population groups or those suffering with certain diseases. In France, for example, the website *Santetresfacile* specifically targets mentally impaired people. The website provides information about health professionals (dentists, ophthalmologists, gynaecologists, psychiatrists and psychologists) to ease access to care, but also provide friendly and understandable information to help people better monitor their health (eat well, sleep well, exercise, etc). In Spain, the Network of Health Schools for Citizenship offers a wide range of programmes, training tools and evidence-based health information to patients, relatives and caregivers, with a special focus on long-term conditions.

Greece, Sweden and the United States have explored specific ways of providing information to foreign and migrant populations on how to navigate the health care system and how to adapt to the cultural environment of their new host countries. Providing clear information about rules for access to care and about available services eases access to primary health care and helps users access services in a more timely and appropriate way. In Greece, for example, a specific website used to offer information on the geographical location of health care services and useful information on specific diseases or symptoms, disease prevention and on legal issues, as well as a list of examination costs. The information was provided in several languages including English, French, Russian, Greek and Montenegrin. In Sweden, information sessions are organised to encourage discussion among immigrants about common problems with navigating the health care system. A registered nurse provides participants with facts about the health care system (phone numbers, details about health facilities and NGOs offering support), specific information on their rights and entitlements to health care, and on frequent migrant health and illness (trauma, cognitive problems, etc.). In the United States, some large networks of providers, such as Kaiser Permanente, have telephone-based interpreter services that can be accessed at all times to provide instant translation. Such tools help make the experience of visiting primary health care facilities easier for foreigners and migrants.

In order to improve the transparency of health information, it is necessary to develop specific training or tools for health professionals to best tailor information to high-risk or priority population groups. In Ireland, the ENGAGE initiative has worked to equip primary health care providers with the skills and resources to best engage and work specifically with men (Jakab et al., 2018[53]). This initiative was launched in response to higher rates of poor lifestyle behaviours among men and low-utilisation of primary health care services. ENGAGE has been found to boost community outreach for better uptake of primary health care prevention and health promotion services among this target group (Jakab et al., 2018[53]). In the Netherlands, to increase access to and use of health information, PHAROS, the Dutch Centre of Expertise on Health Disparities, in co-ordination with other stakeholders, has developed specific tools for primary health care providers to optimise the delivery of primary health care services to migrant groups (EuroHealthNet, 2016[54]). Resources include a website for GPs with frequently asked questions on the provision of services to immigrant patients, a teaching toolkit for education in the prevention of female circumcision, and a programme for refugee children aged 10-12 years old (EuroHealthNet, 2016[54]).

4.4. Conclusions

Ensuring equal access to health care is an important target, most often highlighted in both national health system strategies and global health policy frameworks. The G7 Health Ministers' Meeting held in Paris in May 2019 under the French Presidency is, for example, making the fight against health inequalities a priority objective. The G7 Health Ministers' Meeting encouraged governments to improve primary health care as a lever for fighting health inequalities. As a first point of contact with the health care system, and by providing effective health promotion and prevention interventions, strong primary health care has all the potential to reduce health inequalities.

However, international evidence shows that primary health care is not succeeding in delivering equal access to care across different levels of socio-economic status or geographical location. For example, international figures show that people with a lower income consistently have lower utilisation rates of preventive services in virtually all EU and OECD countries. There are many financial, structural, and personal barriers impeding access to primary health care, which call for policy interventions on both demand and supply sides. On the supply side, this will consist of reorganising primary health care and making it more accessible. These interventions will bring care closer to people and communities that typically are underserved due to distance or because they are otherwise disadvantaged. To improve access to primary health care services, it is important to increase the role of nurse practitioners, community pharmacists and community health workers, to further deploy digital consultations to remove barriers of time and geography, and to develop mobile facilities to reach the most vulnerable and isolated groups of the population. On the demand side, successful levers consist of enabling patients to make the best of their health by addressing social and economic barriers to care. Options for consideration include expanding public coverage for primary health care services, integrating primary health care and social care, conducting primary health care interventions in the workplace and improving health literacy skills for vulnerable populations.

References

Amarasingham, R. et al. (2018), *Using Community Partnerships to Integrate Health and Social Services for High-Need, High-Cost Patients Using Community Partnerships to Integrate Health and Social Services for High-Need, High-Cost Patients 2 BACKGROUND.* [47]

Atherton, H. et al. (2018), "Alternatives to the face-to-face consultation in general practice: Focused ethnographic case study", *British Journal of General Practice*, http://dx.doi.org/10.3399/bjgp18X694853. [39]

Australian Government Department of Health (2019), *Annual Medicare Statistics*, https://www1.health.gov.au/internet/main/publishing.nsf/content/annual-medicare-statistics (accessed on 5 September 2019). [44]

Berchet, C. and C. Nader (2016), "The organisation of out-of-hours primary care in OECD countries", *OECD Health Working Papers*, No. 89, OECD Publishing, Paris, https://dx.doi.org/10.1787/5jlr3czbqw23-en. [12]

Biasio, L. (2017), *Vaccine hesitancy and health literacy*, http://dx.doi.org/10.1080/21645515.2016.1243633. [21]

Bosco, C. and I. Oandasan (2016), *Review of Family Medicine Within Rural and Remote Canada: Education, Practice, and Policy.*, http://www.cfpc.ca/ARFM. [17]

Bostock, S. and A. Steptoe (2012), "Association between low functional health literacy and mortality in older adults: Longitudinal cohort study", *BMJ (Online)*, http://dx.doi.org/10.1136/bmj.e1602. [24]

Bourgueil, Y., F. Jusot and Leleu Henri (2012), "In What Way Can Primary Care Contribute to Reducing Health Inequalities? A Review of Research Literature", *Question d'Economie de la Santé*, http://www.irdes.fr/EspaceAnglais/Publications/IrdesPublications/QES179.pdff. [45]

Buerhaus Peter (2018), *Nurse Practitioners: Nurse Practitioners: A solution to America's primary care crisis*, American Enterprise Institute. [28]

Caffery, L. et al. (2017), *Outcomes of using telehealth for the provision of healthcare to Aboriginal and Torres Strait Islander people: a systematic review*, http://dx.doi.org/10.1111/1753-6405.12600. [38]

Care Quality Commission (2019), *Push Dr Limited : Inspection report*, Care Quality Commission, Manchester, https://www.cqc.org.uk/sites/default/files/new_reports/AAAJ4832.pdf. [35]

Chetty, U. et al. (2016), "The role of primary care in improving health equity: Report of a workshop held by the WONCA Health Equity Special Interest Group at the 2015 WONCA Europe Conference in Istanbul, Turkey", *International Journal for Equity in Health*, http://dx.doi.org/10.1186/s12939-016-0415-8. [1]

Cookson, R. et al. (2017), "Primary care and health inequality: Difference-in-difference study comparing England and Ontario", *PLoS ONE*, http://dx.doi.org/10.1371/journal.pone.0188560. [9]

Cossman, J., W. James and J. Wolf (2017), "The differential effects of rural health care access on race-specific mortality", *SSM - Population Health*, http://dx.doi.org/10.1016/j.ssmph.2017.07.013. [18]

Cravo Oliveira Hashiguchi, T. (2020), "Bringing health care to the patient: An overview of the use of telemedicine in OECD countries", No. 116, OECD, Paris, https://dx.doi.org/10.1787/8e56ede7-en. [34]

Dyer, T., J. Owens and P. Robinson (2016), "The acceptability of healthcare: from satisfaction to trust The increasing importance of acceptability in qual-ity assessment", *Community Dental Health*, Vol. 33, pp. 242-251, http://dx.doi.org/10.1922/CDH_3902Dyer10. [19]

East Melbourne, V. (ed.) (2018), *General Practice: Health of the Nation 2018*, http://www.racgp.org.au. [43]

Eichler, K., S. Wieser and U. Brügger (2009), *The costs of limited health literacy: A systematic review*, http://dx.doi.org/10.1007/s00038-009-0058-2. [26]

Erni, P. et al. (2016), "netCare, a new collaborative primary health care service based in Swiss community pharmacies", *Research in Social and Administrative Pharmacy*, http://dx.doi.org/10.1016/j.sapharm.2015.08.010. [32]

Eurofound (2014), *Access to healthcare in times of crisis*, http://dx.doi.org/10.2806/70615. [11]

EuroHealthNet (2016), *How the Netherlands and PHAROS are reducing health inequalities and improving health literacy*, http://eurohealthnet-magazine.eu/how-the-netherlands-is-reducing-health-disparities-and-ensuring-heath-and-good-quality-care-for-all-thanks-to-pharos (accessed on 6 June 2019). [54]

Golnick, C. et al. (2012), *Innovative primary care delivery in rural Alaska: A review of patient encounters seen by community health aides*, http://dx.doi.org/10.3402/ijch.v71i0.18543. [31]

Hartzler, A. et al. (2018), "Roles and functions of community health workers in primary care", *Annals of Family Medicine*, http://dx.doi.org/10.1370/afm.2208. [30]

Iacobucci, G. (2019), "GP at Hand: patients are less sick than others but use services more, evaluation finds", *BMJ (Clinical research ed.)*, http://dx.doi.org/10.1136/bmj.l2333. [37]

Jakab, M. et al. (2018), *Health systems respond to noncommunicable diseases: time for ambition*, WHO Regional Office for Europe, Copenhagen. [53]

James, C., M. Devaux and F. Sassi (2017), "Inclusive growth and health", *OECD Health Working Papers*, No. 103, OECD Publishing, Paris, https://dx.doi.org/10.1787/93d52bcd-en. [49]

Kringos, D. et al. (2010), "The breadth of primary care: A systematic literature review of its core dimensions", *BMC Health Services Research*, http://dx.doi.org/10.1186/1472-6963-10-65. [4]

Levesque, J., M. Harris and G. Russell (2013), "Patient-centred access to health care: Conceptualising access at the interface of health systems and populations", *International Journal for Equity in Health*, http://dx.doi.org/10.1186/1475-9276-12-18. [10]

Maier, C. and L. Aiken (2016), *Expanding clinical roles for nurses to realign the global health workforce with population needs: A commentary*, http://dx.doi.org/10.1186/s13584-016-0079-2. [29]

Mercer, S. et al. (2017), *Evaluation of the Glasgow 'Deep End' Links Worker Programme*, NHS Health Scotland, Edinburgh. [46]

Moreira, L. (2018), "Health literacy for people-centred care: Where do OECD countries stand?", *OECD Health Working Papers*, No. 107, OECD Publishing, Paris, https://dx.doi.org/10.1787/d8494d3a-en. [20]

Nicholson, P. and J. Gration (2017), "What occupational medicine offers to primary care", *British Journal of General Practice*, Vol. 67/662, pp. 392-393, http://dx.doi.org/10.3399/bjgp17X692213. [50]

OECD (2019), *Health at a Glance 2019: OECD Indicators*, OECD Publishing, Paris, https://doi.org/10.1787/4dd50c09-en. [15]

OECD (2019), *Health for Everyone?: Social Inequalities in Health and Health Systems*, OECD Health Policy Studies, OECD Publishing, Paris, https://dx.doi.org/10.1787/3c8385d0-en. [6]

OECD (2018), "How resilient were OECD health care systems during the "refugee crisis"?", *Migration Policy Debates*, Vol. 17. [52]

OECD (2018), *Policy Survey on the Future of Primary Care*. [27]

OECD (2017), *Tackling Wasteful Spending on Health*, OECD Publishing, Paris, https://dx.doi.org/10.1787/9789264266414-en (accessed on 31 January 2019). [14]

OECD (2016), *Health System Characteristics Survey*, http://www.oecd.org/els/health-systems/characteristics.htm. [5]

Pearl, R. (2014), "Kaiser permanente Northern California: Current experiences with internet, mobile, and video technologies", *Health Affairs*, http://dx.doi.org/10.1377/hlthaff.2013.1005. [40]

Peritogiannis, V. et al. (2017), "Mental healthcare delivery in rural greece: A 10-year account of a mobile mental health unit", *Journal of Neurosciences in Rural Practice*, http://dx.doi.org/10.4103/jnrp.jnrp_142_17. [41]

PriceWaterhouseCoopers (2017), *Voorlopige update PwC rapport 2013: Laaggeletterdheid in Nederland kent aanzienlijke maatschappelijke kosten*. [25]

Quigley, A., N. Hex and C. Aznar (2019), *Evaluation of Babylon GP at hand : Final evaluation report*, Ipsos MORI/York Health Economics Consortium, London, https://www.hammersmithfulhamccg.nhs.uk/media/156123/Evaluation-of-Babylon-GP-at-Hand-Final-Report.pdf. [36]

Reibling, N. and C. Wendt (2013), *Access Regulation and Utilization of Healthcare Services*, http://www.mzes.uni-mannheim.de. [3]

Ruano, A., J. Furler and L. Shi (2015), "Interventions in Primary Care and their contributions to improving equity in health", *International Journal for Equity in Health*, http://dx.doi.org/10.1186/s12939-015-0284-6. [7]

Salmi, L. et al. (2017), "Interventions addressing health inequalities in European regions: the AIR project", http://dx.doi.org/10.1093/heapro/dav101. [8]

Samele, C., Frew Stuart and Urquia Norman (2013), *Mental health Systems in the European Union Member States, Status of Mental Health in Populations and Benefits to be Expected from Investments into Mental Health*. [51]

Scheffler, R. and D. Arnold (2019), "Projecting shortages and surpluses of doctors and nurses in the OECD: What looms ahead", *Health Economics, Policy and Law*, http://dx.doi.org/10.1017/S174413311700055X. [13]

Schillinger, D. et al. (2004), "Functional health literacy and the quality of physician-patient communication among diabetes patients", *Patient Education and Counseling*, http://dx.doi.org/10.1016/S0738-3991(03)00107-1. [22]

Schillinger, D. et al. (2005), *Language, Literacy, and Communication Regarding Medication in an Anticoagulation Clinic: Are Pictures Better Than Words?*. [23]

Starfield, B., L. Shi and J. Macinko (2005), "Contribution of Primary Care to Health Systems and Health", *The Milbank Quarterly*, Vol. 83/3, pp. 457–502. [2]

Wakerman, J. et al. (2017), "Equitable resourcing of primary health care in remote communities in Australia's Northern Territory: A pilot study", *BMC Family Practice*, http://dx.doi.org/10.1186/s12875-017-0646-9. [16]

WHO (2017), *Protecting workers' health Fact sheets*, https://www.who.int/news-room/fact-sheets/detail/protecting-workers'-health. [48]

Yu, S. et al. (2017), *The scope and impact of mobile health clinics in the United States: A literature review*, http://dx.doi.org/10.1186/s12939-017-0671-2. [42]

Zanaboni, P., U. Knarvik and R. Wootton (2014), "Adoption of routine telemedicine in Norway: The current picture", *Global Health Action*, http://dx.doi.org/10.3402/gha.v7.22801. [33]

Notes

[1] In Canada, the Ontario Telehomecare project is also a best practice example of providing co-ordinated support from primary health care to people with complex chronic diseases in their own homes (see Chapter 2).

[2] Push Dr is an online GP service that offers fee-based services to patients. Babylon GP at Hand has two forms in England: One is fee-charging for private patients, and the other is non-fee charging for NHS patients (which is called GP at Hand).

5 Primary health care in low- and middle-income countries

Primary health care has been identified as a crucial health system component, and universal health coverage is now a top priority for the countries. This chapter highlights the major contributors to and components of the primary health care landscape in low- and middle-income countries, and the key strategic approaches to address these fundamental challenges with the aim of ensuring the continued development towards high-quality primary health care systems. The enabling factors of governance in primary health care systems frame the discussion, while a deep dive into primary health care measurement highlights its importance in improving systems. The chapter then discusses how the strengthening of service delivery quality requires considerations of safety, knowledge, and patient perspectives, and how effective financing of primary health care includes the leveraging of the current understanding of primary health care expenditures and the financial tools available. Finally, the chapter shows how with the incorporation of cross-country learning, engagement with the private sector, and leveraging of innovations, primary health care systems can continue to strengthen and advance towards universal health coverage.

Key findings

- The Alma-Ata Declaration promoted the primacy of primary health care (PHC) in the creation of effective and responsive health systems (Declaration of Alma Ata International Conference of Primary Health Care, 1978[1]; The Lancet, 2018[2]), highlighting the importance of a holistic health system development approach
    - In the years and decades following this declaration, vertical and disease-specific approaches continued to be the focal point of the majority of global health service and investment efforts in low- and middle-income countries (LMICs). These approaches led to resources being leveraged for specific diseases, resulting in a series of targeted clinical transformations that saved millions of lives.
    - While an important model of achievement in focused health gains, this was just an early first step in an evolution towards realising Universal Health Coverage (UHC). Now, we are moving forward with the endeavor of promoting comprehensive health and addressing all basic health care needs for populations through PHC (Das et al., 2018[3]).
    - Nearly two decades into the 21st century, major progress cutting deaths from infectious diseases, childhood illnesses, and complications of pregnancy and childbirth has translated into ageing populations and a growing burden of morbidity that make health care needs more complex, and requiring more integrated solutions (Das et al., 2018[3]). PHC serves an important role as a tool to deliver integrated solutions for health, and to deliver on the UHC promise.
- Primary health care has been identified as a major priority across many LMICs, and has been seen to fulfil the functions that play a central role in this report: prioritising the delivery of efficient primary health care, strengthening effective and patient-centred care and reducing inequalities in health care.
- LMICs have the need for a nationally agreed-upon package of PHC services, defined as the guaranteed minimum public health and clinical services provided at the primary level (Rohde et al., 2008[4]).
    - It is crucial that stakeholders are committed to implementing the package, and attention needs to be directed to district management systems with consistent investments in frontline primary health care community health workers.
    - Primary health care systems often lack sufficiently comprehensive data to target weaknesses, understand their causes, and strategically direct resources to address them. Good measurement will be needed to inform understanding of service delivery quality and decisions around PHC financing; to provide the baseline for removing inequalities in care and strengthen provision of evidence-based care.
    - Countries need to mobilise sufficient financial resources to provide or purchase essential primary health care services for their populations, to reduce inequalities in the ability to pay for those services, and to provide financial protection against impoverishment from catastrophic health care costs through three basic health financing functions (revenue generation, resource pooling, and services/goods purchasing).
    - Ensuring high-quality PHC delivery across populations includes improved learning between health care systems and integrated care, developing strategies for engaging the private sector in PHC delivery, and developing and improving technologies aimed at creating opportunities for countries to "leapfrog".

5.1. PHC Governance: Efforts should be stepped up to strengthen PHC governance in LMICs

Strong PHC regulatory frameworks are important contributors to ensuring the essential service delivery mechanisms of PHC. The organisation and delivery of the public primary health care system, and the regulation and accountability components, are key elements of strong governance. Good governance of health system practices also takes shape around the democratic, financial, and performance accountability processes to create transparency. In systems with strong governance – those that are responsible, accountable, transparent, and empowering – national and global PHC goals can be achieved faster, more completely, and more sustainably (USAID, 2017[5]). In these systems, good governance is embedded early in the design phase, and is used to reinforce priorities, deepen a country's sense of ownership, and allow for implementation with a higher likelihood of sustained improvement (Vaz et al., 2018[6]).

In LMIC health systems, the single largest actors are the governments, and in this section, we focus on the role of governments in governance. We describe important aspects of not just the organisation and delivery of the public primary health care system, but of regulation and accountability. We additionally touch on the importance of civil society participation and the role of patient voice, which are major gaps identified by the three recent quality reports (see section 5.3).

5.1.1. The architecture of the health care system can affect the ability of primary health care systems to function effectively

Health system architecture varies across countries, and governance of these health systems – and the delivery of primary health care services – depends on country-specific government roles, mandates, and actions. For example, Uganda has local political councils that appoint a Health Unit Management Committee to oversee the budget, workplan, performance, and other aspects of a Level II facility. Similarly, in Nigeria, Ward Development Committees are designed to govern frontline facilities. Broadly speaking, and especially in decentralised systems like Nigeria or Kenya, PHC is the responsibility of the state.

While this provides each state with flexibility to respond to local needs, it can create challenges for addressing failures around referrals and the care continuum because providers at higher-level facilities do not share the same reporting structure than those at lower-level facilities. Because workers at community, PHC, and district levels often report through and up to different leadership than secondary or tertiary hospitals, referrals and care pathways may be incomplete, suboptimal, and fragmented. The architecture of the system can impact the ability of primary health care systems to function effectively: primary health care systems often include coverage of large territories in rural areas, and local budgets often lack accurate funds to enable managers to conduct adequate routine management of the facility or collaboration with village groups.

5.1.2. Donor-funded projects can accelerate good governance by encouraging oversight, but support for institutional development is required

For donors, higher-functioning systems often include a basket fund and technical assistance collaborations to support the PHC system. The basket funds frequently represent the essential, recurring, fundamental services needed to deliver care. Donors may contribute to this basket fund with the expectation that over time, governments increase the fiscal space to cover these services. Through participation in this basket, donors may have oversight of the essential services. In addition to the basket fund, donors regularly fund technical assistance to address a variety of gaps in service delivery. However, donors can also burden the health system and exacerbate governance challenges with reporting requirements and priorities that may be different and conflicting across donors. Fragmented donors with poorly integrated programs can optimise individual outcomes yet sub-optimise the PHC system. From a governance perspective, this can create strong headwinds for community oversight.

Quality assurance and accreditation programs play important roles in regulating the private sectors

In many LMICs, the private sector is characterised by extreme fragmentation and lack of regulation. It is common for numerous, small-sized private providers to operate clinics, offering a limited number of services at variable levels of quality. Quality assurance and accreditation programs play important roles in regulating private facilities, pharmacies, and non-delivery settings like drug manufacturers, and are among LMIC governments' most effective tools for governing the private sector. It is however a challenge to create systems that can accredit private sector health insurance and other purchasing schemes, as contracting and claims management from numerous small private facilities pose an administrative burden for insurance agencies and government purchasers (Chan et al., 2019[7]). Licensure, performance measurement, monitoring of contractual processes, establishment of public complaints systems, and health insurance schemes are all tools for bringing private sector PHC services and providers into alignment with national policies and minimum standards (Berwick et al., 2018[8]; Ozano et al., 2019[9]). Private sector organisations can be required to demonstrate competence, adhere to minimum standards, and report data on the quality of services delivered in order to be licensed and allowed to operate. Government stewardship of these efforts can be influential (see Box 5.1). For example, in Egypt, a family health fund was established to contract with public and private PHC providers and purchase services for both insured and uninsured users. The fund established accreditation rules and criteria for health facilities, including assessments of patient care and services conducted by the Ministry of Health. Facilities that scored too low on the assessments could not be accredited (Ozano et al., 2019[9]). Increasingly, private sector organisations may also contribute to the development and implementation of national quality strategies (Chan et al., 2019[7]).

Box 5.1. Government stewardship of the for-profit private health sector in Afghanistan

From 2003-08, Afghanistan's private sector for-profit health services went largely unregulated and grew rapidly. Out-of-pocket spending for private sector health services accounted for nearly three-quarters (73.3%) of total Afghan health expenditures by 2011-12, with nearly half of all outpatient visits made to private providers that year. Yet, a 2008 private sector survey showed poor infrastructure, limited formal medical training, and low perceptions of quality among users.

Beginning in 2008, the Ministry of Public Health undertook a long-term stewardship initiative to oversee the sector and bring it into alignment with the country's national health priorities.

Essential stewardship functions:

- *Establish strategic policy directions*: Between 2004 and 2015, national strategies and policies began to define the vision, guiding principles, and detailed plans and objectives for growing and regulating the private sector.
- *Ensure system structures align with strategy and policy goals*: In 2009, an Office of Private Sector Coordination was established to oversee for-profit entities, helping implement policies, facilitate public – private engagement and communication, and advocate within the Ministry of Public Health and other ministries. Efforts to simplify and increase transparency of licensing procedures were undertaken, and relevant staff grew in numbers and training.
- *Establish legal and regulatory policy instruments to guide performance*: For-profit-related regulations and operational policies and procedures were developed, as well as mechanisms for protecting the rights of consumers and providers. Establishment, licensure, and operation of private health care providers came under regulation beginning in 2012, with guidance on minimum required standards covering hospital, clinic, and facility operations issued the following year.

> - *Build and sustain partnerships*: The Ministry of Public Health developed inter- and intra-governmental relationships including with the Ministry of Finance; established a permanent Public Private Dialogue Forum that meets quarterly to review legislative, regulatory, and operational issues; and promoted partnerships with several private sector associations including the Afghanistan Private Hospitals Association and the Afghanistan Medicines Services Union.
> - *Ensure accountability and transparency:* These components were built into the steps taken towards the other stewardship functions. For example, through the creation of an Information and Communications Desk for the Private Sector, within the Ministry of Public Health, the task force and working group materials are posted online, which increased awareness of and participation in the Public Private Dialogue Forum.
> - *Generate actionable intelligence*: The Afghanistan Private Hospitals Association has worked with the Ministry of Public Health and technical experts to develop a functioning Health Management Information System for private hospitals, with a common set of 14 priority indicators to be reported to the Afghanistan Private Hospitals Association and the Ministry of Public Health. Data from 60 hospitals had been reported at least once to the Ministry of Public Health by the end of 2014.
>
> While still at a relatively early stage, the Afghanistan Ministry of Public Health stewardship initiative for the private health sector has been considered a success in part because of its strong policy framework, ongoing political commitment of the government and donors, and efforts to build institutions and systems that focused on increasing the quality of private services.
>
> Source: Cross et al (2017[10]), "Government stewardship of the for-profit private health sector in Afghanistan", https://doi.org/10.1093/heapol/czw130.

Increasing accountability of PHC services requires institutional development

Strong accountability mechanisms are crucial for discouraging corruption, ensuring managers are held responsible to their organisations and the public, and that money meant for delivering quality care does not get diverted (Chan et al., 2019[7]). Performance accountability includes public reporting through monthly or annual scorecards, citizen-provider committees, publication of district and leadership performance, and media coverage. Accountability mechanisms for performance can also include horizontal practices such as performance-based mechanisms (including results-based payment), accreditation, and regulation. Mutual accountability and community engagement play valuable roles in maintaining transparency and accountability in performance (Chan et al., 2019[7]; Brinkerhoff et al., 2017[11]). Specifically, the incorporation of performance management policies into human resources for health systems provides evidence-based insight and accountability for these systems.

In Rwanda for example, the Imihigo system is a strong example of leveraging data for accountability. A performance-based contract is signed between each of the country's mayors and the President, with the goal of using data to hold the mayors accountable to delivering quality primary health care services to their constituents. This Imihigo system is complemented by a nation-wide system to train managers at the national School of Public Health. These data-driven performance tracking efforts accompanied by increased access to management training provide an important example of performance accountability for the health system.

In LMICs, one important route to further strengthening PHC accountability is through supporting the development of legal frameworks of governments, and regulatory measures that protect both the public as well as local-level authorities (Ozano et al., 2019[9]). As complements to legal frameworks, participation, voice, and empowerment of the public are known to increase accountability of PHC services in LMICs. Routes to increased public participation include social accountability efforts, participatory approaches to policy dialogues, decentralisation, performance-based mechanisms, and public financial management tactics (Health Finance and Governance Project, 2018[12]), in addition to social accountability efforts such as citizen scorecards, and user committees (Brinkerhoff et al., 2017[11]).

5.2. Measurement of PHC: A more coordinated approach towards measurement of PHC is needed in LMICs

Measurement is a powerful tool for focusing efforts on improving PHC systems, tracking progress, and creating comparability for peers to learn from. When measurement is lacking – or overly burdensome – it can constrain such progress. Good measurement informs understanding of service delivery quality and decisions around PHC financing; it can provide the baseline for removing inequalities in care and strengthening provision of evidence-based care. The development of PHC systems over the past decades has highlighted the power of measurement and its ability to focus and coordinate effort, track and trend progress, create feedback loops to drive improvement, and create accountability for achieving performance. Significant data gaps remain for key measures, and the absence of clear measures constrains improvement efforts, limits accountability, and limits the ability to focus efforts. As the world's attention turned again to PHC with the Astana Declaration, the critical challenge of quality measurement of PHC systems became acutely evident. However, the global health research community is still determining reliable and validated indicators for measuring key aspects of PHC and, some initiatives, like the Primary Health Care Performance Initiative (PHCPI), are aiming to fill the performance measurement gap and catalyse improvements in LMIC PHC systems to accelerate progress to UHC. Going forward, these efforts will increase in importance as PHC systems aim to strengthen their measurement mechanisms and systems, but a more coordinated approach is needed.

5.2.1. Improvement in primary health care quality is dependent on measurement tools

The evolution from the primary health care-focused Alma-Ata Declaration in 1978 to the vertical- and disease-focused approaches in subsequent years can be traced to an important underlying dilemma: measurement of PHC systems has been a persistent challenge for countries, limiting the ability to monitor progress and create accountability for results. This lack of clear measurement led in part to the global health community prioritising vertical programs where key interventions could be tracked over time and results proven. The Millennium Development Goals grew out of this approach and drove remarkable achievements in specific health areas, but led to a legacy of often fragmented health systems focused on treating specific diseases rather than promotion of comprehensive health. Today, decision makers, researchers, and health providers are still attempting to discern what makes strong, comprehensive PHC health systems, and how to measure and improve on them.

Two lessons have emerged from this global experience:

- The first lesson is the power of measurement and its ability to focus and coordinate efforts, track and trend progress, create feedback loops to drive improvement, and create accountability for achieving performance.
- The second lesson is the inverse of the first: the absence of clear measures constrains improvement efforts, limits accountability, and limits the ability to focus efforts.

These lessons have contributed to a cycle of underinvestment in PHC, as donors and governments have been unable to clearly detect a return on investment in the PHC system, making disease-focused investments much more attractive.

> **Box 5.2. The Salud Mesoamerica Initiative**
>
> The Salud Mesoamerica Initiative, a public-private partnership including the Bill & Melinda Gates Foundation, the Carlos Slim Health Institute, Spain's Cooperation Agency for International Development, and the Inter-American Development Bank (IDB), is an example of a programmethat has made equitable health gains through PHC system investments where measurement played a central role. The initiative, which is a partnership with all eight countries in the region, was built on a national level performance-based financing scheme. The scheme required the donors and country governments to sign onto a performance framework consisting of a short list of population level, time-bound health targets focused on maternal and child health. To receive a performance tranche, the country was required to reach 80% or more of these targets in each phase, which grew in difficulty as phases progressed. This meant that success in only one or two disease areas would result in failure in the programme. This paradigm shift galvanised country efforts to improve the PHC system as the only pathway to achieving the array of health targets – by investing in supply chain improvements, community health platforms, provider competence, and team-based care. Salud Mesoamerica Initiative completed its second phase in 2018 and saw the majority of countries achieve 80% or more of their health targets, as well as increasing government investment in PHC systems. A healthy competition between national governments to achieve the targets introduced additional incentives for improvement. The success of this effort and the central role of measurement highlight the opportunity of having financial incentives linked back to improving the way countries collect their data, leading to the longevity and sustainability of evidence-based policy-making.

5.2.2. There is a crucial lack of data for PHC systems in LMICs

Countries around the world often lack sufficient data on PHC performance; however, in some LMICs, the absence of data is even more severe, given that in some cases there are no basic data on vital registration (such as births, deaths, and pregnancies). Most acutely in LMICs, there is broad agreement that the data necessary for countries to assess their PHC systems, compare their systems across time and to similar countries, and make evidence-informed planning decisions are lacking (Veillard et al., 2017[13]; Kruk et al., 2018[14]).

One legacy of the Millennium Development Goals era that exacerbates this challenge is fragmented data management systems that were developed for specific health programs – such as malaria, HIV, tuberculosis, immunisation – and which often operate in isolation from a comprehensive national data system (Health Data Collaborative, 2019[15]). The current reality is that the global health research community is still shifting away from this vertical approach, and aiming to determine reliable, validated, and comparable indicators for measuring key aspects of PHC in LMICs (Veillard et al., 2017[13]). Further, many interventions are poorly understood, so "even when countries decide to prioritise PHC, they often lack the necessary information to pinpoint weaknesses, identify strengths, and improve their PHC systems" (Veillard et al., 2017[13]).

Data gaps that impact clarity into PHC systems can be found at any level of the health system, including aspects of governance, leadership, and population health management; from the facility level including facility organisation and management, information system existence/use, and local operating funds; and at the outcome level including concepts of responsiveness and resilience. There are both upstream and downstream challenges that can lead to these data gaps:

- First, some phenomena are harder to measure than others or have been generally neglected, therefore new research and development is necessary to create novel indicators and validate tools for their collection.

- Second, some measures exist in developed countries or in similar but separate sectors but have not been adapted for developing countries, so investments are needed to modify and adapt measurement tools to fit new contexts.
- Third, there is a multitude of measurement tools used to collect similar PHC data but are often not harmonised, which results in data that are not comparable. This limits the ability to benchmark and learn across borders, which requires the global measurement community to work together to harmonise and standardise measurement whenever possible.
- Fourth, PHC has not been a visible priority in global health, and therefore corresponding data have often not been collected. As the importance of PHC elevates, so too should the demand for PHC measurement and support to countries to collect the most meaningful and actionable data.

In addition to identifying gaps in data availability, another major concern with PHC measurement is collecting too much data, but not the appropriate type of data needed for improvement. Health system data collection is costly, and often uncoordinated and disconnected from decision-making. For example, according to the Lancet HQSS Commission[1] Report, "26 different bilateral, multilateral, governmental, and non-governmental organisations fund health information systems in Kenya, resulting in duplication of efforts and uneven distribution of resources within the country" (Kruk et al., 2018[14]). Closing these data gaps with appropriate data will require a combination of new investments, and importantly, collaboration between countries, development partners, NGOs, donors, civil society, and others to demand more and better PHC data.

5.2.3. Collecting actionable indicators for performance improvement

There is broad agreement that any new measurements and data collection efforts should not be to generate *more* measures, but rather to create *better* measures, reducing reliance on irrelevant or non-actionable indicators for performance improvement (Veillard et al., 2017[13]). Strategies and new initiatives for PHC measurement and data capacity include shaping internationally comparable datasets such as the System of Health Accounts (see Section 5, Financing PHC); helping to strengthen countries' routine health information systems to produce comparable information; finding acceptable substitute indicators from routine health reporting systems; and imputing data where it is missing (Veillard et al., 2017[13]).

One of the most vexing challenges of measurement for PHC is that of how to appropriately measure service delivery, considered the 'black box' of primary health care. In OECD countries, the black box is more directed on the outcomes of care: we often have visibility into the service delivery, but lack visibility into the outcomes after the services are delivered. In LMICs, the black box encompasses service delivery because of the lack of visibility into the factors influencing the quality of care by providers to patients. Service delivery in LMICs is not well understood, in part because it has received little attention, but it is a critical component to ensuring the PHC system guarantees people receive the care they need, and drives improvements when needed (PHCPI, 2018[16]). Given the causal chain between inputs and outputs in primary health care service delivery, more evidence to better understand PHC patterns and progress mechanisms will help illuminate the process of service delivery, and better allow for planning and implementing whole system interventions and reforms (Randhawa, 2015[17]).

While the gap in sufficient measures is substantial, progress is being made. For example, huge investments over the last decade have improved routine facility reporting systems, considered the cornerstone of PHC monitoring. These systems provide the real-time information about programmeperformance essential to improving service delivery (Kasper et al., 2018[18]). Efforts to address data gaps and open up the black box, through the development of strategies and new initiatives for PHC measurement and data capacity include the Health Data Collaborative, the Primary Health Care Performance Initiative, Vital Signs Profiles, and the collection and reporting of patient-reported experience measures (see Box 5.3). Additionally, the new World Health Organization (WHO) Operational Framework has been introduced for measuring progress towards improving primary health care.

> **Box 5.3. Several initiatives have been implemented to open the black box of PHC**
>
> **Health Data Collaborative**
>
> The Health Data Collaborative was established in 2016 to strengthen country health information systems in anticipation of the monitoring needs associated with the health-related Sustainable Development Goals, aiming to ensure harmonised approaches and methods for data collection in national health information systems (Health Data Collaborative, 2019[15]). The goal is that by 2024, 60 LMICs and supporting donors will have common approaches to strengthening health data systems, and that by 2030, LMICs will no longer need international assistance to sustain strong health data systems (Health Data Collaborative, 2019[15]). One approach the Health Data Collaborative has undertaken is a harmonised survey initiative to reduce the burden of data collection on health workers and improve the efficiency of health investments. A standard toolkit has been developed harmonising disease- and donor-specific data quality tools to assess data quality from routine health information systems with common metrics, methodologies, and tools. This methodology has been integrated into the District Health Information System 2 survey, used in dozens of LMICs (Health Data Collaborative, 2019[15]).
>
> **The Primary Health Care Performance Initiative (PHCPI)**
>
> PHCPI is a collaboration between the Bill & Melinda Gates Foundation, the World Bank, and WHO, in partnership with Ariadne Labs and Results for Development. Launched in 2015, its aim is to fill the performance measurement gap and catalyse improvements in LMIC PHC systems to accelerate progress to UHC (Veillard et al., 2017[13]). PHCPI works with global institutions to align on common measurement frames, approaches, and tools for PHC. The initiative uses evidence-based approaches to determine what is important to measure, and to identify where important data are missing. PHCPI works with countries, donors, and development partners to develop indicators and measurement tools to begin to fill in some of these data gaps to improve PHC system performance. The overarching objective is to closely align its indicators and methodology with the WHO index on the coverage of essential health services, which will be used to monitor progress toward UHC indicators (Veillard et al., 2017[13]).
>
> **The Vital Signs Profiles**
>
> The Vital Signs Profile (VSP) is a new integrated measurement tool launched in 2018 to provide a coherent set of indicators for measuring PHC-oriented performance. The goal of this tool is to provide a "snapshot" of PHC in countries, focusing on financing; capacity including governance, inputs, and population health and facility management; performance including access, quality, and coverage; and equity. The tool is meant to allow decision makers and users to better understand where systems are strong and where they need to improve (PHCPI, 2018[19]).

As mentioned in Chapter 3 of the report, there is growing understanding of the importance of collecting patients-reported indicators, such as experience and outcome measures, in order to better understand how patients perceive their own health care and whether it improves the outcomes they value (OECD, 2019[20]). Patient-reported indicators capture functional and quality of life measures from patients themselves, and measures of their experiences with the health care systems. These indicators positions patients, providers, and policy makers to make choices about the care they receive and provide, and helps care to be more efficient and effective (Gurria and Porter, 2018[21]). These indicators are a core element to the delivery of primary health care explored in this report. More countries have begun collecting this type of information, but they are not typically collected in a way that allows comparison across countries, or is representative of whole populations (Gurria and Porter, 2018[21]). The OECD patient-reported indicators surveys (PaRIS) initiative is meant to address some of these information gaps with a goal of developing international benchmarks of health system performance, as reported by patients themselves (OECD, 2019[20]).

5.3. Service Delivery Quality: Efforts must be strengthened to improve service delivery quality

Evidence has shown that service delivery quality is deeply insufficient at both facility and community levels, and three major reports on service quality address the key challenges (Berwick et al., 2018[8]). The recent quality reports, one a joint report by WHO, the World Bank, and OECD (OECD/WHO/World Bank Group, 2018[22]), the second from the Lancet HQSS Commission (Kruk et al., 2018[14]), and the third from the National Academies of Sciences, Engineering, and Medicine (National Academies of Sciences Engineering and Medicine, 2018[23]), were published in 2018. These reports suggest that features of a system providing high quality care include common elements, such as a skilled and empowered workforce, strong and durable attention from public and private health care leaders as well as an engaged public pushing for accountability, common sense health financing strategies to increase affordable access to health facilities and supplies, and an essential focus on updated measurement and transparency processes. Consensus across these reports suggests alignment within the global health community about what health care quality entails, and the urgent need to improve quality in LMICs (Bollyky, Cowling and Schoder, 2018[24]). The reports agree that poor quality care is especially burdensome in LMICs, where people are particularly vulnerable due to resource limitations and poverty-related threats to health (Berwick et al., 2018[8]). Poor quality care leads to millions of unnecessary deaths and trillions of dollars of economic costs – yet, all three reports agree that quality universal health care could be affordable (Bollyky, Cowling and Schoder, 2018[24]). Authors state, in various ways, that for many populations, universal health coverage "will be an empty vessel unless and until quality improvement, for all nations, becomes as central an agenda as universal health coverage itself" (National Academies of Sciences Engineering and Medicine, 2018[23]). For meaningful progress on quality health care, efforts must be country-led, with political will, accountability, and transparency to be meaningful. The reports also highlight quality gaps in patient safety, and the importance of patient experience (Bollyky, Cowling and Schoder, 2018[24]).

5.3.1. There is no access to care without strong quality

Lack of access to health care services is often assumed to be the key deficit to measuring and improving LMIC health care systems – that people are in poor health because they are unable to reach needed medical services in time. Given this expected association, traditionally, quality in LMICs has been (i) focused on providing and counting physical goods such as clinics and medicine and getting doctors to rural communities that are underserved (Das et al., 2018[3]) and (ii) has been measured structurally, often through inputs such as the condition of infrastructure or the presence or absence of certain drugs (Das, Hammer and Leonard, 2008[25]). However, recent evidence demonstrates little correlation between the availability of inputs (such as medicines) or higher utilisation rates with increased quality of medical care (Das et al., 2018[3]; Randhawa, 2015[17]; Das, 2011[26]). Higher utilisation rates and continued poor outcomes clarify the challenge that there is no access to care without quality: measures that show the fuller array of access to providers show that access is not the issue, but rather the quality of care patients receive when they do come in contact with the health care system (Das et al., 2018[3]).

High quality health care involves the right care, at the right time, in the right place, and by the right care provider, while minimising harm and resource waste and leaving no one behind (Das et al., 2018[3]; Veillard et al., 2018[27]). Getting the right care is at least equal in importance to ensuring access to care is achieved. Available research findings suggest that service delivery quality is deeply insufficient at both facility and community levels, challenging the assumption that qualified providers in well-resourced clinics guarantee quality (Das et al., 2018[3]). Instead, studies find weak links between qualifications and knowledge, and between knowledge and practice. Even fully trained providers with adequate access to infrastructure often fail to deliver high quality care, and approaches such as training doctors have a minimal impact: in Tanzania, three years of medical school were associated with only a 1 percentage point increase in the probability of a correct diagnosis (Das, Hammer and Leonard, 2008[25]). This gap between what providers know to do and how they actually treat patients means that providers with no formal medical training might provide higher quality care than a fully trained doctor (Das et al., 2018[3]); the greater effort of an untrained provider could make up for their lower level of skill (Das, Hammer and Leonard, 2008[25]). These gaps suggest opportunities to dive deep into what constitutes quality for health systems beyond access, and to explore the path forward to improve the quality of service delivery.

5.3.2. Patient safety is a significant concern

The three quality reports reviewed above each highlight quality gaps in patient safety, citing estimates that injuries from failures in patient safety kill as many people as tuberculosis or malaria globally, and that safety failures account for 15% of hospital costs in OECD countries (Berwick et al., 2018[8]). The Lancet Global Health Quality Commission found 15.6 million excess deaths from 61 conditions occurred in LMICs in 2016 (Kruk et al., 2018[14]). After excluding deaths that could be prevented through public health measures, 8.6 million excess deaths were amenable to health care of which 5.0 million were estimated to be due to receipt of poor-quality care and 3.6 million were due to non-utilisation of health care (Kruk et al., 2018[14]). Poor quality of health care was a major driver of excess mortality across conditions, from cardiovascular disease and injuries to neonatal and communicable disorders (Berwick et al., 2018[8]; Kruk et al., 2018[14]). Substandard drugs are estimated to be responsible for hundreds of thousands of deaths each year (Kasper et al., 2018[18]), with costs associated with unsafe medication practices and medical errors estimated to be USD 42 billion annually – or about 1% of all global health expenditure (WHO, 2018[28]; OECD/WHO/World Bank Group, 2018[22]). Estimates suggest that as many as 20% (developed countries) to 25% (developing countries) of the general population experience harm in the PHC setting; yet, up to 80% of harm in primary and ambulatory settings can be avoided (OECD/WHO/World Bank Group, 2018[22]). PHC providers play an important role in promoting patient safety, through steps like preventing inappropriate use of medicines (Nejad, Abrampah and Neilson, 2018[29]).

While patient safety is a universal issue, it poses special challenges for LMICs, where systems face inadequate allocation and use of resources, infrastructure and human resources challenges, lack of respect for patients' rights, and non-compliance with patient safety standards (German Federal Ministry of Health/World Health Organization, 2017[30]). The third WHO Global Patient Safety Challenge – Medication Without Harm – was launched in 2017 with the aim of reducing severe, avoidable medication-related harm by 50% globally in the next five years (WHO, 2017[31]). Ambitious efforts must continue to highlight the threat of safety issues to quality health care.

5.4. Financing PHC: There are too many gaps in the current understanding of PHC financing in LMICs

PHC is recognised as the foundation of any health system and as the most effective, efficient, and equitable approach for delivering essential health services to the majority of the population. In the Astana Declaration, the global community committed to ensuring adequate funding sources for PHC to limit peoples' exposure to financial hardship resulting from lack of access to PHC services (The Lancet, 2018[2]). However, there are massive gaps in the current understanding of PHC financing in LMICs, including how much countries have invested in PHC, how much countries should invest in PHC, and how to address the funding gap if it exists. In addition, the global community has realised that the "mere availability of resources is not enough; conscious and continuous effort is needed to ensure that they are used in ways that are effective, safe and individually tailored to patients' needs" (OECD/WHO/World Bank Group, 2018[22]). However, there is little guidance globally to assist countries to better use their scarce health resources to improve the development and performance of their PHC systems to maximise the health gains of the population.

The financing of health care is composed of three basic functions: revenue generation, resource pooling, and services/goods purchasing. Countries need to mobilise sufficient financial resources to provide or purchase essential health services – most of which are PHC services – for their populations, to reduce inequalities in the ability to pay for those services, and to provide financial protection against impoverishment from catastrophic health care costs through these three basic health financing functions. However, many LMICs, especially those countries in Africa, face tremendous challenges in financing their health systems. These challenges include raising sufficient and sustainable revenues in an efficient and equitable manner to provide individuals with both essential health services and financial protection against unpredictable catastrophic financial losses caused by illness and injury; managing these revenues in a way that pools health risks equitably and efficiently; and ensuring the purchase of health services in an allocatively and technically efficient manner.

5.4.1. Raising sufficient and sustainable revenues for PHC

Measuring PHC expenditure in a comparative and standard manner is a critical first step to understanding why some countries are doing better than others and where extra efforts can be made to perform better.

Recently, the WHO published a paper on PHC expenditure in 27 LMICs (Vande Maele et al., 2019[32]). The data used in this analysis come from the data collected in LMICs using the System of Health Accounts 2011, with funding support from the Bill & Melinda Gates Foundation. The results showed that PHC services compose 54% of total current health care expenditure. Annual per capita PHC expenditure is on average USD 36/year (median of USD 23.8). Of this, about 21% comes from the government, 24% from external resources (i.e. donors), and the remaining 55% from other sources, most of which is from out-of-pocket expenses at the point of services from patients directly. Governments in these LMICs allocate 36% of their total health investment to PHC (Vande Maele et al., 2019[32]). Among the 12 low-income countries, about 60% of their health care expenditure is spent on PHC services. For these countries, annual per capita PHC expenditure is on average USD 22.5/year (median of USD 19.8), with about 15% coming from the government, 39% from external resources, and 46% from other sources (i.e. out-of-pocket). The government allocates on average (mean) about 40% of its health investment to PHC. Across both LMICs and LICs, there are sustainability challenges in this financing, with most of the funding for PHC coming from non-government sources, including substantial out-of-pocket requirements.

In 2017, the WHO financing team estimated the total investment needed to meet the SDGs (Stenberg et al., 2017[33]). The results indicated that an additional USD 3.9 trillion health investment is needed by the 67 LMICs over the next 15 years in order to meet the SDGs. This is about USD 58 per capita per year, which is the average figure during 2026-30[2] (The Lancet, 2018[2]). Estimations show that over two-thirds of the estimated additional resources needs for SDGs are for PHC services, which is an additional (approximately) USD 38 per capita per year during 2026-30, in these 67 LMICs (Stenberg, 2019[34]).

5.4.2. There is a lack of pooled financial resources to cover essential health services equitably across populations

A resource pooling function deals with accumulating and managing prepaid financial resources from individuals so that members who are in a pooled fund can share the health risks collectively, thereby protecting individual pooled members from large, unpredictable health expenditures. In many LMICs, this pooling function is carried out by the government through its health budget. For example, many African countries have embarked on defining or revising an essential package of health care interventions, based on epidemiological analyses of their beneficiary populations. The governments allocate certain proportions of their general revenue to the health budget in order to support government facilities to provide these services to their populations free of charge or at reduced cost, or purchase these services for their populations through some nongovernmental organisations, such as faith-based institutions (Bank, 2016[35]). However, this type of government budgetary pooling mechanism can suffer a series of problems including poor management, lack of accountability, corruption, inappropriate incentives, underfunding to cover the total cost of services and to cover necessary services (resulting in the need for user fees), misallocation of resources, weaker capacity to translate resources into high quality services, challenges reaching the poorest of the poor, and others (Wagstaff and Claeson, 2004[36]). An additional important challenge is that control of government revenue and health allocation is often outside of the control of ministries of health.

In addition to the pooled fund through the government health budgets, many African countries have developed some form of a health insurance scheme. However, only very few countries are building schemes that are able to provide universal coverage for at least a majority of their residents. While Rwanda is one of best examples for providing comprehensive health insurance to its citizens, its system was largely funded through foreign aid in its inception phase. Subsequently, the government of Rwanda has been making great strides to reduce its donor dependency and continue its effort of gradually shifting its funding sources to domestic funding support through premium contributions and government subsidies.

Ghana is another important example of introducing a national health insurance scheme, using employee contributions and national health insurance levies to cover the majority of its citizens with comprehensive health care services. However, this scheme has not been able to reach the entire population, with the issue known as the 'missing middle', where the voluntary enrollment of the informal but non-poor results leaves a gap of coverage. To target this challenge, several countries, such as Nigeria, Tanzania, and Kenya, have introduced a social health insurance scheme. These schemes however only cover public sector workers, who pay monthly premiums. Nongovernment workers in those nations typically do not have, or cannot afford, health insurance except, of course, for the very wealthy in the private sector (Fenny, Yates and Thompson, 2018[37]). Additionally, some of these schemes, such as the Kenya National Hospital Insurance Fund, only focus on hospital services rather than PHC services.

There are additional approaches for insurance schemes, including with community-based health insurance (CBHI) and private insurance. Many African countries, including Nigeria, Tanzania, Kenya, Uganda, Cameroon, DRC, Senegal, Mali, and Burundi, have developed community-based health insurance schemes that cover essential health services and offer financial protection to the people who are in the informal sector. But many of these schemes are small in scale, with limited resources that are not able to avoid catastrophic health spending. There are also challenges with sustainability of these models, as the poorest populations are unable to contribute enough premiums to maintain the schemes. Ethiopia, however, provides an exceptional example. With substantial government subsidies and tireless efforts from local governments and communities, Ethiopia has been able to expand its CBHI scheme coverage from 1% of woredas in 2012/13 to 25% of woredas in 2015/16. The population coverage increased from less than 1% of the population to 13% of its population during the same period (Zelelew, 2017[38]). Additionally, private insurance is another option for pooling; however, there are challenges with coverage and affordability. South Africa is a typical example with private health insurance plans that cover about 16% of the population, although this private insurance is not affordable for the most of population in the country (Crawford and Sachdev, 2018[39]).

In summary, evidence demonstrates that pooled funding mechanisms such as health insurance schemes have strong potential to improve financial protections and enhance utilisation among their enrolled populations, while fostering social inclusion. However, many LMICs, especially those in Africa, are still suffering from a lack of pooled financial resources to cover essential health services equitably across populations.

5.4.3. Purchasing for PHC service is a central component of good public financial management for health

The goal of provider payment mechanisms should be to "help achieve health policy objectives by encouraging access to necessary health services for patients, high quality of care, and improved equity, while promoting the effective and efficient use of resources and, where appropriate, cost containment (Langenbrunner and Cashin, 2009[40]). The three main types of PHC payment methods include line-item or population-based budgeting, fee-for-service, and per-capita or capitation. Although line-item or population-based budget and fee-for-service are still the dominating provider payment methods in LMICs, the capitation payment method has been suggested as the preferred approach, though it is challenging to implement. The Joint Learning Network (see Section 5.5, PHC System Design) has launched a facilitated Learning Exchange on Financing and Payment Models for Primary Health Care in order for countries to share experiences, including technical details and challenges of implementation, for the different models and approaches in their respective country contexts. This process will lead to the development of more deliberative materials that countries will be able to use and learn from (Joint Learning Network, 2019[41]).

Strategic purchasing has been considered as an important approach to guaranteeing high-quality and efficiently allocated service delivery to populations. In general, strategic purchasing needs to identify what and how purchases are made, and by whom, with the goal of assuring the pooled resources of health services are used in an allocatively and technically efficient manner. Purchasers include national health insurance programs, private insurance companies, ministries of health, and other agencies or institutions buying services and medicines on behalf of a population (Cashin, 2017[42]). Strategic purchasing involves active consideration of and transparent decisions about what the purchaser will buy, who will provide those services, and how the services and medicines will be purchased – as well as questions of provider payment methods, rates, and how provider performance will be monitored (R4D, 2019[43]). In addition to national-level purchasers, state-level efforts are also important decision-makers for strategic purchasing. For example, in Nigeria, the design and implementation of prepayment/strategic purchasing schemes for PHC services are managed at the state level in Kaduna and Niger states. In general, strategic purchasing is considered to be a central component of good public financial management for health and efforts toward UHC and, when implemented successfully, creates the right incentives in health systems for quality and efficiency to prevail (R4D, 2019[43]) (see Box 5.4).

> ### Box 5.4. Creating the right incentives through payment systems in Myanmar
>
> PSI, a health-focused non-profit that works with local governments, ministries of health, and local organisations to implement health solutions, piloted a strategic purchasing initiative as part of an implementation research project in Myanmar in 2017. Out-of-pocket expenses for consumers in the pilot location were as high as 70%, resulting in significant financial burden on the poor as well as chronic under-utilisation of health services (Joint Learning Network, 2017[44]).
>
> In the strategic purchasing pilot, PSI simulated the role of purchaser with the expectation, in alignment with the National Health Plan, of eventually being replaced by a national purchaser (Joint Learning Network, 2017[44]). The intervention involved a package of PHC services that would be provided by a local network of GPs serving a population of 2 500 low-income households in two townships in southern Myanmar.
>
> Myanmar is progressing toward UHC, so the pilot service package aligned with the planned Essential Package of Health Services, and was composed of "high impact but cost-effective curative and preventive care interventions in health areas with a high burden of disease, [meant to] be affordable within the project's budget envelope" (Crapper et al., 2017[45]). Services included a primary health care package for children under 5, ante-natal care and post-natal care coverage, infectious disease detection and treatment, and limited management of diabetes and hypertension, as well as a few enhanced services, from some providers, including cervical cancer screening, tuberculose and Human Immunodeficiency Virus treatment, and long-term family planning (Crapper et al., 2017[45]).

> The pilot introduced a blended payment system mixing capitation payments and performance-based incentives in order to increase the range of services provided by private GPs, decrease out-of-pocket expenses, and decrease the time it took people to seek treatment once symptoms began showing (Crapper et al., 2017[45]). Over the first year of implementation, challenges included lower than expected client registration and service utilisation, in part due to distance from households to the GP where they were to receive care. Implementation of the project is ongoing, but this work will provide important insights for pragmatic strategic purchasing.

5.5. PHC Systems Design: Ensuring strong system design capacities for PHC

Comprehensive PHC systems design capacities are one of the essential components to ensuring evidence-based care, chronic disease management, access to person-centred services, and decreased inequalities in health care systems. This includes improved learning between health care systems and integrated care, developing strategies for engaging the private sector in PHC delivery, and developing and improving technologies aimed at creating opportunities for countries to "leapfrog" – to rapidly scale up PHC delivery and quality capabilities, bypassing many of the development challenges that have been historically faced when such supports are lacking. Technology-enabled PHC systems and improved understanding of how governments and private sector can collaborate to ensure high-quality PHC delivery across populations are important mechanisms to accelerating access to PHC across LMICs.

5.5.1. Building integrated PHC systems based on team

Current approaches to health system planning typically do not consider hard trade-offs in service delivery design and do not consider the available fiscal space and political constraints, resulting in aspirational strategic plans that are difficult or impossible to translate into operational plans. Considerations of how to disrupt health planning practices and functions in LMICs are underway, focusing on service delivery, workforce planning, and facility planning. Strategies include helping LMIC governments to develop facility registers and improve human resource information systems to identify how many facilities and workers there are, where they are located, and how the government can optimally distribute them. Additional efforts align around increasing productivity – both quantity and quality of output – of existing facilities and workers in both public and private sectors, rather than encouraging the addition of incremental facilities and workers. Introducing innovations in technology-enabled PHC systems also provides important opportunities.

Truly integrated systems design includes team-based care (WHO, 2018[46]), strong connectivity between community-based and facility-based care (Pesec et al., 2017[47]; WHO, 2018[48]; WHO, 2018[49]), a simultaneous focus on both preventive and curative service delivery (Langenbrunner and Cashin, 2009[40]; Cashin, 2017[42]), and strong community engagement and patient empowerment (Tangcharoensathien et al., 2018[50]; WHO, 2018[51]). Currently, integration mostly takes place at national levels, but not at global or local levels, and there is minimal integration at the global level among donors. At the national level, governments tend to integrate planning across vertical systems, which often most supports siloed decision-making at the local and district levels.

Integrating a PHC system is a complex effort, and there is no single tool to achieve this. To develop and strengthen integrated systems design, we must strengthen the PHC systems design approach, incorporating human resources for health, financing, facilities, private sector, and demand. Management capacity and buy-in are crucial to support the integration of finance systems, data availability, accountability, and other processes, and donors should share the reporting and accountability requirements with governments, rather than having requirements for governments alone.

China provides a unique case study of an integrated PHC system. In China, the city of Xiamen, the Joint Management by Three Professionals reform aimed at improving chronic disease management and to encourage patients' use of community level resources. The reform established multidisciplinary team of a specialist responsible for determining the diagnosis and treatment plan, a general practitioner responsible for implementing the treatment plan, conducting monitoring on a daily basis and providing referral, and a health manager responsible for health education and interventions on patient behaviour. These teams treated patients at the community level, often by conducting home visits, and they encouraged the use of community health centres as a key source of usual care. Several supporting mechanisms have been implemented to enhance the integration of service provision including a financing scheme to improve care coordination. The Joint Management by Three Professionals reform has helped to decrease the overuse of secondary care systems while improving the management of chronic diseases. The proportion of visits to community health centres has risen from 30% in 2012 to 66.5% in 2016. More than 90% of residents enrolled in community health centres were satisfied with the new health service delivery systems. The Joint Management by Three Professionals reform has also reduced the overall cost of care by improving management of chronic diseases using a team-based approach for PHC (WHO, 2018[46]).

As acknowledged throughout of this report, the use of community health team is also crucial to develop and strengthen integrated primary health care systems. LMICs need to adopt a diverse, sustainable skills mix, harnessing the potential of community-based workers in primary health care teams. Community health workers have been found effective in the delivery of preventive, promotional and curative health service (WHO, 2018[52]). The 'Rural Pipeline" project in Guinea aims at deploying community health teams to reduce maternal and infant mortality, fight epidemics and improve well-being.

5.5.2. Strategically involving the private sector can help meet the demand

It is increasing understood that fully functioning PHC systems will require engagement of the private sector for PHC provision. Currently, private sector initiatives are not consistently delivering care in alignment with countries' health system objectives for a range of reasons, including the lack of rigorous evaluation of private sector initiatives, as well as the lack of expectation that the private sector should be aligned with national health objectives (Wadge et al., 2017[53]).

While PHC is the first investment priority for governments trying to achieve UHC, the private sector is capable of filling in gaps in secondary and tertiary care provision – but must be complementary and integrated with local care systems (Wadge et al., 2017[53]). As it stands, in most LMICs the private sector does not have sufficient accountability to guarantee care for patients and protection for health systems in an equitable way. Some approaches to engaging the private sector include interventions that encourage private providers to improve quality and coverage – while advancing their financial interests – such as incentives and subsidies including training, social marketing, social franchising, and purchasing efforts including contracting arrangements and vouchers (Montagu and Goodman, 2016[54]). Many of these efforts are underway in LMICs. Governments and non-governmental organisations use incentives and subsidies, most commonly through offering training to private providers to encourage the use of standard treatment guidelines; social marketing of commodities to create demand for products with high public health value, such as family planning; recruiting of private providers into social franchise networks to enhance delivery of more complex services (see Box 5.5); and providing targeted tax incentives to encourage investments or reduce end-user prices, or offering subsidies to potential clients (Montagu and Goodman, 2016[54]). Purchasing efforts such as contracting are typically used as a temporary solution to assure public service provision, and can include contracting arrangements to leverage private funds for infrastructure investments aimed at expanding capacity faster than government funds alone allow. Contracting is also utilised when private expertise can fill a specialised need better than a government can (for example, dialysis services or pharmaceutical logistics management), or to allow more rapid expansion of service provision (Montagu and Goodman, 2016[54]).

> **Box 5.5. SHOPS Plus initiative in South Africa and India**
>
> The Sustaining Health Outcomes through the Private Sector (SHOPS) Plus project is a private sector health initiative developed by USAID operating in LMICs in Africa, the Caribbean, Asia, and the Middle East. The goal of SHOPS Plus is to harness the potential of the private sector and catalyse public-private engagement in communities to improve health outcomes in areas including family planning, HIV, and child health (SHOPS Plus Project, 2019[55]).
>
> The aim of SHOPS Plus is to increase use of priority health services by:
>
> - Improving the private health sector's enabling environment;
> - Strengthening provision of private sector information, products, and services, with the target of expanded access for underserved populations;
> - Increasing the effectiveness of public-private engagement;
> - Sharing innovative, emerging, and tested private sector models; and
> - Applying a total market approach.
>
> **South Africa**
>
> In South Africa, SHOPS Plus explored a nurse-led social franchise model, the Unjani Clinic Network, a private health care staffing model supporting workforce growth and retention along the HIV clinical cascade (SHOPS Plus, 2019[56]). As the only nurse-led initiative in South Africa, this model shifts PHC tasks to professional nurses, who own and operate individual clinics in their own communities. Their community-level service delivery helps to build local trust while creating permanent jobs for the nurses (SHOPS Plus, 2019[56]; Dominis et al., 2018[57]). The clinics are sited strategically in low-income communities with high need, with each provider responsible for a standard set of PHC services, including those across the HIV diagnoses and treatment process (SHOPS Plus, 2019[56]). The cost of establishing the clinics was fairly low, and covered by corporate social investments and enterprise development funding focused on small- to medium-sized black-owned businesses in South Africa. The Unjani Clinic Network is working to become a national service provider under the country's National Health Insurance Policy, which is focusing on re-engineering PHC, with a goal of lower costs and improved health outcomes (SHOPS Plus, 2019[56]).
>
> **India**
>
> In India, SHOPS Plus is implementing evidence-based interventions to change the behaviours of public sector health care providers and beneficiaries in an effort to increase the use of maternal, neonatal and child health, family planning, and tuberculosis treatment products and services (SHOPS Plus, 2019[58]). With a goal of harnessing the potential of the private sector, and catalysing public-private engagement in servicing the health needs among the urban poor, the project is employing four approaches:
>
> 1. A media platform to send targeted messaging through diverse channels;
> 2. Workplace interventions to reach underserved youth populations;
> 3. Engagement with private and public sector networks to amplify messaging;
> 4. Use of technology-based systems to improve quality of service provision

5.5.3. Digital technologies have potential to optimise the delivery of PHC

In the development and strengthening of PHC systems, there are promising opportunities to leapfrog by incorporating digital innovations. These opportunities will continue to grow, as mobile health (mHealth) and other innovations are adopted, leveraged, and improved. In particular, mHealth is expected to have a large impact on health care quality and efficiency. As the main targets for mHealth and eHealth initiatives, the Astana operational framework highlights the potential for individuals, health providers, health information systems, and medical devices (Kasper et al., 2018[18]), finding that advances in information and communication technology in particular are having broad-based impacts in the PHC sector.

In health information systems, traditional paper-based records have been partially or fully replaced by electronic systems in many countries, improving both timeliness and accuracy of data collection and reporting systems (Kasper et al., 2018[18]). Electronic health records are being adopted in many places, and "big data" approaches to analysing patterns and trends in PHC are thought to be particularly relevant in the coming years (Kasper et al., 2018[18]). New medical devices increasingly come embedded with technology to increase their precision while recording clinical data – and even providing electronic data to health records, facilitating diagnoses, and enabling systems supporting health care decisions (Kasper et al., 2018[18]).

Digital health technologies are critical to optimising health systems and improving quality of care for individuals and populations but must be used judiciously; these technologies are also capable of deepening inequities among populations if not developed and studied carefully (National Academies of Sciences Engineering and Medicine, 2018[23]). An important aspect of health planning efforts includes planning for infrastructure to be "future-fit," supporting the adoption of innovative service delivery options such as virtual consultations, telemedicine, remote prescriptions, and evaluation of system impacts. Innovation in the hardware (e.g. diagnostics, devices), enablers (e.g. data, HRIS, connectivity, geo data), and software (e.g. triage, EMR, quality) will require new considerations in planning. This has implications for all PHC domains, for example in human resources for health, in terms of planning for training, and in facilities, anticipating smaller, more mobile facilities.

Technology-enabled PHC systems are one route to focusing on innovation to help leapfrog the PHC system. One example of technology-enabled PHC is Babyl Rwanda, which links telemedicine, artificial-intelligence-powered diagnosis and triage, longitudinal care records linking public health centres, a call centre, and labs and pharmacies via remote prescriptions and digital payments. Babyl provides nurse and GP appointments, prescriptions, and referrals to laboratory tests and specialists. The national insurance provider pays (Burki, 2019[59]). As the country has around 1 200 doctors for 12 million people, Rwanda is well placed to take advantage of digital technology. The Rwandan government has invited Babyl to integrate with PHC health centres nationwide, and Babyl and government stakeholders are evaluating the costs and benefits of an integrated digital health throughout the health system. Global partners including the Bill & Melinda Gates Foundation, the Rockefeller Foundation, USAID, the World Bank, and DFID are aligning to support the ecosystem for tech-enabled PHC systems, through alignment on an evidence agenda and policy and regulatory guidance for countries looking to broaden their horizons away from traditional PHC delivery systems.

5.6. Conclusions

Recognising the challenges of the implementation of the original Alma-Ata declaration to realise UHC, the 40th anniversary was a pivotal opportunity for leaders to reconvene and recommit to primary health care as a central path to UHC with the Astana Declaration. Universal health coverage is now the top priority for the World Health Organization[3], with PHC as cornerstone of a sustainable health system for universal health coverage. This chapter highlighted the major contributors to and components of the PHC landscape in LMICs, and the key strategic approaches to address these fundamental challenges with the aim of ensuring the continued development towards high-quality PHC systems. The enabling factors of governance in LMIC PHC systems are crucial framing, while measurement provides a critical tool for focusing efforts on improving systems. The strengthening of service delivery quality includes the considerations of safety, knowledge, and patient perspectives. The effective financing of PHC includes the leveraging of the current understanding of PHC expenditures and the financial tools available. By incorporating cross-country learning, engagement with the private sector, and leveraging of innovations, PHC systems can continue to strengthen and advance towards universal health coverage.

References

Bank, W. (2016), *Universal Health Coverage in Africa: A Framework for Action*, https://www.worldbank.org/en/topic/universalhealthcoverage/publication/universal-health-coverage-in-africa-a-framework-for-action (accessed on 2 September 2019). [35]

Berwick, D. et al. (2018), *Three global health-care quality reports in 2018*, http://dx.doi.org/10.1016/S0140-6736(18)31430-2. [8]

Bollyky, T., K. Cowling and D. Schoder (2018), *Three More Billboards On The Long Road To Global Quality Health Care*, Health Affairs, http://dx.doi.org/DOI: 10.1377/hblog20181011.858188. [24]

Brinkerhoff, D. et al. (2017), *Accountability, Health Governance, and Health Systems: Uncovering the Linkages*, https://www.hfgproject.org/accountability-health-governance-health-systems-uncovering-linkages/. [11]

Burki, T. (2019), "GP at hand: a digital revolution for health care provision?", *The Lancet*, Vol. 394, https://doi.org/10.1016/S0140-6736(19)31802-1. [59]

Cashin, C. (2017), *Results for Development Institute. Aligning public financial management and health financing: sustaining progress toward universal health coverage*, World Health Organization, http://apps.who.int/iris/bitstream/10665/254680/1/9789241512039-eng.pdf. [42]

Chan, B. et al. (2019), "Stewardship of quality of care in health systems: Core functions, common pitfalls, and potential solutions", *Public Administration and Development*, http://dx.doi.org/10.1002/pad.1835. [7]

Crapper, D. et al. (2017), *Myanmar Strategic Purchasing 1: Package of Services*, Health Finance and Governance, https://www.hfgproject.org/myanmar-strategic-purchasing-1-package-services/. [45]

Crawford, S. and R. Sachdev (2018), *Global analysis of health insurance in Sub-Saharan Africa*, Ernst & Young, https://www.ey.com/Publication/vwLUAssets/EY-global-analysis-of-health-insurance-in-sub-saharan-africa/$File/ey-global-analysis-of-health-insurance-in-sub-saharan-africa.pdf. [39]

Cross, H. et al. (2017), "Government stewardship of the for-profit private health sector in Afghanistan", *Health Policy and Planning*, http://dx.doi.org/10.1093/heapol/czw130. [10]

Das, J. (2011), "The quality of medical care in low-income countries: From providers to markets", *PLoS Medicine*, http://dx.doi.org/10.1371/journal.pmed.1000432. [26]

Das, J., J. Hammer and K. Leonard (2008), *The quality of medical advice in low-income countries*, http://dx.doi.org/10.1257/jep.22.2.93. [25]

Das, J. et al. (2018), "Rethinking assumptions about delivery of healthcare: Implications for universal health coverage", *BMJ (Online)*, http://dx.doi.org/10.1136/bmj.k1716. [3]

Declaration of Alma Ata International Conference of Primary Health Care (1978), *DECLARATION OF ALMA-ATA, International Conference of Primary Health Care*, http://dx.doi.org/10.1016/S0140-6736(79)90622-6. [1]

Dominis, S. et al. (2018), *Driving Innovation at the Community Level | Sustaining Health Outcomes through the Private Sector (SHOPS) Plus*, https://www.shopsplusproject.org/resource-center/driving-innovation-community-level. [57]

Fenny, A., R. Yates and R. Thompson (2018), "Social health insurance schemes in Africa leave out the poor", *International Health*, http://dx.doi.org/10.1093/inthealth/ihx046. [37]

German Federal Ministry of Health/World Health Organization (2017), *Second Global Ministerial Summit on Patient Safety – A Global Movement on Patient Safety*. [30]

Gurria, A. and M. Porter (2018), *Putting People at the Centre of Health Care*, Huffpost, https://www.huffpost.com/entry/putting-people-at-the-cen_b_14247824?guccounter=1 (accessed on 2 July 2019). [21]

Health Data Collaborative (2019), *Who we are*, https://www.healthdatacollaborative.org/who-we-are/ (accessed on 2 March 2019). [15]

Health Finance and Governance Project (2018), *Better Health? Composite Evidence from Four Literature Reviews*, https://www.hfgproject.org/better-health-composite-evidence-from-four-literature-reviews/. [12]

Joint Learning Network (2019), *Financing and Payment Models for Primary Health Care*, http://www.jointlearningnetwork.org/PHC_learning_exchange. [41]

Joint Learning Network (2017), *Myanmar Strategic Purchasing Brief Series*, http://www.jointlearningnetwork.org/resources/the-strategic-purchasing-brief-series-myanmar-strategic-purchasing-brief-se. [44]

Kasper, T. et al. (2018), *Operational Framework draft for consultation: Primary health care: transforming vision into action.*, World Health Organization, Geneva. [18]

Kruk, M. et al. (2018), "Mortality due to low-quality health systems in the universal health coverage era: a systematic analysis of amenable deaths in 137 countries", *The Lancet*, http://dx.doi.org/10.1016/S0140-6736(18)31668-4. [14]

Langenbrunner, J. and C. Cashin (2009), "How-To Manuals Designing and Implementing Health Care Provider Payment Systems How-To Manuals", *Development*. [40]

Montagu, D. and C. Goodman (2016), *Prohibit, constrain, encourage, or purchase: how should we engage with the private health-care sector?*, http://dx.doi.org/10.1016/S0140-6736(16)30242-2. [54]

National Academies of Sciences Engineering and Medicine (2018), *Crossing the global quality chasm: Improving health care worldwide*. [23]

Nejad, S., N. Abrampah and M. Neilson (2018), *Technical Series on Primary Care: Quality in Primary Health Care*, World Health Organization, Geneva. [29]

OECD (2019), *Patient-Reported Indicators Surveys (PaRIS)*, http://www.oecd.org/health/paris.htm (accessed on 2 March 2019). [20]

OECD/WHO/World Bank Group (2018), *Delivering Quality Health Services: A Global Imperative*, WHO, Geneva, https://doi.org/10.1787/9789264300309-en. [22]

Ozano, K. et al. (2019), *Discussions around Primary Health Care and the Private Sector during the Global Symposia on Health Systems Research 2018*, https://www.healthsystemsglobal.org/upload/other/Discussions-around-Primary-Health-Care-and-the-Private-Sector.pdf. [9]

Pesec, M. et al. (2017), "Primary health care that works: The Costa Rican experience", *Health Affairs*, http://dx.doi.org/10.1377/hlthaff.2016.1319. [47]

PHCPI (2018), *Measuring Primary Health Care Performance*, https://improvingphc.org/measuring-primary-health-care-performance (accessed on 2 July 2019). [16]

PHCPI (2018), *Vital Signs Profiles*, https://improvingphc.org/vital-signs-profiles (accessed on 2 March 2019). [19]

R4D (2019), *Strengthening Strategic Purchasing Expertise in Africa. Results for Development*, https://www.r4d.org/projects/toward-health-strengthening-strategic-purchasing-expertise-africa/. [43]

Randhawa, H. (2015), *Report of the Expert Consultation on Primary Care Systems Profiles & Performance (PRIMASYS)*, Alliance for Health Policy and Systems Research, Geneva. [17]

Rohde, J. et al. (2008), *30 years after Alma-Ata: has primary health care worked in countries?*, http://dx.doi.org/10.1016/S0140-6736(08)61405-1. [4]

SHOPS Plus (2019), *Examining a nurse-led social franchise model in South Africa | Sustaining Health Outcomes through the Private Sector (SHOPS) Plus*, https://www.shopsplusproject.org/article/examining-nurse-led-social-franchise-model-south-africa. [56]

SHOPS Plus (2019), *India | Sustaining Health Outcomes through the Private Sector (SHOPS) Plus*, https://www.shopsplusproject.org/where-we-work/asiamiddle-east/india. [58]

SHOPS Plus Project (2019), *Overview*, https://www.shopsplusproject.org/project-overview. [55]

Stenberg, K. (2019), *Current expenditure on PHC and projected resource needs for PHC in low and middle income countries*. [34]

Stenberg, K. et al. (2017), "Financing transformative health systems towards achievement of the health Sustainable Development Goals: a model for projected resource needs in 67 low-income and middle-income countries", *The Lancet Global Health*, http://dx.doi.org/10.1016/S2214-109X(17)30263-2. [33]

Tangcharoensathien, V. et al. (2018), *Health systems development in Thailand: a solid platform for successful implementation of universal health coverage*, http://dx.doi.org/10.1016/S0140-6736(18)30198-3. [50]

The Lancet (2018), *The Astana Declaration: the future of primary health care?*, http://dx.doi.org/10.1016/S0140-6736(18)32478-4. [2]

USAID (2017), *Quality of Health Service Consensus Statement*, https://www.hfgproject.org/employing-governance-to-improve-health-sector-performance/ (accessed on 2 July 2019). [5]

Vande Maele, N. et al. (2019), "Measuring primary health care expenditure in low and lower-middle income countries", *BMJ Global Health*, http://dx.doi.org/10.1136/bmjgh-2019-001497. [32]

Vaz, P. et al. (2018), *Strengthening Governance for Improved Health Sector Performance*, HFG Series: Advances in Health Finance & Governance. [6]

Veillard, J. et al. (2017), "Better Measurement for Performance Improvement in Low- and Middle-Income Countries: The Primary Health Care Performance Initiative (PHCPI) Experience of Conceptual Framework Development and Indicator Selection", *Milbank Quarterly*, http://dx.doi.org/10.1111/1468-0009.12301. [13]

Veillard, J. et al. (2018), *Universal quality healthcare coverage—a commitment to building a healthier and more productive society*, Thebmjopinion, https://blogs.bmj.com/bmj/2018/07/05/universal-quality-healthcare-coverage-a-commitment-to-building-a-healthier-and-more-productive-society/ (accessed on 2 March 2019). [27]

Wadge, H. et al. (2017), *How to harness the private sector for universal health coverage*, http://dx.doi.org/10.1016/S0140-6736(17)31718-X. [53]

Wagstaff, A. and M. Claeson (2004), *The millennium development goals for health - rising to the challenges*, The World Bank; 2004 Jan. Report No.: 29673, Washington, http://documents.worldbank.org/curated/en/875031468329973611/The-millennium-development-goals-for-health-rising-to-the-challenges. [36]

WHO (2018), *China: Multidisciplinary teams and integrated service delivery across levels of care; The Global Conference on Primary Health Care.*, https://www.who.int/docs/default-source/primary-health/case-studies/china.pdf. [46]

WHO (2018), *Ghana: Community engagement, financial protection and expanding rural access. Country case studies on primary health care.*, World Health Organization, https://www.who.int/docs/default-source/primary-health/case-studies/ghana.pdf. [51]

WHO (2018), *Jamaica: Development of workforce for first level of care. Country case studies on primary health care.*, World Health Organization, https://www.who.int/docs/default-source/primary-health/case-studies/jamaica.pdf. [48]

WHO (2018), *Sri Lanka: Community-based workforce development for maternal and child health. Country case studies on primary health care.*, World Health Organization, https://www.who.int/docs/default-source/primary-health/case-studies/sri-lanka.pdf. [49]

WHO (2018), *WHO | 10 facts on patient safety*, World Health Organisation. [28]

WHO (2018), *WHO guideline on health policy and system support to optimize community health worker programmes,*, World Health Organization, https://www.who.int/hrh/community/guideline-health-support-optimize-hw-programmes/en/. [52]

WHO (2017), *The third WHO Global Patient Safety Challenge: Medication Without Harm.*, http://www.who.int/patientsafety/medication-safety/en/ (accessed on 2 March 2019). [31]

Zelelew, H. (2017), *Community Health Financing: Lessons from Ethiopia.* [38]

Notes

[1] The Lancet Global Health Commission on High Quality Health Systems.

[2] The reason why the WHO team reports the average for 2026-30 is that this is the more mature scale-up phase so it is less dependent on the speed of scale-up for the initial years, where a slower scale-up would mean lower additional costs.

[3] See "Director-General Dr Tedros takes the helm of WHO: address to WHO staff", available at http://www.who.int/dg/speeches/2017/taking-helm-who/en/.

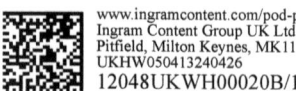
www.ingramcontent.com/pod-product-compliance
Ingram Content Group UK Ltd.
Pitfield, Milton Keynes, MK11 3LW, UK
UKHW050413240426
12048UKWH00020B/1491

9 789264 933330